Theory and Practice in
Novel Drug
Delivery System

Theory and Practice in
Novel Drug Delivery System

S.P. Vyas

M Pharma Ph D Post-Doc (London, UK)
Director-PG studies
Professor and Head
Department of Pharmaceutics Sciences
ISF College of Pharmacy, Moga, Punjab
Formerly: Head Department of Pharmaceutical Sciences
Dr HS Gour University, Sagar (MP)

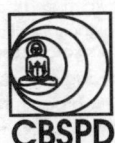

CBSPD

CBS Publishers & Distributors Pvt Ltd

New Delhi • Bengaluru • Chennai • Kochi • Kolkata • Lucknow • Mumbai
Hyderabad • Jharkhand • Nagpur • Patna • Pune • Uttarakhand

Theory and Practice in Novel Drug Delivery System

ISBN: 978-81-239-1689-7

Copyright © Author & Publisher

First Edition: 2009

Reprint: 2011, 2018, 2020, 2024 2025

Published by Satish Kumar Jain and produced by Varun Jain for

CBS Publishers & Distributors Pvt Ltd

4819/XI Prahlad Street, 24 Ansari Road, Daryaganj, New Delhi 110 002, India
Ph: 011-23289259, 23266861   Website: www.cbspd.com
                              e-mail: delhi@cbspd.com
Corporate Office: 204 FIE, Industrial Area, Patparganj, Delhi 110 092
Ph: 011-4934 4934   Fax: 011-4934 4935   e-mail: publishing@cbspd.com
                                           publicity@cbspd.com

Branches

- **Bengaluru:** Seema House 2975, 17th Cross, KR Road, Banasankari 2nd Stage, Bengaluru 560 070, Karnataka, India
  Ph: +91-80-26771678/79   Fax: +91-80-26771680   e-mail: bangalore@cbspd.com
- **Chennai:** 7, Subbaraya Street, Shenoy Nagar, Chennai 600 030, Tamil Nadu, India
  Ph: +91-44-26680620, 26681266   Fax: +91-44-42032115   e-mail: chennai@cbspd.com
- **Kochi:** 42/1325, 1326, Power House Road, Opp KSEB, Power House, Ernakulam 682 018, India
  Ph: +91-484-4059061–65   Fax: +91-484-4059065   e-mail: kochi@cbspd.com
- **Kolkata:** 147, Hind Ceramics Compound, 1st Floor, Nilgunj Road, Belghoria, Kolkata 700 056, West Bengal, India
  Ph: +91-9096713055/56   e-mail: kolkata@cbspd.com
- **Lucknow:** Basement, Khushnuma Complex, 7-Meerabai Marg (behind Jawahar Bhawan), Lucknow 226 001, India
  Ph: +91-522-4000032   e-mail: tiwari.lucknow@cbspd.com
- **Mumbai:** PWD Shed. Gala no. 25/26, Ramchandra Bhatt Marg, Next to JJ Hospital Gate no. 2, Opp. Union Bank of India
  Noorbaug Mumbai 400 009, Maharashtra, India
  Ph: +91-22-66661880/89   e-mail: mumbai@cbspd.com

Representatives

- **Hyderabad** 0-9885175004
- **Jharkhand** 0-9811541605
- **Nagpur** 0-8692091830
- **Patna** 0-9334159340
- **Pune** 0-9664372571
- **Uttarakhand** 0-9716462459

Printed at SRK Graphics, Shahdara, Delhi, India

Preface

Novel and controlled release technology is an area of current interest to pharmaceutical academicians and working research scientists. It involves a myriad of approaches based on different physical, chemical, and strategic concepts such as osmotic pressure; and osmotic pumps; bioadhesion and site retentive systems; ultraemulsion and multiemulsion; enzyme/microbioflora of colon and colon targeted therapy, polymers and design of transdermal drug delivery systems; spherical crystallization with bearance on tablet compression and characteristics; microemulsions for topical and parenteral delivery, sustained release and bioresponsiveness for implants and inserts for long-term hormonal therapy, micellar solubilization for improved bioavailability potentials, surface modified liposomes, microparticles, nanoparticles, erythrocytes, ethosomes, dendrimers, etc. as nanosystems for controlled and targeted drug delivery. Also including niosomes, organogels, SLNs for improved therapeutics application. It is thought that the experimental protocols with concepts and therapeutic details relating to these systems be provided to the students, technicians and teachers so that they can be much more familiar with the concepts, systems and preparation methods. The present book, therefore, presents experimental protocols with details, which have been developed by various research laboratories. This will provide real support to the students for their practical classes and also to the teachers for preparations to the classes. I am really thankful to my academic friends who motivated me for authorship of such a book that deals with both theory and practice on the subject and this is how it is named as *Theory and Practice in Novel Drug Delivery System*.

This is probably the first book on such a title which has otherwise remained as a resolute need for long. The sources of the protocol described in the book have been acknowledged and references are given at the end of each chapter under suggested readings. Some of the protocols are based on publications from our group. The total compilation is a great at a source reading material for pharmacy professionals and postgraduates, especially those who are involved in work on controlled and targeted drug delivery.

I thank my students who demanded for such a readable source, my friends who encouraged me and supported me to bring the manuscript in this printed form. I am also thankful to CBS Publishers & Distributors, New Delhi, for their quickly publishing work inputs to the book. I am thankful to my wife Vasundhara, son Eng. Himanshu and daughters Sonal and Anchal for convictively supporting me during my involvement with the book. I owe my sincere thanks to Dr. Amit Rawat, Dr. Sunil Mahor, Dr. Kapil Khatri, Dr. Swati Gupta, Mr. Amit K. Goyal, Mr. Bhuvanehswar Vaidya, Mr. Abhinav Mehta, Dr. PN Gupta, Mr. Neeraj Mishra, Ms. Shailja Tiwari, Ms. Madhu Gupta, Ms. Shivani, Mr. Rishi Paliwal, Mr. Sharad Mangal, Mr. Arvind Jain, and my other students and friends who helped me during the preparation of the manuscript of the book. The constructive suggestions are invited from students and teachers so that they can be incorporated to make the source further enriched.

SP Vyas

Contents

Floating Drug Delivery Systems
Floating Tablet/Microspheres/Density Based Systems

Several approaches are currently utilized in the prolongation of the gastric retention time (GRT), including floating drug delivery systems (FDDS), also known as hydrodynamically balanced systems (HBS), swelling and expanding systems, polymeric bioadhesive systems, modified-shape systems, high-density systems, and other delayed gastric emptying devices.

LOW DENSITY OR FLOATING DRUG DELIVERY SYSTEMS

This approach exploits the floating property of substances with density lower than the fluid medium. Floating drug delivery systems either float due to their low density than stomach contents or due to the gaseous phase formed inside the system after they come in contact with the gastric environment. Various floating dosage forms are reported in the literature (Fig. 1.1). Depending upon the working principle of floating drug delivery systems they are divided into two main categories: non-effervescent and effervescent floating drug delivery systems.

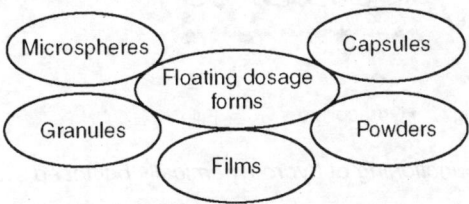

Fig. 1.1: *Various floating dosage forms*

NON-EFFERVESCENT FDDS

The FDDS belonging to this class are usually prepared from gel-forming or highly swellable cellulose type hydrocolloids, polysaccharides or matrix forming polymers like polyacrylate, polycarbonate, polystyrene and polymethacrylate. In one approach, gel-forming hydrocolloid swells in contact with gastric fluid after oral administration and maintains relative integrity of shape and bulk density of less than unity within gastric environment (Hilton and Deasy, 1992). The air thus trapped by the swollen polymer imparts buoyancy to the dosage form. Nevertheless, the gel structure acts as a reservoir for sustained drug release. Sheth and Tossounian, 1984, suggested that when these dosage forms come in contact with an aqueous medium, the hydrocolloids imbibe water and start to hydrate thereby forming a gel at the surface. The resultant gel layer subsequently controls the trafficking of drug out and passage of solvent into the dosage form. With the passage of time the exterior surface of the dosage form goes into solution and immediate adjacent hydrocolloid layer becomes hydrated and maintains the gel structure. The drug in dosage form dissolves in and diffuses out with the diffusing solvent forming a 'receding boundary' within the gel structure. Fig. 1.2 illustrates the working principle of a hydrodynamically balanced system (HBS).

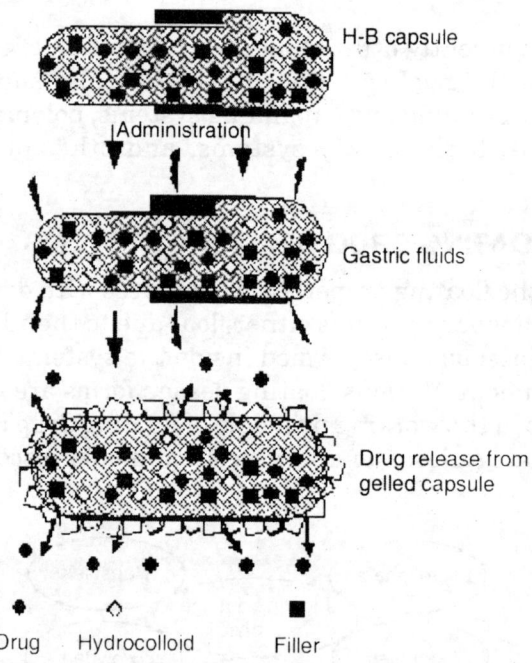

Fig. 1.2: Functioning of hydrodynamically balanced system (HBS)

EFFERVESCENT FDDS

These floating delivery systems employ matrices from swelling polymers like Methocel® or chitosan and effervescent components such as sodium bicarbonate and tartaric or citric acid (Desai, 1984) or matrices having chambers of liquid components that gasify at body temperature (Ritschel, 1991; Michaels *et. al,* 1975; Michaels, 1974). The matrices are prepared in such a manner that when they come in contact with stomach fluid, carbon dioxide is generated and retained entrapped in the hydrocolloid gel. This leads to an upward drift of the dosage form and maintains it in a floating condition. A single layer tablet can be produced by intimately mixing the carbon dioxide generating component in tablet matrix (Hashim and Li Wan Po, 1987). A bilayer tablet may be compressed (Ingani *et al.*, 1987) in which gas liberating component is present in hydrocolloid layer and the drug is compressed in other layer for sustained release. The concept has been judiciously utilized to develop floating capsule system consisting of a mixture of sodium alginate and sodium bicarbonate. Recently, a multiple unit-floating pill has been developed based on the concept of effervescence (Ichikawa *et al.*, 1991b).

In this system carbon dioxide gas is generated from reaction of sodium bicarbonate and tartaric acid. The system consisted of sustained release pill surrounded by an effervescent layer. This coated system is further coated with swellable polymers like polyvinyl acetate and purified shellac (Fig. 1.3). Moreover, the effervescent layer is divided into two sub layers to prevent direct contact between tartaric acid and sodium bicarbonate.

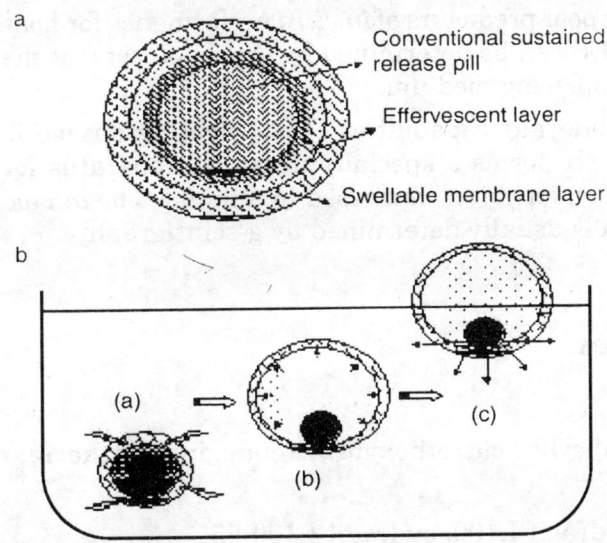

Fig. 1.3: *(A) multiple-unit oral floating drug delivery system. (B) working principle of effervescent float-ing delivery system: (a) Penetration of water (b) generation of carbon dioxide and buoyancy (c) Swellable layer*

In Vitro and *in Vivo* Evaluation

The various parameters that need to be evaluated for their effects on GRT of buoyant formulations can mainly be categorised into following different classes.

1. *Galenic parameters:* Diametric size ('cut-off size'), flexibility and density of matrices.
2. *Control parameters:* Floating time, dissolution, specific gravity, content uniformity and hardness and friability (if tablets).
3. Geometric parameters: Shape.
4. *Physiological parameters:* Age, sex, posture, food, and bioadhesion.

The test for buoyancy and *in vitro* drug release studies are usually carried out in simulated gastric and intestinal fluids maintained at 37°C. In practice, floating time is determined by using the USP disintegration apparatus containing 900 ml of 0.1 N HCl as a testing medium maintained at 37°C. The time required to float the HBS dosage form is noted as floating (or floatation) time. Dissolution tests are performed using the USP dissolution apparatus. Samples are withdrawn periodically from the dissolution medium, replenished with the same volume of fresh medium each time, and then analysed for their drug contents after an appropriate dilution. Recent methodology as described in USP XXIII states "The dosage unit is allowed to sink to the bottom of the vessel before rotation of the blade is started. A small, loose piece of nonreactive material such as not more than a few turns of a wire helix may be attached to the dosage units that would otherwise float". However, standard dissolution methods based on the USP or British Pharmacopoeia (BP) have been shown to be poor predictors of *in vitro* performance for floating dosage forms. The specific gravity of FDDS can be determined by the displacement method using analytical grade benzene as a displacing medium.

Determining the buoyant capabilities of the floating dosage forms and the sinking characteristics of the NF forms a specially designed apparatus for measuring the total force acting vertically on an object immersed in a liquid. The *in vivo* gastric retentivity of a floating dosage form is usually determined by g-scintigraphy.

PROTOCOL: 1.1
Floating Microspheres

Materials

Drugs (Aspirin, salicylic acid, ethoxybenzamide, indomethacin, riboflavin)	0.1–1 g
Polymers	1.0 g
Eudragit S100, eudragit L100, eudragit L100-55	
Ethylcellulose (N-10-F)	
Hydroxypropylmethylcellulose (TC-5R)	
Hydroxypropylmethylcellulosephthalate (HP-55)	
Monostearin (wall membrane reinforcing agent)	0.5 g
Polyvinyl alcohol (PVA-120, dispersing agent)	
Dichloromethane	8 ml
Ethanol	8 ml

Principle
Emulsion solvent diffusion method

Procedure
1. Weigh drug (0.1–1.0 g), polymers (1.0 g), monostearin (0.5 g) and dissolve or disperse in a mixture of dichloromethane (8 ml) and ethanol (8 ml) at room temperature.

2. Introduce solution or a suspension of drug (depending on solubility) into an aqueous solution of polyvinyl alcohol (0.75 % w/v, 200 ml) at 40°C, forming an oil-in-water (o/w) type emulsion.

3. Stir the resultant emulsion, employing a propeller type agitator at 300 rpm. The finely dispersed droplets of the polymer solution of drug were solidified in the aqueous phase via diffusion of the solvent.

4. Evaporate the dichloromethane from the solidified droplet by using an aspirator, leaving the cavity of the microsphere filled with water.

5. After agitating the system for 1 h, sieve the resulting polymeric particulate systems between 500 and 1000 mm and dry overnight at 40°C to produce microballoons (Scheme 1.1).

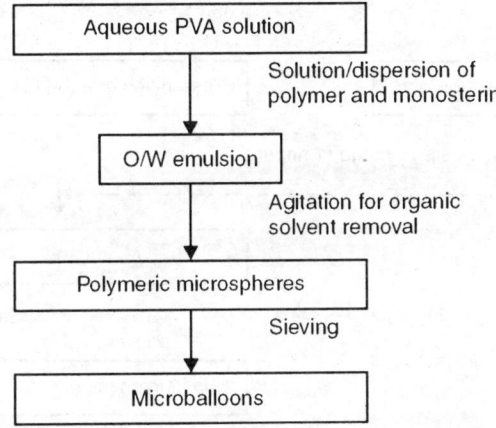

Scheme 1.1: *Preparation of floating drug delivery systems by emulsion solvent diffusion method*

PROTOCOL: 1.2

Floating Chitosan Microcapsules for Oral Use

Principle

Capillary Extrusion Method

Materials

Chitosan (MW /750, 000, deacetylation degree: 83.5%)

Drug

Sodium dioctyl sulfosuccinate (DOS)

Pentasodium tripolyphosphate (TPP)

Procedure

1. Take 1.5–4.5% w/v of drug and disperse in a stirred solution of 2% w/v chitosan in 2% v/v acetic acid until a uniform dispersion is obtained.

2. Mix bubble free dispersion of chitosan through a disposable syringe (with a nozzle of 1 mm inner diameter) into 20 ml of a gently agitated solution of the crosslinking agent (DOS or TPP). The dropping rate is 30 beads/min and the falling distance 5 cm.

3. Separate the gelled microcapsule after a reaction time of 2 h, wash with deionised water and then air dry the microcapsule for 48 h.

4. A number of variables such as stabilisation time, chitosan and crosslinking agent concentrations as well as drug/polymer ratio can also be used to prepare microcapsule of different size (Scheme 1.2).

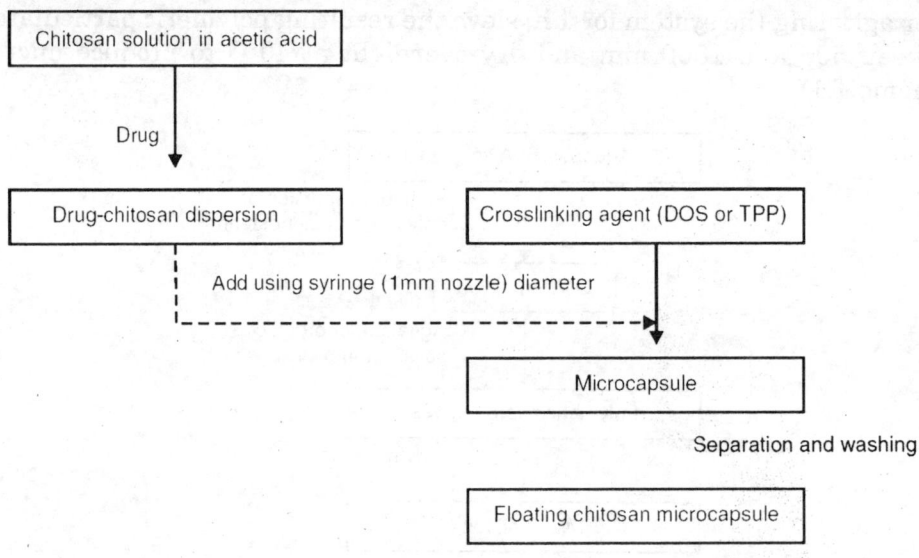

Scheme 1.2: *Floating chitosan microsphere preparation by capillary extrusion method*

PROTOCOL: 1. 3
Floating Microspheres (Controlled) Drug Delivery System

Materials

Drug	0.1 g
Polymer (Eudragit S-100 or hydroxypropyl methyl cellulose)	1.0 g
Monostearin (membrane-reinforcing agent)	0.5 g
Dichloromethane	8 ml
Polyvinyl alcohol (PVA-120 as a dispersing agent)	0.75%
Ethanol	8 ml

Procedure

- Dissolve the drug, polymers (1.0 g), and monostearin in a mixture of dichloromethane (8 ml) and ethanol (8 ml) at room temperature.

- Add this drug solution to the aqueous solution of polyvinyl alcohol (0.75% w/v, 200 ml) at 40°C.
- Stir the resultant emulsions at 300 rpm with a propeller-type agitator for 1 h.
- Separate the resulting polymeric spheres by centrifugation and sieve between 500 and 1000 μm and dried overnight at 40°C.

PROTOCOL: 1.4
Floating Multiple-unit Capsule

Materials

Hydroxypropylmethylcellulose (Methocel)
Eudragit N30D/ RS (70:30)
Hydroxypropylcellulose (Klucel)
Sodium bicarbonate

Procedure

- The nominal composition of the floating and the high-density minitablets is as given above. Prepare the floating minitablets by wet granulation with a solution of 10%m/v Klucel® LF in ethanol. Compress the minitablets.
- Then, coat with a solution of Eudragit NE30D/ RS : 70:30. The tablets retain a density of 1.3 g/cm³, but float due to the reaction of sodium bicarbonate with the acidic contents of the test medium. The buoyancy of these floating minitablets is satisfactory for more than 6 h in artificial gastric fluid containing 0.05% polysorbate 80.
- Prepare high-density minitablets by wet granulation with methylene chloride. Compress using the same device as used to prepare the floating minitablets. The apparent density of these minitablets is 2.6 g/cm³. Each size 1 gelatin capsule can be filled with 10 minitablets.

In vitro Drug Release Testing

The dissolution tests is performed at 37°C using the USP xxiii paddle apparatus containing 500 ml of artificial gastric fluid. Assay the samples spectrophotometrically at 274 nm using an automated dissolution system. The stirring rate is set at 50 rpm. Repeat the experiment 6 times to assess the reproducibility of the prepared tablets.

PROTOCOL:1.5
Floating Matrix Tablets Based on Low Density Foam Powder

Materials

Polypropylene foam powder (Accurel MP 1002 and MP 1000)
Chlorpheniramine maleate
Diltiazem HCl
Theophylline anhydrous

Verapamil HCl

Hydroxypropyl methylcellulose (HPMC; Methocel E5, E50 and K15M)

Carrageenan (type CHP-2),

Corn starch

Gum guar

Gum Arabic

Polyacrylic acids [Carbopol 934P (polymerised in benzene, highly cross-linked with allyl sucrose), Carbopol 971P (polymerised in ethyl acetate, lightly cross-linked with allyl pentaerythritol), Carbopol 974P (polymerised in ethyl acetate, highly cross-linked with allyl pentaerythritol), Noveon AA1 (polycarbophil (polymerised in ethyl acetate) cross-linked with divinyl glycol)]

Sodium alginate

Dibasic calcium phosphate

Lactose (α-lactose monohydrate, Flowlac 100)

Microcrystalline cellulose (MCC, Avicel PH-101)

Magnesium stearate

The polypropylene foam powder is sieved to obtain different size fractions.

Tablet Preparation

Prepare tablets containing 0.5% w/w magnesium stearate as lubricant by direct compression. Then blend the respective powders [drug, foam powder, polymer(s) and optional additives, compositions listed in Table 1.6 thoroughly with a mortar and pestle.

Weigh 500 mg of the mixture and feed into the die of an instrumented single-punch tableting machine to produce tablets using flat-faced punches (2, 9, 12, or 16 mm in diameter). Adjust the pressure to keep the hardness of the tablets constant (approximately 80 N) and measure with a hardness tester (Scheme 1.3).

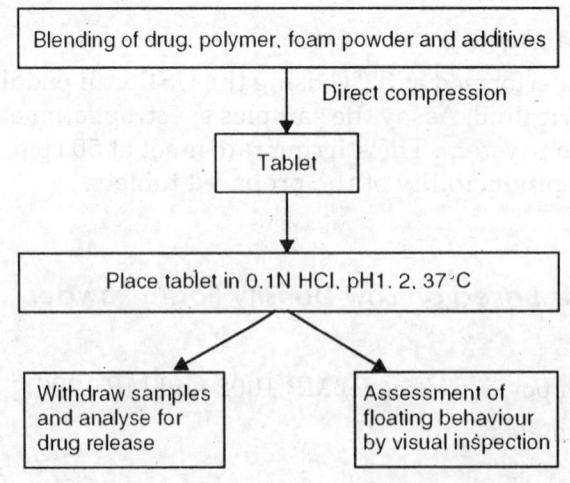

Scheme 1.3: *Floating tablet preparation and evaluation*

Floating Behaviour of the Tablets

The *in vitro* floating behaviour of the tablets is studied by placing them in 500 ml plastic containers filled with 300 ml preheated 0.1 N HCl (pH 1.2, 37°C), followed by horizontal shaking for 8 h (37°C, 75 rpm). The floating lag times (time period between placing the tablet in the medium and tablet floating) and floating durations of the tablets can be determined by visual observation.

In vitro Drug Release

Place the tablets in 500 ml plastic container filled with 300 ml preheated release medium (0.1 N HCl, pH 1.2, 37.8°C), followed by horizontal shaking for 8 h (37°C, 75 rpm). Analyse the amount of drug released by appropriate spectrophotometric method (wavelengths for drug estimation that can be used in the current protocol: CPM, 264 nm; Diltiazem HCl, 236 nm; Theophylline, 270 nm; Verapamil HCl, 278 nm).

Density Measurements

Calculate the apparent densities of the tablets from their volumes and masses (n should be large). The volumes V of the cylindrical tablets is calculated from their heights h and radii r (both determined with a micrometer gauge) using the mathematical equation for a cylinder $V = \pi r^2 h$. Determine the density of 0.1 N HCl at 37°C with a pycnometer (Scheme 1.4).

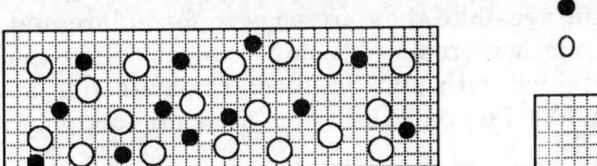

Scheme 1.4: *Schematic presentation of the structure of the low density, floating matrix tablets*

SUGGESTED READINGS

- Desai S, (1984), A novel floating controlled release drug delivery systems based on a dried gel matrix, M.S. Thesis, St. John's University, Jamaica, New York.
- Hashim H and Lee Wan Po A, (1987), Int. J. Pharm. 35, 201.
- Hilton AK, and Deasy PB, (1992), Int. J. Pharm. 86.
- Ichikawa M, Watanave S, and Miyake Y. (1991), J. Pharm. Sci. 80, 1062.
- Ingani HM, Timmermans J, and Moes AJ, (1987), Int. J. Pharm. 35, 157.
- Michaels AS, (1974), US Patent 3, 786, 813.
- Michaels AS, Bashwa JD, Zaffaroni A, (1975), US Patent 3, 901, 232.
- Ritschel WA, Menon A, and Saki A, (1991), Exp. Clin. Pharmacol. 13, 629.
- Rouge N, Allemann E, Gex-Fabry M, Balant L,. Cole ET, Buri P, Doelker E, (1998), Pharm. Acta Helv. 73 1998 81.
- Sheth PR and Tossounian JL, (1984), Drug Dev. Ind. Pharm. 10, 313.
- Streubel A, Siepmann J, Bodmeier R, (2003) Eur. J. Pharm. Sci. 18,37.

2

Oral Osmotic Pumps

INTRODUCTION

Osmotic pumps are controlled drug delivery devices based on the principle of osmosis. Wide spectrums of osmotic devices are in existence, out of them osmotic pumps are unique, dynamic and widely employed in clinical practice (Santus and Baker, 1995; Singh *et al.*, 1999). Osmosis is an aristocratic phenomenon, which is exploited for development of delivery systems with every desirable property of an ideal controlled drug delivery system. Osmotic pumps offer many advantages like they are easy to formulate and simple in operation, improved patient compliance with reduced dosing frequency, more consistent and prolonged therapeutic effect is obtained with uniform blood concentration and moreover they are inexpensive and their industrial adaptability vis-a-vis production scale up is easy.

Elementary osmotic pumps essentially contain an active agent having suitable osmotic pressure, contained into a tablet, coated with a semipermeable membrane usually of cellulose acetate (Theeuwes, 1975). A small orifice is drilled through the coating by using LASER or high-speed mechanical drill. In fact, this system represents a coated tablet with an aperture. When exposed to an aqueous environment, the osmotic pressure of the soluble drug within the tablet draws water through the semipermeable coating, resulting in formation of a saturated aqueous drug solution within the device. The membrane is non-extensible and increase in volume due to imbibition of water raises inner hydrostatic pressure, eventually leading to flow of saturated solution of active agent out of the device through small orifice. Solubility of drug in water plays a critical role in functioning of osmotic pump. Typically the solubility of drug delivered by these pumps should be at least 10 to 15% w/v.

The drug is pumped out of the system through the orifice at a controlled rate dm/dt, which is equal to the multiple of volume flow rate of water (dv/dt) into the core and drug concentration C_S.

$$dm/dt = (dv/dt) \, C_S$$

In principle, this delivery system dispenses drug continuously at a zero order rate until the concentration of the osmotically active salt in the system decreases below saturation solubility, where upon a non-zero order release pattern results. Recently, controlled release oral osmotic pump of naproxen sodium (Ramakrishna and Mishra, 2001) and ibuprofen (Ozdemir and Sahin, 1997) have been developed.

OSMOSIS: AN OVERVIEW

Osmosis refers to the process of movement of solvent from lower concentration of solute towards higher concentration of solute across semipermeable membrane. Abbe Nollet first reported osmotic effect in 1748, but Pfeffer is the pioneer of quantitative measurement of osmotic effect. He measured the effect in 1877 by utilising a membrane, which is selectively permeable to water but impermeable to sugar (Fig. 2.1). This membrane separated sugar solution from pure water. Pfeffer observed a flow of water into the sugar solution that was halted when a pressure π was applied to the sugar solution. Pfeffer postulated that this pressure, the osmotic pressure π of the sugar solution is directly proportional to the solution concentration and absolute temperature.

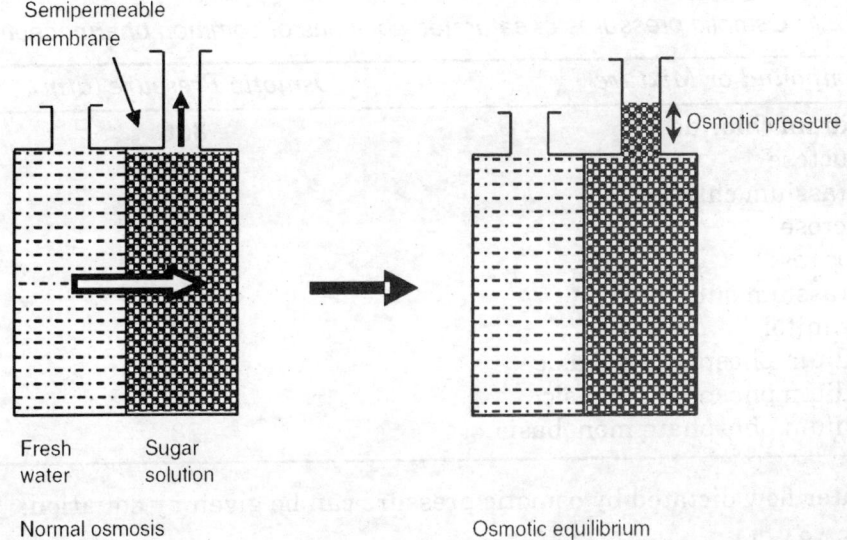

Fig. 2.1: *A scheme illustrating osmotic flow and the attainment of osmotic equilibrium*

Van't Hoff established the analogy between the Pfeffer results and the ideal gas laws by the expression

$$\pi = n_2RT \tag{1}$$

Where n_2 represents the molar concentration of sugar (or other solute) in the solution, R depicts the gas constant, and T the absolute temperature.

The Van't Hoff equation presents a good means for calculating the osmotic pressures of solutes across perfect semipermeable membranes and is accurate for low solute concentrations. But in case if the membrane is not completely semipermeable and permits passage for solute along with solvent, the osmotic pressure calculated by equation (1) will be more when compared with experimental value. Concentrated solutions also show deviations from these ideal equations. A number of researchers have discussed, modified and a more accurate expressions of this equation has been brought about.

Another method of obtaining a good approximation of osmotic pressure is by utilising vapour pressure measurements by using the expression:

$$\pi = RT \ln (Po/P)/v \tag{2}$$

Where Po represents the vapour pressure of the pure solvent, P is the vapour pressure of the solution, and v is the molar volume of the solvent. As vapour pressures can be measured with less effort than osmotic pressure, this expression is frequently used.

Osmotic pressure for soluble solutes are extremely high, as displayed in Table 2.1, showing osmotic pressures of solutes commonly used in controlled release pharmaceutical formulations. This high osmotic pressure is responsible for high water flow across semipermeable membrane.

Table 2.1: *Osmotic pressures of saturated solutions of common pharmaceutical solutes*

Compound or Mixture	Osmotic Pressure (atm)
Sodium chloride	356
Fructose	355
Potassium chloride	245
Sucrose	150
Dextrose	82
Potassium sulphate	39
Mannitol	38
Sodium phosphate tribasic	36
Sodium phosphate dibasic	31
Sodium phosphate monobasic	28

The water flow dictated by osmotic pressure can be given by equation:

$$dV/dt = A\theta\Delta\pi / l \tag{3}$$

Where dV/dt represents the water flow across the membrane area A and thickness l with permeability θ. Δπ depicts the difference in osmotic pressure between the two solutions on either side of the membrane.

This equation is strictly applicable for perfect semipermeable membrane, which is completely impermeable towards solute. Staverman reflection coefficient is included in equation to negotiate deviation from complete semipermeability character of membrane.

ROSE NELSON PUMP

The present day osmotic devices are modified versions of Rose Nelson pump, which was introduced by two Australian physiologists Rose and Nelson, who were interested in the delivery of drugs to the sheep and cattle gut. The original pump proposed by these workers was never patented.

The pump composed of three chambers: a drug chamber, a salt chamber holding solid salt, and a water chamber (Fig. 2.2). A semipermeable membrane separates the salt from water chamber. The movement of water from the water chamber towards salt chamber is influenced by difference in osmotic pressure across the membrane. Conceivably, volume of salt chamber increases due to water flow, which distends the latex diaphragm dividing the salt and drug chambers, eventually the drug is pumped out of the device.

The kinetics of pumping from Rose Nelson pump is presented by equation:

$$dMt/dt = (dV/dt) . C \qquad (4)$$

Where dMt/dt is the drug release rate, dV/dt is the volume flow of water into the salt chamber, and C represents the concentration of drug in the drug chamber. Combining equation (3) and (4) results in

$$dMt/dt = A\theta\Delta\pi \, C \, / \, l \qquad (5)$$

These basic equations are applicable to the osmotically driven controlled drug delivery devices.

The saturated salt solution created a high osmotic pressure compared to that pressure required for pumping the suspension of active agent. Therefore, the rate of water entering into the salt chamber remains constant as long as sufficient solid salt is present in the salt chamber to maintain a saturated solution and thereby a constant osmotic pressure driving force is obtained.

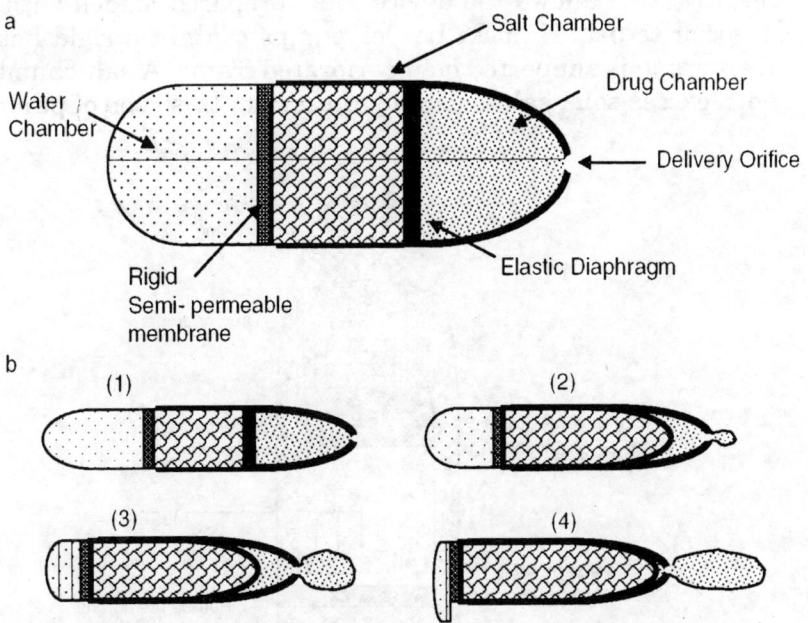

Fig. 2.2: a. Essential features of the three-chamber Rose-Nelson osmotic pump
b. Four stages of drug delivery from Rose-Nelson pump

The major problem associated with Rose Nelson pumps was that the osmotic action began whenever water came in contact with the semipermeable membrane. This reflects that pumps had to be stored empty and water was ought to be loaded prior to use, an inconvenient and maladroit procedure. The Pharmetrix device described in patent 89-1 overwhelmed this drawback. This device is composed of impermeable membrane placed between the semipermeable membrane and the water chamber. This seal permits the storage of pump in fully loaded condition; the pump is activated when the seal is broken. Water is then drawn by a wick to the membrane surface, and the pumping action begins. This modification allows improved storage of the device, which on demand can be easily activated. There have been a large number of Rose Nelson patents, most of these patents describe the use of Rose Nelson pumps as miniature infusion systems to be strapped to the patient, delivering drug via an indwelling catheter. Cyanamid has patented a Rose Nelson pump 71-1. This patent includes, in place of elastic diaphragm of Rose and Nelson's device movable pistons. This was the first device utilising osmotic pressure as a driving force.

HIGUCHI LEEPER OSMOTIC PUMP

Higuchi and Leeper have proposed a series of variations of the Rose Nelson pump and these designs have been described in U.S. patents 73-1, 73-2 and 73-3, which represents the first series of simplifications of the Rose Nelson pump made by the Alza corporation. One of these pumps is illustrated in Fig. 2.3. The Higuchi Leeper pump, has no water chamber, and the activation of the device occurs after imbibition of the water from the surrounding environment. This variation allows the device to be prepared loaded with drug and can be stored for long prior to use. Higuchi Leeper pumps contain a rigid housing, and the semipermeable membrane is supported on a perforated frame. A salt chamber containing a fluid solution with excess solid salt is usually present in this type of pump.

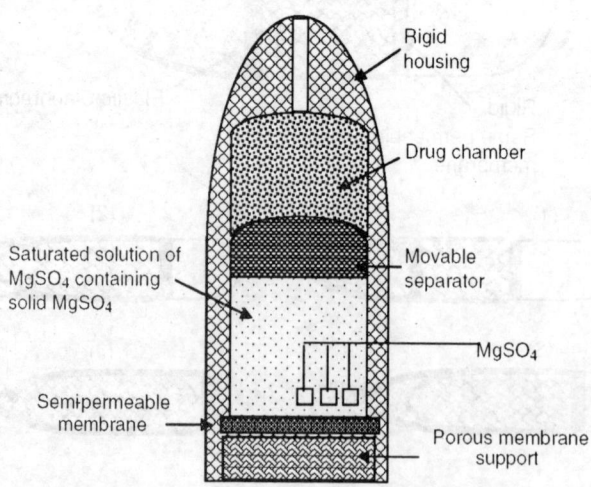

Fig. 2.3: Higuchi-Leeper pump design

Higuchi Leeper pump is widely employed for veterinary use. This type of pump is either swallowed or implanted in body of an animal for delivery of antibiotics or growth hormones to animals. This presents advantage over other medications, which ought to be taken repeatedly, which is inconvenient in case of animals. This problem is overcome by using this device, which can be loaded with full dose and swallowed once, eventually leading to delivery of full course of medication in rumen.

HIGUCHI THEEUWES OSMOTIC PUMP

Higuchi and Theeuwes in early 1970s developed another variant of the Rose Nelson pump, even simpler than the Higuchi Leeper pump. This device is illustrated in Fig. 2.4. In this device, the rigid housing is provided by the semipermeable membrane. This membrane is strong enough to withstand the pumping pressure developed inside the device due to imbibition of water. The desired drug is loaded in the device only prior to its application, which extends advantage for storage of the device for longer duration. The release of the drug from the device is dictated by the salt used in the salt chamber and the permeability characteristics of the outer membrane. Small osmotic pumps of this form are available under trade name Alzet®. They are used frequently as implantable controlled release delivery systems in experimental studies requiring continuous administration of drugs. Diffusional loss of the drug from the device is minimised by making the delivery port in the shape of a long thin tube as shown in Fig. 2.5.

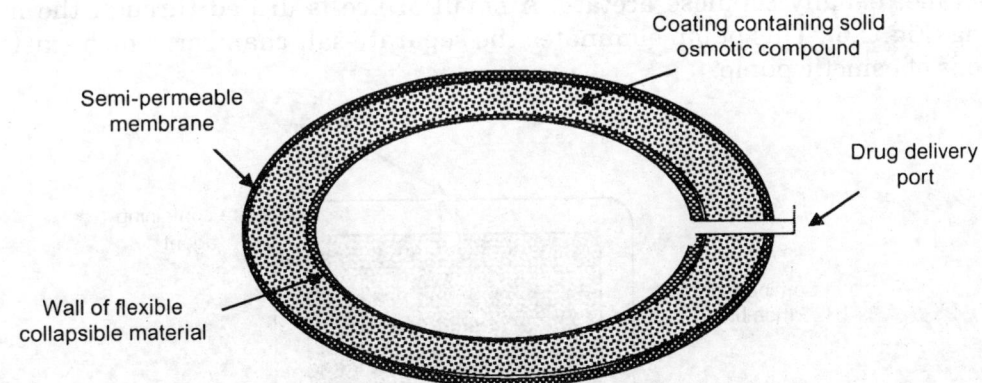

Fig. 2.4: *Higuchi Theeuwes pump design*

One modification of Higuchi Theeuwes pump utilises a mixture of citric acid and sodium bicarbonate in the salt chamber (patent 80-2) to generate the pressure required for delivery of drug. When contacted with water, the mixture produces carbon dioxide gas, which then exerts a pressure on the elastic diaphragm, eventually delivery of drug from device is obtained.

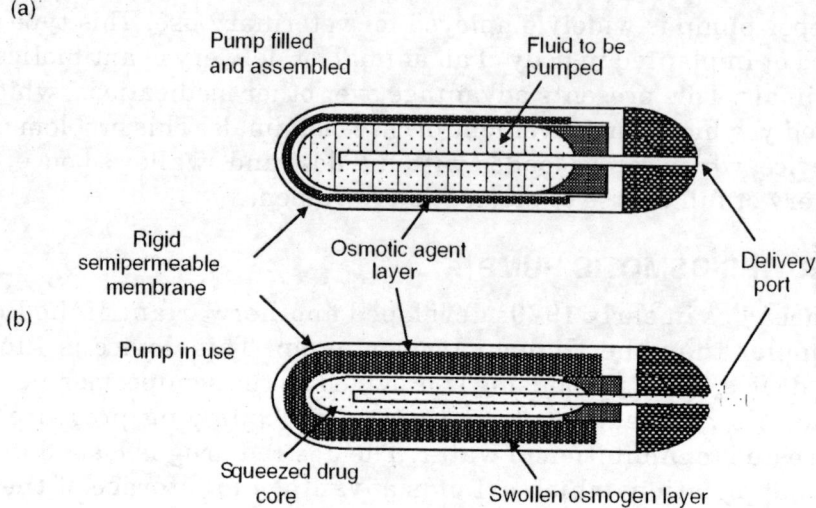

Fig. 2.5: *Theeuwes miniature osmotic pump*

ELEMENTARY OSMOTIC PUMP

Rose Nelson pump was further simplified in the form of elementary osmotic pump, which made osmotic delivery as a major method of achieving controlled drug release. Elementary osmotic pump was invented by Theeuwes in 1974 and it essentially contains an active agent having a suitable osmotic pressure, formed into a tablet coated with semipermeable membrane, usually cellulose acetate. A small orifice is drilled through the membrane coating (Fig. 2.6). This pump eliminates the separate salt chamber, which exists in other versions of osmotic pump.

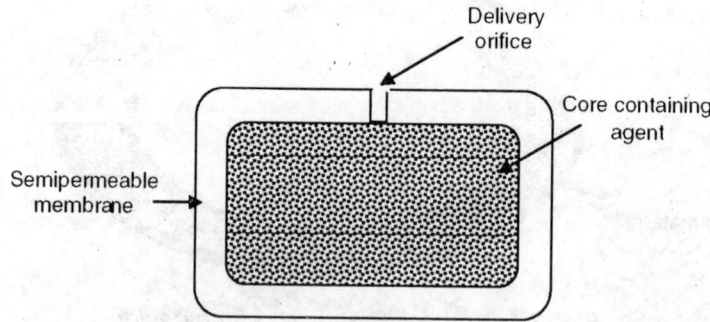

Fig. 2.6: *The elementary osmotic pump*

This device in fact represents a coated tablet with a hole and perhaps, represents the ultimate simplification of the original Rose Nelson device. When this coated tablet is exposed to an aqueous environment, the osmotic pressure of the soluble drug inside the tablet draws water through the semipermeable coating, resulting in formation of a saturated aqueous solution inside the device. The membrane is non-extensible and the increase in volume due to imbibition of water raises the hydrostatic pressure inside the tablet, eventually leading to flow of saturated solution of active agent out of the device through the small orifice. In other words, this tablet functions as a small pump withdrawing water from external environment through the membrane wall and expelling water as a saturated agent solution via the orifice. This process of pumping continues at a constant rate till the entire solid drug inside the tablet has been eliminated leaving only solution filled shell. This residual dissolved drug is delivered at decline rate to attain equilibrium between external and internal drug solution.

The pump initially releases the drug at a rate given by equation (4)

$$dM_t/dt = (dV/dt) \cdot C_s \tag{4}$$

Where dV/dt depicts the water flow into the tablet and C_s is the solubility of the agent inside the tablet. Substituting the value for the water flux from equation (3) gives (5) as

$$dM_t/dt = A\theta\Delta\pi\, C_s\, /\, l \tag{5}$$

This equation reflects that constant release of drug is maintained as long as amount of solid drug is above saturation level and $\Delta\pi$ is maximum. This zero order delivery is followed by decline or non-zero order delivery rate M_{nz} expressed as

$$M_{nz} = C_s\, V_p \tag{6}$$

Where V_p depicts the internal volume of the membrane component. The initial drug content of the device, M_o, is given by

$$M_o = \rho V_p \tag{7}$$

Where ρ is the density of solid drug. The fraction of drug delivered at a non zero order rate is expressed as

$$M_{nz}/M_o = C_s/\rho \tag{8}$$

Since M_o represents initial drug content, it must be equal to the drug delivered at zero and non-zero order release,

$$M_o = M_z + M_{nz} \tag{9}$$

This can further be modified as

$$1 = M_z/M_o + M_{nz}/M_o \tag{10}$$

Substituting values of equation (8) in this equation yields

$$M_z/M_o = 1 - C_s/\rho \tag{11}$$

Extinction of last traces of solid drug leads to fall in both $\Delta\pi$ and C_s and decline in rate of release follows parabolic pattern. It has been suggested that the non-zero order rate after dissolution of last solid drug can be described by the expression

$$dM/dt = (dM/dt)z/[1 + (1/C_sV_p)\,(dM/dt)z\,(t - t_z)]^2 \tag{12}$$

Where (dM/dt) represents the zero-order rate, V_p depicts the internal volume of the membrane and t_z is the time the device is delivering drug at a zero-order rate.

Solubility of drug in water plays a critical role in functioning of osmotic pump. Typically the solubility of drugs delivered by these pumps are at least 10 to 15 wt%, example of drugs with this property are sodium indomethacin, potassium chloride, metoprolol and acetazolamide.

The elementary osmotic pump was developed by Alza under the name OROS®, for controlled release oral drug delivery formulations. The conventional high-speed tabletting machinery and coating machinery are utilised for producing the devices, and laser-drilling system contacted to a conventional tablet-labelling machine is used for drilling small hole in coated tablet. Controlled oral drug delivery offers many advantages like they are easy and self-medication can be done, no need of trained personnel, and avoidance of pain, better patient compliance and treatment of some local gastrointestinal infections. Antigen delivery can also be done by oral route, which leads to the elicitation of systemic as well as mucosal immune response. Antigens enter the systemic circulation through M cells present on the Peyer's patches located in the intestinal tract.

The first elementary osmotic pump that hit the market was Osmosin® (controlled release indomethacin) but withdrawn from the market due to side effects. After little episodes of minor products a mega success was attained from controlled release nifedipine (Procardia XL). Other related products include acutrim® (phenyl propanolamine), minipress XL® (Prazosin), and volmax® (Salbutamol). A number of other products are reported to be on the verge of entry into the market which includes diltiazem, glipizide, verapamil, gemfibrozil and isradipine. For OROS® tablets, the semipermeable membrane coating the device must be 200–300 microns thick to withstand the pressure generated within the device. These thick coverings lower the water permeation rate, particularly for moderately water-soluble drugs. In general we can predict that these thick coating devices are suitable for highly water-soluble drugs. The delivery rate attained with moderately soluble drugs is usually low, even with the most water-permeable membranes. Theeuwes has solved this problem by firstly utilising a coating material with very high water permeability. For example, addition of plasticisers and a water-soluble additive to the cellulose acetate membranes increased the permeability of latter up to tenfold.

The second approach of Theeuwes involves the use of multilayer composite coating around the tablet (Fig. 2.7). The first layer is made up of thick microporous film that provides the strength required to withstand the internal pressure, while second layer is composed of thin semipermeable membrane that produces the osmotic flux. The support layer is formed by various approaches; one novel approach includes coating the tablets with a layer of cellulose acetate containing 40 to 60 % of pore-forming agent such as sorbitol. This layer in turn is coated with the semipermeable layer. When contacted with water, the water-soluble sorbitol leaches out from the membrane, leaving a microporous structure behind.

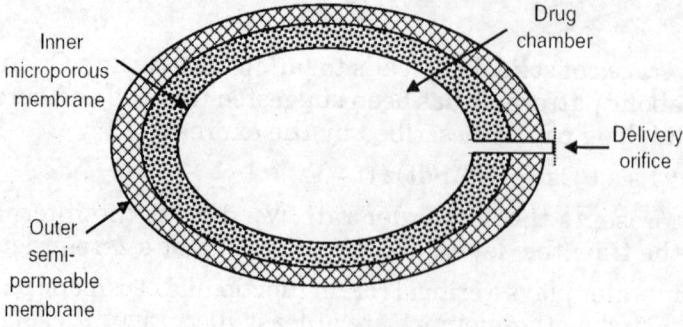

Fig. 2.7: *The composite membrane coating used to deliver moderately soluble drugs*

Another variation in the membrane material includes use of a bioerodable coating, which acts as an enteric coating, moderating drug release patents (77-5, 78-2 and 78-1). One more modification includes the addition of a carbonate or bicarbonate salt to the drug chamber, which eventually leads to effervescence when exposed to water due to formation of carbon dioxide at the stomach pH. This effervescent action prevents the precipitated drug like indomethacin, from blocking the delivery passage from the tablet. Solubility of the agent can be controlled by incorporating buffer compounds in the formulation.

Salbutamol presents unique example of drug with unusual solubility properties. Patents 88-11 and 89-8 describe an interesting tablet for delivery of salbutamol, which possesses a solubility of 270 mg/ml in pure aqueous media, but upon addition of NaCl, the solubility of only 11 mg/ml in a saturated salt solution. The tablet is similar to elementary osmotic pump, with a mixture of salbutamol and NaCl in the tablet core. Then exposed to aqueous environment water imbibition takes place at a rate controlled by the osmotic pressure of saturated solution of salbutamol and NaCl. As excess salbutamol is present, the NaCl is exhausted first, and the rate of water inflow decreases due to decrease in osmotic pressure of the solution inside the tablet. However, solubility of salbutamol increases very quickly with the decrease in NaCl concentration, eventually causing an increased salbutamol delivery although tablet is pumping less solution. The release profile of the device is constant for salbutamol until the sodium chloride becomes exhausted, afterwards the remaining drug is delivered as a large pulse. This release pattern is exploited for nocturnal asthma in which pulsatile delivery of salbutamol is required.

Theeuwes *et al.,* 1981, 1980 has devised a large number of modifications in simple elementary osmotic pump. The simple elementary pump suffers from the disadvantage that it can only deliver relatively soluble drugs, which are capable of developing an osmotic pressure greater than physiological body fluids. Incorporation of water soluble compound into the tablet formulation, which serves as osmotic attractants overcomes this limitation but partially. NaCl, sucrose, fructose or other common tabletting aids can be utilised. However, ultimately saturated solution of both the drug and osmotic attractant are left in the device. This constrains the amount of drug that can be delivered at a constant rate. For example, consider a 500 mg tablet containing NaCl as an osmotic attractant (solubility 26 wt%) with drug (solubility 1 wt%), it reflects that the ratio of NaCl to drug in the tablet is 26:1 and the osmotic device would deliver only 18 mg of drug. Osmotic attractant of lower solubility permits for incorporation of more drug into the tablet but diminishes the release rate. Thus, in order to obtain desired or meaningful delivery rates with elementary osmotic pump, solubility of drug must be relatively high.

Delivery of insoluble drug is achieved by a method illustrated in Fig. 2.8. In this approach osmotic agent is coated with an elastic, semipermeable film. These particles are then mixed with the insoluble drug substance and the resultant mixture is coated with the rigid semipermeable membrane. Osmotic agent tend to draw water across two membranes eventually swells and hydrostatically force the insoluble drug out of the orifice made in the device. Several coated tablets have been reported in which the exit hole, through which the drug escapes, is formed following leaching of water soluble component, such as lactose or poly (ethylene glycol), from the coating material. Once the tablet has been swallowed, water-soluble component dissolves in external fluid, resulting in initiation of pumping system. In early 1970s, several slow release tablet formulation were popular, which utilises osmotic component in their release mechanism.

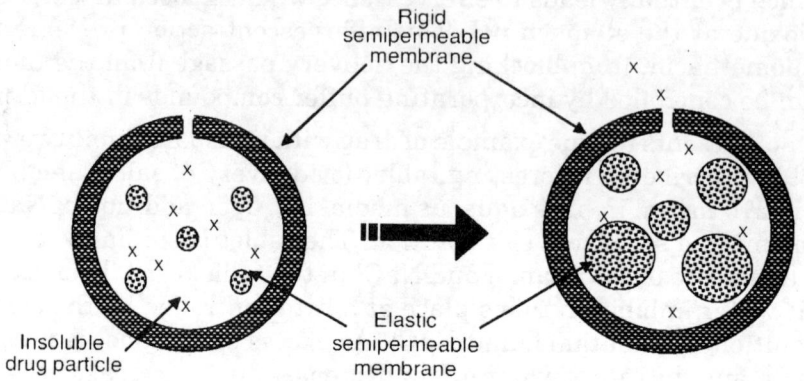

Fig. 2.8: *A proposed method of delivering insoluble drugs*

General Considerations and Materials Used

Osmotic pumps are essentially contains drug and semipermeable membrane. In this case, drug itself act as an osmogen and shows good aqueous solubility (e.g. potassium chloride pumps). If the drug does not possess any osmogenic property, the osmogenic salt and other sugars can be incorporated in the formulation. Osmogens are freely water soluble and capable of producing osmotic pressure. Single osmogen can be used for the formulations and in some case combination of osmogens have been used.

Apart from these essential components, other materials such as hydrophilic and hydrophobic polymers and hydrogel (either swellable or non-swellable nature), wicking agents, solubilising agents and surfactants have been used depend on the type of formulations. The coating semipermeable membrane usually contains a plasticiser and in some cases surfactants, flux regulating agents and pore forming agents. Apart from the above materials, common tabletting aids such as lubricants, binders, diluents, glidants, wetting agents, etc. can be used for the development of osmotic systems. The wall thickness is in between 1–1000 μm, but 200–500μm is desirable. The percentage weight increase of the tablets after coating should be around 10–15%. One aperture is usually made in the system, in some cases more than one delivery passages can be made with the diameter of 200–600μm.

Semipermeable Membrane

The choice of a rate-controlling membrane is an important aspect in the formulation development of oral osmotic systems. Since the membrane in osmotic systems is semi permeable in nature, any polymer that is permeable to water but impermeable to solute can be selected. Some of the polymers that can be used for above purpose include cellulose esters such as cellulose acetate, cellulose diacetate, cellulose triacetate, cellulose propionate, cellulose acetate butyrate, etc.; cellulose ethers like ethyl cellulose and eudragits. Cellulose acetate is commonly employed semipermeable polymer for the preparation of osmotic pumps. It is available in different acetyl content grades. Particularly acetyl content 32 and 38% are widely used. Cellulose acetate is having degree of substitution (DS), i.e., the average number of hydroxyl groups on the anhydro-glucose unit of the polymer replaced by substituting group. If it is up to 1, the acetyl content up to 21%. Cellulose diacetate is having a DS of 1–2 and an acetyl content of 21–35%. Cellulose triacetate is having a DS of 2–3 and an acetyl content of 35–44.8%. Apart form cellulose derivatives, some other polymers such as agar acetate, amylose triacetate, betaglucan acetate, poly (vinyl methyl) ether copolymers, poly (orthoesters), poly acetals and selectively permeable poly (glycolic acid) and poly (lactic acid) derivatives can be used as semipermeable film forming materials. The permeability is the important criteria for the selection of semipermeable polymers.

Hydrophilic and Hydrophobic Polymers

These polymers are used in the formulation development of osmotic systems for making drug entrapped matrix core inside the pumps. The highly water soluble compounds can be entrapped in hydrophobic matrices and moderately water soluble compounds can be entrapped in hydrophilic matrices to obtain more controlled release. Generally mixtures of both hydrophilic and hydrophobic polymers have been used in the development of osmotic pumps of water-soluble drugs. The selection is based on the solubility of the drug as well as the amount of drug should be released from the pump. The polymers are either swellable or non-swellable nature. Mostly swellable polymers have been used for the pumps containing moderately water-soluble drugs, since they increase the hydrostatic pressure inside the pump by swelling nature. The non-swellable polymers are used in case of highly water-soluble drugs. Ionic hydrogels such as sodium carboxymethyl cellulose is preferably used because of its osmogenic nature. More precise controlled release of drugs can be achieved by incorporating these polymers into the formulations. Hydrophilic polymers such as hydroxy ethyl cellulose, carboxy methylcellulose, hydroxy propyl methylcellulose, high molecular weight poly (vinyl pyrrolidine) and hydrophobic polymers such as ethyl cellulose and wax materials can be used for this purpose (Rudnic *et al.*, 2000).

Wicking Agents

A wicking agent is defined as any material with the ability to draw water into the porous network of a delivery device. A wicking agent is either swellable or non-swellable nature. They are characterised by having the ability to undergo physisorption with water. Physisorption is a form of absorption in which the solvent molecules can loosely adhere to surfaces of the wicking agent via van der Waals' interactions between the surface of the wicking agent and the adsorbed molecule. The function of the wicking agent is to carry water to surfaces inside the core of the tablet, thereby creating channels or a network of increased surface area. For bioactive agents with low solubility in water, the wicking agent aids in the delivery of partially solubilised bioactive agent through the passageway in the semipermeable coating. Materials suitable for acting as wicking agents include colloidal silicon dioxide, kaoline, titanium dioxide, alumina, niacinamide, sodium lauryl sulfate (SLS), low molecular weight poly (vinyl pyrrolidine) (PVP), m-pyrol, bentonite, magnesium aluminum silicate, polyester and polyethylene. SLS, colloidal silica and PVP are non-swellable wicking agents.

Solubilising Agents

Non-swellable solubilising agents are classified into three groups,

- Agents that inhibit crystal formation of the drugs or otherwise act by complexation with the drugs (e.g. PVP, poly (ethylene glycol) [PEG 8000] and α, β, γ - cyclodextrins)
- A high HLB micelle-forming surfactant, particularly anionic surfactants (e.g. Tween 2C, 60 and 80, poly oxyethylene or poly ethylene containing surfactants and other long chain anionic surfactants such as SLS)
- Citrate esters and their combinations with anionic surfactants (e.g. alkyl esters particularly triethyl citrate)

Above all, combinations of complexing agents and anionic surfactants such as PVP with SLS and poly (ethylene glycol) and SLS are mostly preferred.

Osmogens

Osmogens are essential ingredient of the osmotic formulations. Table 2.1 shows some osmogenic agents commonly used in preparation osmotic pumps. They include inorganic salts and carbohydrates. Generally combinations of osmogens are used to achieve optimum osmotic pressure inside the system.

Surfactants

Surfactants are particularly useful when added to wall forming material. They are producing an integral composite that is useful for making the operative wall of the device. The surfactants act by regulating the surface energy of materials to improve their blending in to the composite and maintain their integrity in the environment of use during the drug release period. Typical surfactants such as poly oxyethylenated glyceryl recinoleate, polyoxyethylenated castor oil having ethylene oxide, glyceryl laurates, glycerol (sorbiton oleate, stearate or laurate), etc.

Coating Solvents

Solvents suitable for manufacturing the wall of the osmotic device include inert inorganic and organic solvents that do not adversely harm the core, wall and other materials. The typical solvents include methylene chloride, acetone, methanol, ethanol, isopropyl alcohol, butyl alcohol, ethyl acetate cyclohexane carbon tetrachloride, water, etc. The mixtures of solvents such as acetone-methanol (80:20), acetone-ethanol (80:20), acetone-water (90:10), methylene chloride-methanol (79:21), methylene chloride-methanol-water (75:22:3), etc. can be used and express as weight: weight.

Plasticisers

Plasticisers lower the temperature of the second order phase transition of the wall or the elastic modules of the wall and also increase the workability, flexibility and permeability of the fluids. Generally from 0.001 to 50 parts of a plasticiser or a mixture of plasticisers are incorporated into 100 parts of wall forming materials. Suitable polymers should have a high degree of solvent power for the materials, are compatible with the materials over both the processing and the temperature range, exhibit permanence as seen by their strong tendency to remain in the plasticised wall, impart flexibility to the materials and are non-toxic. Exemplary plasticisers include dialkyl phthalates and other phthalates, trioctyl phosphates and other phosphates, alkyl adipates, triethyl citrate and other citrates, acetates, propionates, glycolates, glycerolates, myristates, benzoates, sulfonamides and halogenated phenyls.

Flux Regulators

Flux regulating agent of flux enhancing agent or flux decreasing agents is added to a wall forming material, assists in regulating the fluid permeability of flux through wall. This agent can be pre-selected to increase or decrease the liquid flux. Agents that produce a marked increase in permeability to fluid such as water are essentially hydrophilic, while those produce a marked decrease to fluids (water) are essentially hydrophobic. They also increase the flexibility and porosity of the lamina. Polyhydric alcohols such as poly alkylene glycols and low molecular weight glycols such as polypropylene, poly butylene and poly amylene, etc. can be used as flux regulators. The amount of flux regulator added to a material generally is an amount sufficient to produce the desired permeability, and it will vary according to the lamina forming materials. Usually from 0.001 parts to 50 parts or higher of flux regulator can be used to achieve the desired results.

Pore Forming Agents

These agents are particularly used in the pumps developed for poorly water-soluble drug and in the development of controlled porosity or multi-particulate osmotic pumps. These pore-forming agents cause the formation of microporous membrane. The microporous wall may be formed *in situ* by a pore-former being removed by dissolving or leaching it during the operation of the system. The pores may also be formed in the wall prior to operation of the system by gas formation within coating polymer solutions which result in void and pores in the final form of the wall. The pore-formers can be inorganic or organic and solid or liquid in nature. For example, alkaline metal salts such as sodium chloride, sodium bromide, potassium chloride, potassium sulfate, potassium phosphate, etc., alkaline earth metals such as calcium chloride and calcium nitrate, carbohydrates such as sucrose, glucose, fructose, mannose, lactose, sorbitol, mannitol and, diols and polyols such as polyhydric alcohols and polyvinyl pyrrolidine can be used as pore forming agents.

Pores may also be formed in the wall by the volatilisation of components in a polymer solution or by chemical reactions in a polymer solution which evolves gases prior to application or during application of the solution to the core mass resulting in the creation of polymer foams serving as the porous wall. The pore-formers should be non-toxic, and on their removal, channels are formed that fill with fluid. The channels become a transport path for fluid. pH insensitive pore-formers are usually preferred.

Modified Multichamber Elementary Osmotic Pump

Elementary osmotic pump is limited to the delivery of relatively soluble drugs, generally with solubilities more than 2–5 wt%. Multichamber tablet approach solved the problem and practically and commercially proved the worth in the form of major product Procardia XL (controlled release nifedipine).

These multichamber tablets can be divided into two major classes based on whether one chamber expands into the other or they have got rigid walls and maintain their volume for the whole course of operation. The classes of tablets with expanding chamber are more important and are frequently employed by manufactures to produce osmotic devices and therefore will be discussed in priority.

TABLETS WITH A SECOND EXPANDABLE OSMOTIC CHAMBER

Tablets with two chambers separated by an elastic or movable barrier are particularly interesting and valuable because they allow delivery of drugs with limited solubility. This class of osmotic pump can further be classified into two groups one with internal film that moves from a rest to an expanded state or the volumes of the chambers communicating through opening provided in between.

In the tablets with a second expandable osmotic chamber, the water is simultaneously drawn into both the chambers in proportion to the osmotic gradient, eventually causing the increase in volume of the chamber and subsequently forcing the drug out from the drug chamber. Fig. 2.9 illustrates the mechanism of action of these devices. Conceptually, the device is related to Higuchi-Leeper pumps described earlier but in these devices, the semipermeable membrane forms the entire shell, and water is drawn simultaneously into both the chambers. The selection of matrix in which the drug is to be suspended presents a challenge in front of product formulation people. The matrix should have a sufficient osmotic pressure to draw water through the membrane into the drug chamber. Under hydrated conditions matrix have to be fluid enough to be pushed easily through a small hole by the little pressure generated by the elastic diaphragm.

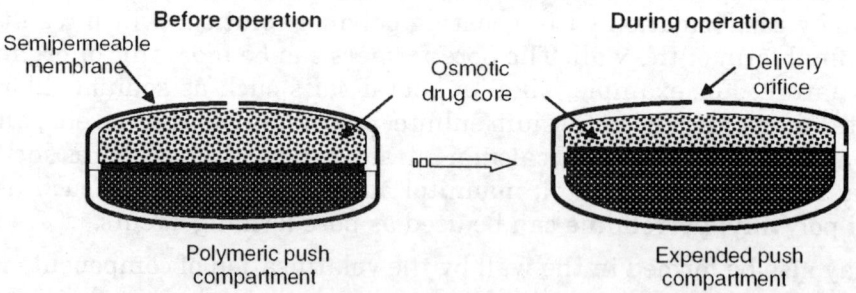

Fig. 2.9: *Drug delivery process of two-chamber osmotic tablet*

Among the successful approaches, incorporation of finely dispersed drug in hydrogel presents a most valuable alternative. Many of the useful hydrogel polymers were ionic materials such as sodium carboxy methylcellulose, which contains ionisable groups, which provide most of the osmotic pressure required to draw water through the semipermeable membrane. These polymers possesses dual property of being compressed in dry conditions and becomes fluid gels easily extrudable through the small delivery hole in hydrated conditions.

The controlled release nifedipine (Procardia XL) device is illustrated in Fig. 2.10. The device contains an external semipermeable membrane made up of cellulose acetate bearing a laser drilled small orifice. The drug chamber possesses the drug, nifedipine, hydroxy propyl methylcellulose, poly (ethylene oxide) along with small amount sodium chloride to assist in drawing water into the chamber. A mixture of poly (ethylene oxide) and hydroxy propyl methyl cellulose constitute the swellable hydrogel chamber. The two layered tablet is made with a special tablet press, such as the Manesty layer press.

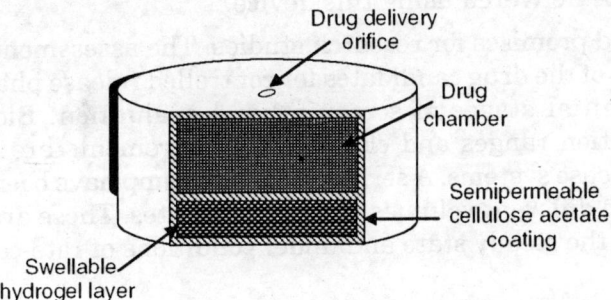

Fig. 2.10: *Osmotic tablet of nifedipine*

The working principle of the nifedipine osmotic device involves the imbibition of fluid by the drug chamber composition to form a fluid composition *in situ,* and the delivery of the suspension through the passageway. Concurrently, imbibition of fluid by the hydrogel layer causes this second layer to swell and assists with the first composition to drive the drug through the orifice. The osmotic device may be considered as a cylinder, with the second hydrogel composition expanding like the movement of a piston to aid in delivering the agent from the device.

Devices with a Non-Expanding Second Chamber

The second class of multichamber devices comprises of systems containing a non-expanding second chamber. This class can be further divided into two groups, based on the function of the second chamber.

In one group of these devices, the second chamber serves for the dilution of the drug solution leaving the device. This is important in cases where the drug leaves the oral osmotic device as a saturated solution; irritation of the gastrointestinal tract is a risk. This was the reason behind the withdrawal of Osmosin®, sodium indomethacin. The device essentially contains a normal drug containing OROS® tablet from which drug is released as a saturated solution. However, before the drug can exit from the device, it must pass through a second chamber. Water is also drawn osmotically into this chamber either due to the osmotic pressure of the drug solution or because the second chamber bears a water-soluble diluents such as sucrose or sodium chloride.

The second group of non-expanding multichamber devices essentially contains two separate simple OROS® tablets formed into a single tablet as shown in Fig 2.11. Two chambers contains two separate drugs and both are delivered simultaneously.

A more sophisticated version of these devices consists of two rigid chambers, one contains biologically inert osmotic agent such as sugar or a simple salt like NaCl, and the second chamber contains the drug. When exposed to aqueous environment, water is drawn into both chambers across the semipermeable membrane as shown in Fig. 2.11. The solution of osmotic agent formed in the first chamber then passes to the drug chamber through the connecting hole where it mixes with the drug solution before escaping through the microporous membrane that forms part of the wall around the drug chamber. Relatively insoluble drug could be delivered using this device.

These systems hold promises for research studies. The assessment of the pharmacology and pharmacokinetics of the drug candidates for controlled release pharmaceutical products is essential during initial stages of screening and evaluation. Bioavailability studies, therapeutic concentration ranges and clearance measurements are of great value in the design of controlled release systems. A series of osmotic pump have been developed (as shown in Table 2.2) to provide different volumes and delivery rates. These are useful in evaluating drug pharmacology in the steady state and under conditions of rate-controlled drug inputs.

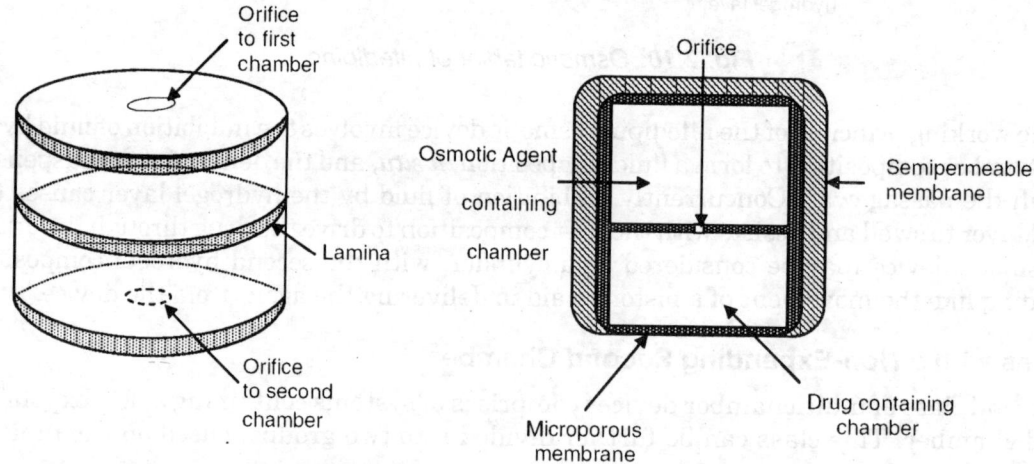

Fig. 2.11: *Example of multichamber osmotic devices with chambers separated by rigid non-expanding walls*

Table 2.2: *Characteristics of osmotic pumps*

Research use	Route of administration	Duration of steady-state delivery (hr)	Fill volume (ml)	Steady-state delivery rate (ml/hr)	Distinguishing terminology
Clinical research	Oral	12	0.2	15	Oral pump
Clinical research	Oral	24	0.2	8	Oral pump
Clinical research	Rectal/vaginal	30	2	60	Rectal pump
Animal research	Implant	168	0.2	1	Mini-osmotic pump
Animal research	Implant	336	0.2	0.5	Mini-osmotic pump
Animal research	Implant	168	2	10	Osmotic pump
Animal research	Implant	336	2	5	Osmotic pump

The range of sizes and pumping capabilities is from 0.2 to 2 ml in fill volume; study state pumping rates of 0.5 to 60 microlitres/hr can be achieved and duration of delivery of 12 to 336 hr, depending upon the devices fill volume and pumping rate.

PROTOCOL: 2.1
Preparation of Controlled Porosity Osmotic Pump (CPOP) Materials

Core Components of Optimised Formulations
Diltiazem Hydrochloride (DLTZ)
Polyvinyl pyrrolidine
Mannitol
Hydroxy propyl methyl cellulose (200–300 cps, medium viscosity grade)
Sodium carboxy methyl cellulose (NaCMC – medium viscosity 400–800 cps)
Talc
Mg stearate

Components of Coating Solutions
Cellulose acetate (320 S)
Polyethylene glycol (PEG) 400
Sorbitol

Preparation of Tablet and Coating
- For small scale preparations of these osmotic pumps, the components are blended for 20 min in a Terbula mixer and the blend is then milled using a Quadromini Comil 193AS, blend again for 20 min lubricated with magnesium stearate and blended for an additional 4 min.
- The tablets are then compressed using a Manesty single station Type "F" tablet press with 13/32-in. standard round concave (SRC) tooling. The average tablet weight is kept approx. 500 mg and average hardness is maintained typically 8–10Kg.
- The tablet cores are sprayed with a coating solution made from Cellulose acetate, polyethylene glycol, acetone and water. In some formulation the ratio of CA/PEG may be changed in order to study the effect of the coating permeability on drug release performance.
- In case of bilayer tablets a small quantity of a red or blue dye (generally 0.1w/w) is added to the swellable layer with appropriate adjustment in the quantity of other excipients. This will help to identify the drug layer side after the coating was completed.
- Then delivery ports are then made on the drug side of the coated bilayer tablets. Holes are generally 0.9mm in diameter and drilled mechanically or by laser, on the face of the tablets.
- Two different types of delivery ports are made on the tablets. 0.9mm slits were made either on the face of the tablets or the land (sometimes referred to as the band of the tablet).

Swellable Core Containing Osmotic Pumps

In this class of osmotic pumps different types of core configuration is prepared and their descriptions are shown as:

- Homogeneous cores, consisting of single layer.
- Tablet in tablet (TNT) cores, consisting of a water swellable central core surrounded by the drug formulations.
- Bilayer cores consisting of water swellable layer and a drug containing osmotic layer adjacent to each other.
- Trilayer cores, consisting of a water swellable layer sandwiched between two drug containing layers.

PROTOCOL: 2.2

Preparation of Swellable Core Containing Osmotic Pumps

Materials

Atenolol

NaCl

Tartaric acid

Polyvinyl pyrrolidon k30

Ethyl cellulose (EC)

Polyethylene glycol 400 (PEG 400)

Methanol (HPLC grade)

Preparation of Core Tablets

- Mix the composition of core tablet atenolol powder, tartaric acid, NaCl and PVP and then the mixture is granulated through a 1000 µm sieve using wet method.
- Dry the granules at 50°C for 4 h. After that pass the granules by a 1250 µm sieve and compress into core tablets with an indentation using single-punch tabletting machine with upper concave faced punch.
- Keep the diameter and the deepness of the indentation 1.00 mm and 1.50 mm, respectively. Maintain weight of each tablet within the range of (250 ± 5) mg.

Coating and Drying of Core Tablets

- The prepared core tablets are coated with EC (3%, w/v) in 95% ethanol containing PEG400 (33%, PEG400/EC, v/w) as coating solution.
- Perform the coating in a pan coater. Pan-rotating rate is adjusted to 33 rpm; spray rate is 3 ml/min. The coated tablets are dried overnight at 50°C to remove the residual solvent.
- After coating, the indentation remains of sufficient size at least partly uncoated as the orifice for drug release.
- Keep the prepared osmotic pump tablets in a dessicator for future experiments (Scheme 2.1).

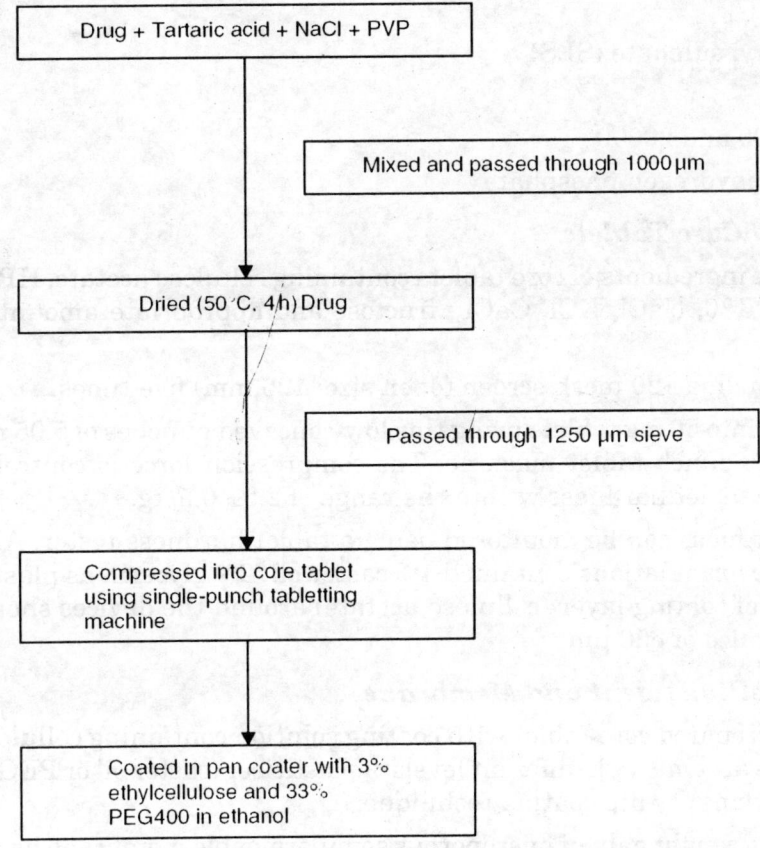

Scheme 2.1 *preparation of swellable core containing osmotic pumps*

PROTOCOL: 2.3

Preparation of Swellable Elementary Osmotic Pump for Delivery of Poorly Water-soluble Drugs

Materials

Cellulose acetate with 40% acetyl groups (CA)

HPMCs (K100M, E50LV, E15LV and E5LV)

Carbopols 940 and 934 (B.F. Goodrich)

Sodium carboxy methyl cellulose (NaCMCs) 200 and 1500 cps

Poly vinyl pyrrolidone (PVP K30)

NaCl

KCl

Magnesium stereate

Fructose

Sodium lauryl sulphate (SLS)

Caster oil

PEG 300, 600 and 20000

Potassium dihydrogen phosphate

Preparation of Core Tablets

- Mix all the ingredients of core tablets containing cellulose acetate, HPMCs, carbopols 940, PVP K30, NaCl, KCl, $CaCl_2$, fructose and appropriate amount of magnesium stearate.

- Sieve through a 120 mesh screen (open size: 125 mm) five times.

- Compress into 50 mg tablets using this low-concaved punches of 5.05 mm in diameter on a single punch tablet machine. The compression force is controlled in order to obtain the tablet hardness within the range of 2.5± 0.5 kg.

- Tablet hardness can be monitored using a tablet hardness tester. All devices made from these formulations contained 1% caster oil, 2% glycerin as plasticisers and the thickness of coating layer (cellulose acetate) around the devices should be 0.13 mm with an orifice of 650 μm.

Coating of Swelling Agent and Membrane

- Coat the prepared core tablet with coating solution containing cellulose acetate (CA, 4%, w/v) in acetone with different levels of plasticiser (caster oil or PEGs with different concentrations) by dip coating technique.

- Control the weight gain of microporous semipermeable membrane by adding variable amount of PEG 400 (25% of total coating materials), which acts as a hydrophilic plasticiser and enhances the physical-mechanical property of CA membrane.

- The coating conditions are variable: stainless steel pan, 200 mm diameter; 4 baffles; rotation rate of the pan, 40 rpm; nozzle diameter of spray gun, 1 mm; spray rate, 3 ml/min; spray pressure, 2 bar; drying temperature, 40°C.

- Dry the coated tablets at room temperature for 12 h at 50°C.

- Drill the dry coated tablet by microdriller on both the sides of the tablets. For coated tablets, a small orifice can be drilled through one side of each coated tablet by standard mechanical micro-drills with various diameters (ranging from 250 to 800 μm).

PROTOCOL: 2.4

Preparation of Monolithic Osmotic Tablet System for Water-insoluble Drug

Materials

Naproxen powder

Gum Arabic

Cellulose acetate (CA, 54–56.0 wt.% acetyl content)

Polyethylene glycol 400 (PEG 400)

Preparation of Tablet Core

- Manually mixing of Naproxen powder and gum Arabic
- Compression of the resultant power mixture into tablets on 12-mm concave punches under a pressure of 8–10 Pa

Coating and Drilling of Tablet Core

- Coat the prepared core tablet with coating solution containing cellulose acetate (CA, 4%, w/v) in acetone using a coating pan. The diameter of the coating pan is 230 mm, pan-rotating rate is 50 rpm and spray rate of CA solution is 4 ml/min.
- Dry coated tablets at room temperature for 24 h.
- Drill the dry coated tablet by microdriller on both sides of the tablets with 1.25 mm orifice.
- Composition of tablet materials, amount of plasticiser, membrane thickness, coating solution can be changed as per requirement.

PROTOCOL: 2.5

Preparation of Novel Pulsed-release Osmotic Pump Systems

Materials

Terbutaline sulfate (TB)

Eudragit (RS-PO and RL-PO)

Milayers: microcrystalline cellulose (MCC)

Starch

Sodium carboxylmethyl starch (CMS-Na)

Triethylcitrate (TEC)

Hydroxypropylmethylcellulose E5 (Methocel E5)

Sodium chloride

Preparation of Core Tablets

- Mix all the ingredient of core tablets containing 10% (w/w) TB, 30% sodium chloride, 20% milayers: microcrystalline cellulose (MCC), 20% starch, 20% sodium carboxylmethyl starch (CMS-Na) and appropriate amount of magnesium stearate.
- Mix all excipients for 15 min and sieve through a 120 mesh screen (opening size: 125 mm) five times.
- Compress into 50 mg tablets using this low-concaved punches of 5.05 mm in diameter on a single punch tablet machine. The compression force is controlled in order to obtain the tablet hardness within the range of 2.5 ± 0.5 kg. Tablet hardness can be monitored using a tablet hardness tester.

Coating of Swelling Agent and Membrane

- After warming core tablets for 15 min, coat core tablets by conventional pan-spray method under the variable operating conditions. The ratio of Eudragit RS to RL is different but the total amount of Eudragit polymer is constant in the dispersion formulation.
- Dry tablets at 50°C for 5 h to remove residual solvent after coating.
- Determine the surface morphology and *in vitro* release kinetics of coated tablets.

PROTOCOL: 2.6

Preparation of Chitosan-based Controlled Porosity Osmotic Pump Tablets for Colon-specific Delivery System

Materials

Budesonide

Chitosan (deacetylation degree 96%)

Silicified microcrystalline cellulose (SMCC, Pro-Solv® 90)

Citric acid

Cellulose acetate (CA, 54.5–56 wt.% acetyl content)

Eudragit® L100-55

Triethylcitrate (TEC),

Polyethylene glycol (PEG) 400

Talc and magnesium stearate (Mg-St)

Preparation of Core Tablets

- Mix budesonide, chitosan and other ingredients by spatulation
- Sieve the resultant powder mixture through 100-mesh screen
- Compress into tablets using 8.0 mm standard concave punches on a single punch tablet machine. The weight of each tablet should be maintained within the range of 200±5 mg in order to maintain the relatively constant volume and surface area.

Coating and Drilling of Tablet Core

- Coat the prepared core tablet with coating solution containing cellulose acetate (CA, 4%, w/v) in acetone with different levels of pore forming agent (chitosan) using a coating pan. The weight gains of microporous semipermeable membrane can be controlled by adding variable amount of PEG 400 (25% of total coating materials) that acts as a hydrophilic plasticiser and enhances the physical–mechanical property of CA membrane. The coating conditions are variable: stainless steel pan, 200 mm diameter; 4 baffles; rotation rate of the pan, 40 rpm; nozzle diameter of spray gun, 1 mm; spray rate, 3 mL/min; spray pressure, 2 bar; drying temperature, 40°C.
- Dry coated tablets at room temperature for 12 h at 50°C.

- Drill the dry coated tablet by a microdriller on both the sides of the tablets with 1.25-mm orifice. Composition of tablet materials; amount of plasticiser, membrane thickness, and coating solution can be changed as per requirement.

SUGGESTED READINGS

- Abrahamsson, B., Alpstrn, M., Bake, B., Jonsson, V. E., Eridsson-Lepdowska, M. and Larsson, A. (1998), J. Control. Rel. 52(3), 301.
- Ayer, A. D., Theeuwes, F., (1980). US Patent No. 4, 200, 098.
- Ayer, A. D., Theeuwes, F., (1981). US Patent No. 4, 285, 987.
- Baker, R.W. and Lonsdale H.K. (1975), Chem. Tech. 5, 668.
- Bauer, K., Kaik, G. and Kaik, B. (1994), Hypertension 24(3), 339.
- Bonson, P., Wong, P. S. and Theeuwes, F. (1982), U. S. Patent 4, 344, 929.
- Bosker, F. J., Van Esseveldt, K. E., Klompmakers, A. A. and Westenberg, H. G. (1995), Psychopharmacology (Berl) 117(3), 358.
- Catellani, P. L., Colombo, P., Peppas, M. A., Santi, P. and Bettini, R. (1998), J. Pharm. Sci. 87(6), 726.
- Chaffman M., Brogden R.N. (1985) Drugs. 29, 387–454.
- Chandrasekaran, S.K., Theeuwes, F. and Yum, S. I. (1979) ; In: Drug Design, vol. 8, E. J. Ariens (Ed.), Academic, New York, 134.
- Di Joseph, J. F., Russo, R. J. and Cochran, D. W. (1993), Transplantation 55(2), 450.
- Eckenhoff, B. and Wright, R. M. (1983); In: Controlled Drug Delivery, S. D. Bruck (Ed.), vol. 2nd, CRC Press, Inc., Florida, 76.
- Encarnacion, M. and Chin, I. (1994), Eur. J. Clin. Pharmcol. 46(6), 533.
- Florence, A. T. and Jani, P. U. (1994), Drug Saf. 10(3), 233.
- Grundy, J. S. and Foster, R. T. (1996), Clin. Pharmacokinet. 30(1),28.
- Haslam J.L., Rork G.S.,U.S. patent 4, 880, 631, Nov. 14, 1989.
- Higuchi, T. and Leeper, H. M. (1976), U. S. Patent 3, 995, 631.
- Higuchi, T. and Leeper, H. M. (1973), U.S. Patent 3, 760, 804.
- Higuchi, T. (1973), U.S. Patent 3,760, 805.
- Hopkins, S.P., Bulgrin, J. P., Sims, R. L., Bowman, B., Donovan, D. L. and Schmidt, S. P. (1998), J. Vasc. Surg. 27(5), 886.
- Ikeda, Y., Carson, B. S., Lauer, J. A. and Long, D. M. (1993) J. Neurosur. 79(5), 716.
- Katz, B., Rosenberg, A. and Frishman, W. H. (1995), Am. Heart J. 129(2), 359.
- Keith, A. D. (1984) , U. S. Patent 4, 428, 926.
- Kendall, M.J., Jack, D. B., Woods, K. L., Laugher, S. J., Quarterman, C. P. and John, V. A. (1982), British J. Clin. Pharmacol. 13, 393.
- Lia X., Pana W. S., Niea S. F., Wub L. J.(2004) Journal of Controlled Release, 96,359.
- Liu H, Yang XG, Nie SF, Wei LL, Zhoub LL, Liu H, Tang R, Pan WS, (2007) International Journal of Pharmaceutics, 332, 115.
- Lu EX, Jiang ZQ, Zhang QZ, Jiang XG, J Control Rel., 92 (2003) 375.

- Makhija S.N., Vavia P.R., (2003) Journal of Controlled Release 89, 5.
- McClelland G.A., Sutton S.C., Engle K., Zentner G.M., Pharm. Res. 8 (1991) 88.
- McKellar, Q. A. (1994), Vet. Parasitol. 54(1–3), 249.
- Nakano, M., Higuchi, T. and Hussain, A. (1976), U.S. Patent 3, 995, 632.
- Okimoto, K., Rauewski, R. A. and Stella, V. J. (1999) J. Control. Release, 58, 29.
- Ozdemir, N., Sahin, J., (1997) Design of a Controlled Release Osmotic Pump System of Ibuprofen, Int., J. pharma, 158, 91–97
- Pastore, C. J., Isner, J. M., Bacha, P. A., Kearney, M. and Pickering, J. G. (1995), Circ. Res. 77(3), 519.
- Polli, G. P., Shoop, C. E. and Grim, W. M. (1970), U. S. Patent 3, 538, 214.
- Prabakaran D., Singh P., Kannaujia P., Vyas S.P, Int. J. Pharm. 259 (2003) 173.
- Ramakrishna, N., Mishra, B., 2001 Design and Evaluation of Osmotic Pump Tablet of Naproxen Sodium Pharmazie, 56, 958–962.
- Reid, C.E. (1966); In: Desalimation by Reverse Osmosis, U. Merten (Ed.), MIT Press, Cambridge, MA,1.
- Rose, S. and Nelson, J.F. (1955), Australian J. Exp. Biol. 33, 415.
- Sandberg, A., Abragamsson, B., Svenheden, A., Olofsson, B. and Bergstrand, R. (1993), Pharm. Res. 10(1), 28.
- Santus G., W.R. Baker, J. Control. Release 35 (1995) 1.
- Santus, Giancarlo and Baker, R. W. (1995), J. Control. Rel. 35, 1.
- Staverman, A.J. (1951), Rec. Trav. Chim. 10, 344.
- Theeuwes F., J. Pharm. Sci. 64 (1975) 1987–1991.
- Theeuwes, E., Swansm, D., Wong, P., Bonsen, P., Place, L., Heimlich, K. and Kwan, K. C. (1983), J. Pharm. Sci. 72(3),253.
- Theeuwes, F. and Ayer, A. D. (1978), U. S. Patent 4, 256, 108.
- Theeuwes, F. and Bayne, W. (1981); In: Controlled Release Pharmaceuticals, J. Urquhart (Ed.), American Pharmaceutical Association, Washington, DC.
- Theeuwes, F. and Higuchi, T. (1974), U. S. Patent, 3, 845, 770.
- Theeuwes, F. and Yum, S. I. (1976), Annals of Biomedical Engineering 4(4), 343.
- Theeuwes, F. (1973), U.S. Patent 3, 760, 984.
- Theeuwes, F. (1978), U. S. Patent 4, 256, 108.
- Theeuwes, F. (1985); In: Rate Control in Drug Therapy, L. F. Prescott and W. S. Nimmo (Eds.), Churchill Livingstone, Edinburgh, 116.
- Theeuwes, F., Bayne, W. and McGuire, J. (1978), Arch. Ophthalmol. 96, 2219.
- Theeuwes, F., Bayne, W. and Mefford, W. S. (1978), U. S. Patent. 4, 088, 864.
- Verma R.K., Krishna D.M., Garg S., (2002), J. Control. Release 79, 7.
- Walduck, A. K. and Opdebeeck, J. P. (1997), J. Control. Rel. 43, 75.
- White, W. B., Anders, R. J., MacIntyre, J. M., Black, H. R. and Sica, D. A. (1995), Am. J. cardiol. 76(5), 375.
- Wyatt, I., Coutts, C. T., Foster, P. M., Davies, D. T. and Elcombe, C. R. (1995), Toxicology 95(1–3), 51.

- Yum, S. I. and Wright R. M. (1983); In: Controlled Drug Delivery, S. D. Bruck (Ed.), vol. 2nd, CRC Press, Inc., Florida, 76.
- Zenter, G. M., Rork, G. S. and Himmelstein, K. J. (1985), J. Control. Rel. 1, 269.
- Zentner G.M., McClelland G.A., Sutton S.C., (1991).J. Control. Release 16, 237.
- Zentner G.M., Rork G.S., Himmelstein K.J., (1990) U.S. patent 4, 968, 507.
- Zentner G.M., Rork G.S., Himmelstein K.J(1985), J. Control. Release 2, 217.
- Zhang Y, Zhang Z, Wu F, (2003),Journal of Controlled Release 89,47.

3

Bio/mucoadhesive Systems

BIO/MUCOADHESIVE DRUG DELIVERY

Bioadhesives is the term that describes the adhesion of a polymer to a biological substrate. More specifically, when adhesion is restricted to the lining of the mucous layer of mucosal surface it is termed as mucoadhesion. This has gained considerable interest in the concept of bioadhesion since the immobilisation of drug carrying particles at the mucosal surface would result in,

- A prolonged residence time at the site of action or absorption;
- A localisation of the drug delivery system at a given target site;
- An increase in the drug concentration gradient due to the intestine contact of the particles with the mucosal surface;
- Direct contact with intestinal cells, which is the step earlier to particle absorption.

Bioadhesion can be obtained by building up either non-specific interactions, driven by the physicochemical properties of the particles and the intestinal surfaces or specific interactions when a ligand attached to the particle is used for the recognition and attachment to a specific site at the mucosal surface.

An alternative approach is to employ bioadhesive polymers that adhere to the mucin/epithelial surface. Such polymers could be applied to any mucous membranes as well as non-mucous membranes. Thus, bioadhesive polymers would find application in the eye, nose, vagina and GIT including the buccal cavity and rectum (Park and Robinson, 1984).

EVALUATION OF BIOADHESIVE DRUG DELIVERY SYSTEMS

In vitro Evaluation

The morphological evaluation of the drug carrier (especially microcarriers) systems includes Scanning Electron Microscopy (SEM), Transmission Electron Microscopy (TEM) and Fourier Transform Infrared Spectroscopy (FTIR). *In vitro* release studies of various bioadhesive drug delivery systems are carried out by using dissolution apparatus either paddle or basket type, diffusion membrane method and simple incubation of the formulation in the medium. Bioadhesion is the exclusive and important property to be evaluated for the bioadhesive systems.

EVALUATION OF VARIOUS BIOADHESION PROPERTIES

Shear Stress Measurement of Bioadhesive Polymers

Two smooth, polished plexi glass blocks are selected fix one block with adhesive 'Araldite' on a glass plate, which is fixed on a levelled table. The level is adjusted with a spirit lamp. To the upper block a thread is tied and the thread is passed down through a pulley. The length of the thread from pulley to pan is 12 cm. At the end of the thread a pan of weight 17g is attached into which the weights can be added (Rao and Chary, 1998).

Different polymer solutions of 3% w/v strength are prepared using water as a solvent. A fixed amount (one drop) of polymer solution is kept on the center of the first block with a pipette and then the second block is placed on the first block and pressed by applying 100g weights such that the drop of polymer spreads as a uniform film in between in the two blocks. After keeping it for fixed time intervals of 5, 10, 15 and 30 min, the weights are added to the pan. The weights just sufficient to pull the upper block or to make it slide down from the base block represent the adhesion strength, *i.e.* the shear stress required.

Ishida *et al.*, 1983, have developed one more shear tester that measures the force required to separate two polymer coated glass slides joined by a thin film of natural or synthetic mucous. The results of this technique correlate well with *in vivo* test results (Chen and Cyr, 1970).

Detachment Force Measurement

This method is used to measure *in vitro* mucoadhesive capacity of different polymers. It is a modified method developed by Martti Marvola to assess the tendency of mucoadhesive to adhere to the oesophagus. The assembly consists of single organ bath, a stand, glass rod, a pan for keeping beaker and a reservoir for addition of water into beaker (Rao and Chary, 1998).

Immediately after slaughter, the intestine is removed from the sheep and transported to laboratory in tyrode solution (composition: sodium chloride 8 g/L, potassium chloride - 0.2 g/L, $CaCl_2. 2H_2O$ 0.134 g/L, sodium bicarbonate 1.0 g/L, sodium dihydrogen phosphate 0.05 g/L and glucose H_2O 1.0 g/L). During the experiment the solution is aerated with pure oxygen and kept at 37°C and 6–7 cm long segments of intestine are cut. The lower end of the intestine segment is tied off and then tied to the aerator tube; the upper end is tied around a glass tube of diameter 15mm. 6mm plain tablets, tablets layered on one side with mucoadhesive polymer and polymer matrix (2:1 ratio) tablets of the given drug are prepared. A fine hole drilled in the tablets to be tested with a fine needle at the centre. A thread is passed through it and tied around the tablet. The other end of the thread is tied to the glass rod suspended from the stand. The length of the thread is such that in resting state the tablet should be at the middle of the intestinal piece. To the other end of the glass rod tie a pan in which a beaker is placed. After inserting the tablet into intestinal segment and lightly pressing the intestinal segment with tablet by a forceps, the assembly should be kept undisturbed for a fixed time interval of one hour and 30 min. Then add water with a burette slowly drop by drop into the beaker. The amount of water required to pull out the tablet from the intestinal segment represents the force required to pull the tablet against the adhesion. The force in Newton is calculated by the equation,

$$F = 0.00981 \text{ W}/2$$

Where   W = amount of water.

Following characteristics can be studied from the experiment

- The effect of the contact time for which the product remains in intestine and the force needed to detach it.
- The strength of different mucoadhesive polymers and the effect of amount of polymer in the formulation on the force needed to detach it.

Wilhelm Plate Technique

This technique has traditionally been used for dynamic contact angle measurement and involves a microbalance or tensiometer. A glass slide is coated with the polymer of interest and then dipped into a beaker of synthetic or natural mucous. The surface tension, contact angle and adhesive force can be automatically measured using available software (Smart *et al.,* 1984).

Tensile Studies on Mucoadhesive Polymer Conjugates

The lyophilised polymer conjugates (30mg), controls and unmodified polymer were compressed to flat-faced discs (Bernkop-Schnurch and Steininiger, 2000). Tensiometer studies with these discs were carried out on native porcine intestinal mucosa. Test discs were therefore attached to the mucosa with a force of 2.5mN. After a contact time of 30 min. between test disc and mucosa in 100 mM Tris-HCl buffered saline (TBS), pH 6.8 at 25°C, pull mucosa at a rate of 0.1 mm s^{-1} from the disc. The total work of adhesion (TWA) representing the area under the force/distance curve and the maximum detachment force (MDF) can be determined using the WINWEDGE software (TAL Technologies, Inc., Philadelphia, PA) in combination with EXCEL 5.0 (A Microsoft software).

Mucoadhesion Studies

In order to evaluate the binding of the mucosa as well as the cohesiveness of the tablet, an appropriate new method has been established. The prepared tablets (flat-surface discs) are attached to freshly excise intestinal porcine mucosa, which has been spanned on a stainless steel cylinder (diameter: 4.4 cm, height: 5.1 cm, apparatus 4-cylinder, USP XXII). Thereafter, place the cylinder in the dissolution apparatus according to the USP containing 100 mM TBS pH 6.8 at 37±0.5°C and fully immersed cylinder is agitated with 250 rpm. The detachment, disintegration and/or erosion of test tablets are observed and recorded within a time period of 10 h (Bernkop-Schnurch and Steininger, 2000).

Measurement of Tablet Bioadhesion

The maximum adhesion force and the work of adhesion-shear to separate the tablet from freshly excised rabbit stomach tissue or small intestine are measured by using a modified tensile tester (Instron, model 1122) adapted for bioadhesion measurements. A section of tissue is cut from fundus of the rabbit stomach (or first portion of the small intestine) and secured, mucosal side out, onto a polyacrylic cylinder (3 cm diameter) using a rubber band to adequately fix the tissue onto the cylinder without deforming it. The polyacrylic cylinder is fastened to the wall of a polyacrylic square vessel (13 cm). In addition, a rectangular aluminum piece with a hole in the middle is used as support for the tablets. This hole has a diameter of 2 mm greater than that of the tablets to allow swelling of tablet due to absorption of medium. The experiment is carried out in a constant volume of test medium (USP simulated gastric or intestinal fluid). After 30 min, the adhesion and shear forces required to separate two parallel surfaces (tablet-tissue) are recorded as a function of time, until the tablet has crossed the tissue surface (cross head speed 1 mm/min; chart speed 20 mm/min; full scale load 1 kg). The mechanical parameters are then calculated (Rhodes *et al.*, 1994).

Adhesion Force Measurement

The adhesion properties of bioadhesive polymer tablets can be evaluated by measuring the force required to separate the tablet from an adherent (Takayama *et al.*, 1990). The tablet is attached to the holder with cyanoacrylate type adhesives. Buffer solutions (2 ml; pH 2.0, 3.5 and 5.0) are gently added on the tablet to hydrate the tablet surface for 5 min at 25°C. A lyophilised porcine dermis and rabbit peritoneal membrane excised from male New Zealand white rabbits (3.0–3.5 kg) are used as adherents. The rabbits are killed by pentobarbital injection; the peritoneal membrane is extracted and stored at 10°C before the experiment and thawed at 4°C in an isotonic saline solution before it is used. The residual water on the surface is removed with the help of a filter paper. The porcine dermis of rabbit peritoneal membrane, which is cut into round shape with a diameter of 5mm, is attached to the tip of an adapter in tensiometer with cyanoacrylate type adhesive. The adherents are then immersed in buffer solutions (pH 2.0, 3.5 and 5.0) for 5 min at 25°C before the measurement. The holder bearing the sample tablet is lifted up in contact with the adherent, which is primarily hydrated in the buffer solutions by applying a loading pressure of 250g/cm^2. The tablet and the adherent are kept in contact with each other for 3 min. The tablet is then stretched from the adherent at an extension rate of 4 mm/s and the force required to detach the tablet from the adherent is recorded.

Adhesion Studies of Hydrogels

The adhesion capacity of hydrogels is determined by applying the tensile-tester. The hydrogel is adhered to the upper support and the substrate to the lower support using a cyanoacrylate adhesive. Upon contact of hydrogel and substrate a defined force is applied for certain time (Blanco-Fuente *et al.*, 1996). This is followed by an extension phase at a defined rate until total separation of components is achieved.

The optimum conditions including two hydration environments influencing the adhesion are:

- An applied force of 0.5 N and a contact time of 20 min.
- *Assays where water is limited:* Studies are carried out using dry tanned leather as substrate. Water (25 ml) is homogeneously extended on the hydrogel situated on the upper support of the tension apparatus.
- *Assays where there is no water limitation:* The same assays and conditions, but as before used, the substrate and hydrogel previously introduced into 25 ml of water at 37°C.

Bioadhesion Measurement of Tablets

This experiment determines the colonic bioadhesion of the tablets. The GIT of male Wister rats (200–300 g) is used as the biological substrate in these experiments (Kakoulides, 1998). Animals are allowed free access to food and water until they are sacrificed by carbon dioxide asphyxia. Immediately after the death of the animal, the carcass is opened. The GIT is isolated and divided into 4 segments namely; stomach, proximal small intestine (PSI), distal small intestine (DSI), and the colon. The sections are opened laterally to expose the mucosal surface, washed gently with physiological (pH 7) phosphate buffer to remove the luminal contents, flash-frozen in liquid nitrogen and stored at –18°C. The control experiments employing fresh tissue are conducted in order to confirm the validity of the approach and utilised within 24h of dissection. It behaves similar to biomaterial obtained immediately after isolation from the animal.

The tissue under test is allowed to thaw to room temperature before it is fixed onto a tissue clamp so as to expose a $3.8cm^2$ circular area. The clamped tissue is then immersed in 75 ml of an isotonic solution, buffered at a predetermined pH (depending on the intestinal section tested) and kept at 37, where it is further allowed to stand for 5 min before each measurement. The water bath is placed on a vertically moving platform that is positioned beneath the sensor arm of the balance (GEC-Avery, UK).

Using a pestle and mortar mill the polymeric materials under test. The powdered fraction that passes through a 55 mm sieve is collected and used for the adhesion studies. Circles of 6 mm diameter are cut from double-sided adhesive film and one is attached to a 1.4 g weight. The protective film is peeled off through the free side and the weight is repeatedly placed against a sample of the test powder until its surface is completely covered with particles. The surface is cleared of loosely held particles, by exposing it to compressed air for 2 min, and then attached to the sensor arm, which is positioned directly above the mucosal surface. The platform is raised at maximum speed until the disk and the weight are completely immersed in the buffer. The balance is tared and the platform is raised slowly until the negative reading of the balance remained constant for 5 seconds. The surfaces are allowed to interact for 2 min and then the platform is lowered at a rate of 1 mm min^{-1} until adhesive joint failure occur. The maximum detachment force and the work of adhesion are calculated as the mean of six set of measurements. The tissue is also examined in order to identify the position at which the fracture of the adhesive joint has occurred.

Unique Flow Chamber Technique

A polymer microsphere is placed on the surface of a natural mucous layer and fluid, moving at physiological rate, is introduced into the chamber, and movement of the microsphere is monitored by video equipment. By measuring the size and speed of the microsphere, it is possible to calculate the bioadhesive force (Peppas *et al.*, 1994)

Everted Sac Technique

- Everted sac experiments are performed using viable segments of rat jejunum. Unfasted rats (400 g, male) are sacrificed and intestinal tissue is excised and flushed with 10 ml of ice-cold phosphate buffered saline, pH 7.2 containing 200-mg/dl glucose (PBSG).

- Evert the segments of jejunum (6 cms) with help of stainless steel rod and wash with PBSG to remove the contents. Ligatures are placed at both ends of the segment and the sac is filled with 1–1.5 ml of PBSG. Tissue is maintained at 4°C prior to incubation and the sacs are introduced into a 15 ml tube containing 60 mg of bioadhesive microspheres and 5 ml of PBSG.

- The sacs are incubated at 37°C and agitated end-over-end and after 30 min, the sacs are removed and the solution of PBSG and unbound microspheres is centrifuged for 30 min.

- Discard the supernatant fluid and wash sedimented microspheres three times with 5 ml distilled water and again centrifuge and discard the supernatant fluid then freeze dry the microsphere by lyophilisation for 24–48 h.

- The weight of the bound spheres is determined by subtraction of the tared weight of the tube and lyophilised spheres from the initial tare weight of tube and spheres and can be reported as percent binding (Santos *et al.,* 1999).

CAHN FORCE MEASUREMENT TECHNIQUE

Experimental Design and Methods of Microbalance

Cahn Dynamic Contact Angle Analyzer (Model DCA, 322 CAHN Instruments, IN., Ceritos, CA) has been modified and used to measure adhesion. The equipment is designed for measuring contact angles and surface tensions using the Wilhelmly plate technique and serves essentially as an extremely accurate microbalance. The DCA 322 system essentially includes a microbalance stand assembly a Cahn DACS IBM-compatible computer, and an Okidata microline 320 dot matrix printer. The microbalance unit consists of stationary sample and tare loop and a z-translation stage powered by a stopper motor. The balance can be operated with samples weighing up to 3 g and has sensitivity as low as 1×10^{-5} mN. The stage speed can be varied from 20 to 264 mm/s (Chickering *et al.,* 1995; Chickering and Mathiowitz, 1995).

To develop an automated, reproducible method for bioadhesion measurements, it is necessary to modify the operation of the balance and stage. The standard DACS IBM-computer compatible system was replaced with an Apple Macintosh II computer. A modem port is used to interface the computer and microbalance. Lab view II software is used to write a user-friendly, menu-driven package to automatically run tensile experiments, with easily adjustable settings for stage speed, applied load time of adhesion. After each run, graphs of load versus stage position and load versus time are plotted and 11 parameters are automatically calculated: they include, (1) Compressive deformation, (2) Peak compressive load, (3) Compressive work, (4) Yield point, (5) Deformation to yield, (6) Returned work, (7) Peak tensile load, (8) Deformation to peak tensile load, (9) Fracture strength, (10) Deformation to failure, and (11) Tensile work.

Tissue Chamber

A temperature-controlled tissue chamber is constructed to maintain physiological temperature and pH. The chamber is fabricated of plexi glass and consist of a 3 ml tissue cell jacketed by a circulating water bath connected to a Fisher Scientific Isotemp refrigerated circulator (model 9000). Two stainless steel clamps with thumbscrews are used to secure tissue samples to the bottom of the tissue cell.

Mounting Microspheres

The microspheres are melt-mounted on the balance by using a red-hot, 280 μm diameter, iron wires of 2 cm length for piercing of microspheres. Hydrogel microspheres are attached to the same wires using cyanoacrylate glue (Super Glue Corp., Hollis, NY). After mounting, wires are suspended from a sample clip in the microbalance enclosure).

Microbalance Operation

Cahn system is simpler in operation. The temperature of circulating water bath is adjusted to physiologic temperature (37 °C), freshly excised tissue is placed, submerged in phosphate-buffered saline (PBS) in the chamber and the microsphere is suspended from the sample loop. The stage rises until the applied load between microsphere and tissue reaches the programmed set point. At this juncture, motion is stopped for the duration of the adhesion time, and then the stage is lowered. Once the stage returns to its initial position, parameters are calculated and graphs are plotted. The interpretation of the microbalance recordings is well explained by Chickering *et al.*, (1995) and Mathiowitz (1999).

LIMITATIONS OF THIS SYSTEM

The microbalance-based system has several limitations,
- Microspheres smaller than 300 μm are difficult to mount
- Overshoot of the applied load must be accounted
- Very small and very large applied loads are difficult to control
- Changes in applied load over time due to tissue relaxation or contraction are not accounted after stage stops moving.

In vivo Evaluation Methods

In vivo methods used for evaluation of mucoadhesive systems are based on the administration of polymers to a laboratory animal and tracking their transit through the GI system. Administration methods include forced oral lavage, surgical stomach implantation and infusion through a loop placed *in situ* in the small intestine. Tracking generally followed with the help of X-ray studies, radio-opaque markers, radioactive elements and fluorescent dyes. Various animals including rats, rabbits, guinea pigs, mice and sheeps have been used for the studies.

X-RAY STUDIES FOR MONITORING GI TRANSIT
X-ray Studies on Bioadhesive Tablets

- Barium sulfate ($BaSO_4$) tablets of 8 mm diameter are prepared in 3 different types of polymers.
- Control or plain tablets of $BaSO_4$.
- $BaSO_4$ tablets layered on one side with mucoadhesive polymer.
- $BaSO_4$ and polymer as matrix mixture in the ratio of 2:1.

Ten healthy rabbits of same age and weight are taken as subjects. They are fasted overnight and the next day morning the tablets are administered to them followed by 25 ml of water. At different intervals of 1, 3, 5 and 8 h, the rabbits are X-ray photographed and observed for the nature and position of the tablet for 8 h after administration of the tablets. During the study, the rabbits are fed after 5 h of tablet administration, so that the effect of food can be assessed (Rao and Chary, 1998).

X-RAY GI TRANSIT MONITORING OF RADIO-OPAQUE MICROSPHERES

Prior to administration, 200 mg of barium sulphate loaded microspheres are suspended in one ml of 0.9% sodium chloride (Chickering *et al.*, 1997). Male rats (250–300 g), fasted overnight, are anaesthetised with methoxyflurane and a silicone feeding tube (2 mm OD) is used to administer microsphere suspensions into their stomach. Following administration rats are allowed to recover from anaesthesia. Since, it is difficult to assure that 100% of the intended microspheres dose has been delivered, a post-administration counting method should be used. Animals are reanesthatised and X-rayed, thereby verifying the presence of microspheres in lumen of the stomach. From these X-rays it is possible to determine the number of microspheres initially administered to each animal.

After X-ray treatment, animals are placed in metabolic cages positioned above a custom-designed automatic faeces-collecting machine. Faeces are separated from the urine and collected at 2 h 50 min intervals over a three-day period. During this time the animals are provided with food and water *ad libitum*. Faeces are X-rayed and microspheres are counted to determine their rate of passage from stomach to anus, and the percentage of remaining microspheres in the animal at each point.

Bioavailability Studies of Radiolabelled Nanoparticles

The radiolabelled nanoparticles are mixed with non-labelled nanoparticles (Sakuma *et al.*, 1999). The final nanoparticle concentration and the radioactivity in this mixture are adjusted to 10 mg/ml and 0.3–0.5 kBq/ml, respectively. An aqueous solution of PEG is prepared as a control. The concentration of non-labeled PEG is adjusted to 10 mg/ml and a small amount of tritiated PEG is added to this solution, to yield 0.3–0.5 kBq/ml radioactivities. The prepared dosing solution is given orally to male rats simultaneously fasted overnight (200–250 g) at a dose of 25 mg of nanoparticles in a 2.5 ml solution/kg of body weight. The aqueous solution of PEG is administered to rats under the same conditions at 5, 30 and 60 or 120 min after administration, rats are sacrificed by ether inhalation overdose and both stomach and small intestine are removed. The intestine is cut into 10 cm sections and radioactivity in each segment is measured with the gamma counter or a beta counter (GM Counter).

BIOAVAILABILITY STUDIES OF DRUG ENCAPSULATED BIOADHESIVE MICROSPHERES
Blood Sampling Set-Up

- Bioavailability studies require catheters for repeated blood sampling. Male rats (200–250 g) are anaesthetised with an intraperitoneal injection of sodium phenobarbital

(60 gm/kg) (Chickering *et al.,* 1997). With the animals supine, midline incision is made from the top of the neck to the clavicle. Blunt dissection is used to locate and isolate the external jugular vein. Three ligatures are placed around the vessel and one ligature is used to tie off the cranial end of the isolated segment, a small incision is made in the side of the vessel, and a silicone catheter [Bio-Sil medical grade silicone tubing (500 µm inside diameter, 940 µm outside diameter and 53 cm length), Sil-Med Corp. Taunton, MA, USA] filled with heparin (666 U/ml) is inserted into the vessel lumen and advanced towards the heart. The other two ligatures are tied off around the vessel and catheter, caudal to the point of insertion, while being careful not to deform and restrict the catheter.

- Animals are turned prone, and second incision is made from the base of the skull to the midpoint between the scapulae. Forceps are used to tunnel subcutaneously to the opening of the ventral incision. The free end of the catheter is pulled beneath the skin to emerge from the dorsal incision at the base of the neck. The ventral incision is sutured. The free end of catheter is fed through a 30.5 cm long stainless steel spring tethered with 22-gauge swivel. The button-end of the tether is sutured to the facial covering of the muscles in the back of the neck, and a pure-string stitch is used to close the dorsal incision.

- Tall cages are constructed for untangled movement of the tether. To produce an enclosure 33 cm high, two rat cages (36 × 30 × 16 cm) are joined; one inverted on top of the other, with 4 derlin spacers (1 cm thick) to allow adequate airflow. Additional air holes are drilled, and a derlin collar is glued into the centre of the top cage. The swivel-end of the tether is passed through the top of the upper cage and secured in the collar with a setscrew. A three-way stopcock is attached to the swivel on the outside of the cage with a small section of silicone tubing (8 cm) to facilitate syringe changes without breaking the closed-catheter system. The set up allows blood samples to be drawn from outside the cages without handling or anesthetising the animals. Moreover, animals are seen in near normal mobility.

Formulation Administration and Drug Estimation

Intra-gastric administration: Following surgery, the animals are anesthetised with methoxyflurane; a flexible silicone feeding tube introduced via oesophagus or stomach. Bioadhesive microspheres are suspended in 1.5 ml of syrup and administered to the animals through the silicone tube. A positive displacement plunger is passed through the tube to ensure proper storage. After the drug is administered, blood samples are withdrawn from the animals approximately at the interval of 1 h for the first 4 h and approximately every 4 h after that point for the next 68 h. Samples are centrifuged and 100 µl of serum is separated and blood cells are suspended in 100 µl of saline (0.9 % NaCl) and returned to the animals. Catheters are flushed with saline and plugged with heparin (1000 U/ml) after returning to the blood cells. The drug from the serum is estimated by appropriate method.

PROTOCOL: 3.1

Mucoadhesive Microcapsules of Alginate by Ionic Gelation Method

Materials

Model drug

Sodium carboxymethylcellulose (NaCMC viscosity 1500–3000 cps) – 1%w/v solution in double distilled water at 25°C.

Hydroxy propylmethylcellulose (HPMC viscosity 50 cps)

2%w/v solution in double distilled water at 25°C.

Carbopol 934P

Sodium alginate

Calcium chloride (CaCl$_2$)

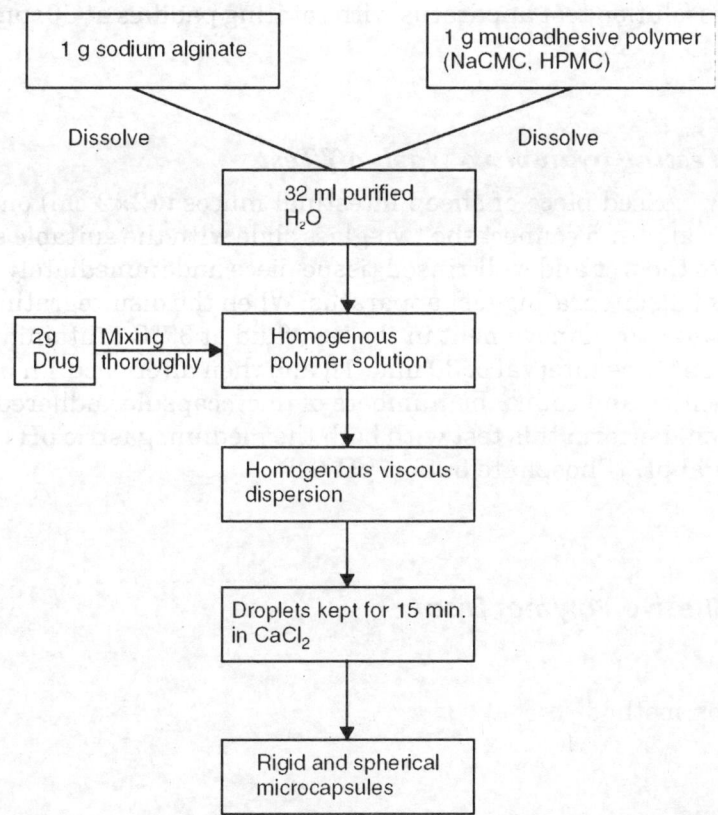

Scheme 3.1 *Preparation of alginate mucoadhesive microparticles*

Procedure

- Dissolve 1.0 g sodium alginate and 1.0 g mucoadhesive polymer (NaCMC, HPMC, Carbopol) in 32 ml of purified water to get homogenous polymer solution.

- Add 2.0 g drug in this polymer solution and mix thoroughly using magnetic stirrer to form homogenous viscous dispersion.
- Add this drug containing solution manually drop wise in 40 ml 10% w/v **CaCl₂ solution** through a syringe with a needle of size no. 18.
- Keep these added droplets in CaCl₂ solution for 15 minutes to complete the curing reaction and to produce solid rigid spherical microcapsules.
- Collect the prepared microcapsules by decanting. Wash the collected microsphere repeatedly with distilled water and dry at 45°C for 12hr (Scheme 3.1).

Characterisation of Mucoadhesive Microcapsules

Microencapsulation efficiency (*Refer Chapter Microspheres*)

In vitro drug release study

By the USP dissolution test apparatus with rotating paddles at 50rpm at 37±1°C using PBS medium.

SEM Microscopy

Mucoadhesion Testing by in vitro Wash-off Test

Mount the freshly excised piece of sheep intestinal mucosa (2×2 cm) onto the glass slide using cynoacrylate glue and connect the two-glass slide with the suitable support. Spray 50 microcapsules onto the wet and well-rinsed tissue piece and immediately hang the support onto the USP tablet disintegrating test apparatus. When the disintegrating machine starts, provide a slow up and down movement in the test fluid at 37°C containing 1L vessel of the machine, at different time interval of 30 min, 1h and then after each 1 h interval up to 12h. Then stop the machine and count the numbers of microcapsules adhered to the surface of the tissue specimen. Perform this test with both the medium gastric pH (0.1N HCl pH 1.2) as well as intestinal pH (Phosphate buffer, pH 6.2).

PROTOCOL: 3.2
Buccal Mucoadhesive Polymer Disc

Principle
Direct compression method

Materials
Polyoxyethylene

Polyethyleneglycol (Carbowax)

Polyisobutylene (Vistanex)

Chlorpheniramine maleate

Anhydrous lactose

Procedure
Preparation of Chlorpheniramine Maleate Buccal Adhesive Devices

- The drug loaded buccal devices of 10mm diameter can be prepared using a Carver® press either by direct compression or the compression molding process.
- Fill the sufficient amount of the mixture (drug, polymer, plasticiser, and/or elastomer polyisobutylene) in a die of 1mm thickness having a 5cm internal diameter and a 6cm external diameter.
- Then compress this mixture under a 4,500 kg force between the two heated platens at 70°C for 5 min.
- Cut the polymer disks in 10mm diameter from the above compression-molded mixture with the help of a cork borer.

Characterisation of Polymer Discs

Bioadhesive Strength

- A commercial bench-mounted vertical tensile/compression tester may be used for the quantitative measurements of bioadhesive bond strength. The samples between the stationary lower compression platen mounted to the main frame of the machine and the upper compression anvil fixed via the load cell to the moving crosshead, may be tested.
- Take glass plate or bovine sublingual tissue and store at – 20°C as model mucosal substrate surface. Thaw the tissue to room temperature in normal saline solution and then cut into the dimensions of approximately 20 cm^2 surfaces.
- Fix the substrate surface (bovine sublingual mucosa or a glass plate) to the stationary base compression platen using cyanoacrylate adhesive.
- Use constant volume of water to wet the above substrate surfaces (20 ml for the glass plate and 40 ml for the bovine tissue).
- Then adhere the compressed disks to the wet substrate by applying a constant force (1 N for glass plate and 5 N for the bovine tissue) for 5 min.
- Move the compression anvil at a constant speed (0.2 mm/min for glass plate and 5 mm/min for bovine tissue).
- Data representing force as a function of displacement at 1sec intervals, until the compressed disks is detached from the substrate surface (break point).
- Calculate the maximum force required to initiate the detachment and area under the force-displacement curve for the quantification of the bioadhesive strength.

Elasticity Evaluation

Use the tensile tester with a standard 3 mm diameter puncture probe-chuck assembly at a crosshead speed of 0.2 mm/min for the quantitative measurement of elasticity of the prepared devices. The elasticity of the device characterised by measuring the maximum penetration force and corresponding displacement required by the probe to cause failure of the device. Based on the design, apparatus can be fabricated.

Drug Release Kinetics

- Use a standard USP dissolution apparatus I without the basket fixture to evaluate drug release kinetics from the prepared device formulations. In order to mimic the *in vivo* adhesion of the devices to the gum area, affix the each prepared device to the bottom flat end of the stirring rod instead of the basket fixture.

- The wet adhesive properties of the bioadhesive devices are utilised to affix the prepared bioadhesive devices. Moisten the flat bottom surface of the rod with the deionised water and attach the devices onto this moistened surface by maintaining a gentle fingertip pressure for 5 minutes. Use deionised water at $37 \pm 0.5°C$ as the dissolution medium, and operate the dissolution apparatus at 100 rpm.

- Collect the samples representing 10 ml aliquots at predetermined time intervals and replace with an equal volume of fresh dissolution medium. Filter the samples through a 0.45 µm filter and then estimate for drug content using spectrophotometric method.

PROTOCOL: 3.3

Bioadhesive Polyethylene Glycol Gels

Materials

Carbopol 934P

Polyvinylpyrrolidone K-90 (PVP)

Polyethylene glycol 400 (PEG 400)

Polyethylene glycol 4000 (PEG 4000)

Oral Gel

PEG 400 and PEG 4000 combine in an evaporating dish at $70\pm1°C$ and cool to room temperature. Transfer the resulting gel onto a glass slab and levigate homogeneously with a known amount of CP and PVP. Formulations comprising constant amounts of PEG 400 and PEG 4000 (6 parts to 2 parts) but different ratios of CP and PVP can be prepared. Narrow concentration ranges of CP and PVP should be used, because the PEG gels become hard and are difficult to spread at higher concentrations.

Rheological Studies

- The rheograms of the bioadhesive gels can be obtained at $28\pm0.1°C$ using a rheometer equipped with a cone and plate measuring system. The dimension of the measuring cone CP 6 is 50 mm and the angle of the cone is generally 2°.

- The sample is applied carefully onto the plate using a spatula, avoiding the shearing of the formulation.

- The following parameters such as flow profile, zero-rate viscosity, and thixotropy are to be investigated. Pre-shearing time of 5 seconds, followed by ascending curve time of 120 seconds at a maximum shear rate of 100 s^{-1} followed by a hold time of 10 seconds at a minimum shear rate of 0 s^{-1} and then a descending time of 120 seconds. The rheogram obtained is an average of at least 2 determinations (readings).

PROTOCOL: 3.4

Pelleted Bioadhesive Polymeric Nanoparticles for Buccal Delivery of Proteins

Principle

Emulsion internal phase evaporation method.

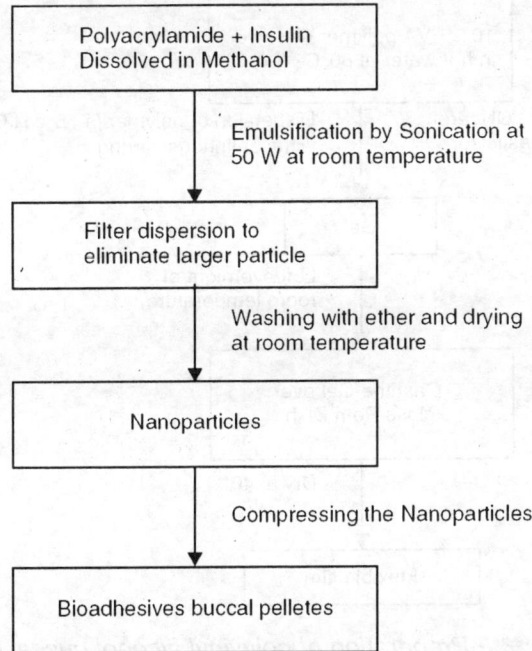

Scheme: 3.2 *Preparation of the buccal pellet for delivery of the proteins*

Materials

Insulin (model protein)

Polyacrylamide (Mw 10,000)

Span 80

Procedure

- Dissolve polyacrylamide and insulin in acidified methanol and emulsify this polar phase with light paraffin oil containing span 80 by sonication at 50 W at room temperature for complete evaporation of the internal phase (methanol).

- Filter the dispersion through a membrane filter (0.45µm) to eliminate larger particles.

- Filter the prepared nanoparticles and those retained over 0.22µm are washed with ether and dried at room temperature.
- Compress the prepared nanoparticles into pellets and the final bioadhesive buccal pellets are obtained as in form of disc of 1 cm (Scheme 3.2).

PROTOCOL: 3.5

Preparation of Mucoadhesive Buccal Patches

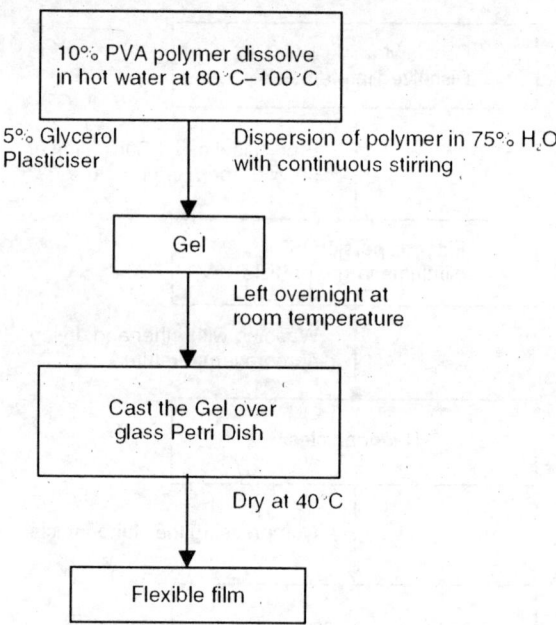

Scheme: 3.3 Preparation of polyvinyl alcohol buccal patches

Materials

Chitosan (maximum granule size 0.2 mm, degree of acetylation > 80%)

Polyvinyl alcohol (PVA)

Hydroxyethyl cellulose (15000 MPAS, HEC)

Polyvinyl pyrrolidone (PVP, Povidone®)

Gelatin powder

Polyvinyl Alcohol Buccal Patches

- The PVA polymer powder is dissolved in 10% w/v concentration in hot water at 80 to 100 °C, and for HEC, disperse the calculated amount of the polymer in a 75% water volume under continuous stirring using a mechanical stirrer.
- 5% v/v glycerol may be added as a plasticiser and adjust the final volume with distilled water.

- Leave the prepared gels overnight at room temperature to obtain the clear, bubble-free gels. Cast the prepared gels over a glass petri dish and allow to dry in an oven maintained at 40 °C to get a flexible film (Scheme 3.3).

Hydroxyethyl Cellulose Buccal Patches

- Dissolve or disperse the HEC polymer powder in 10%w/v concentration in hot water at 80 to 100°C using a mechanical stirrer under continuous stirring.
- Add 5% v/v glycerol as a plasticiser gradually and the final volume was adjusted with distilled water.
- Leave the prepared gels overnight at room temperature to obtain the clear, bubble-free gels. Cast the prepared gels over a glass petridish and allow to dry in an oven maintained at 40°C to get a flexible film (Scheme 3.4).

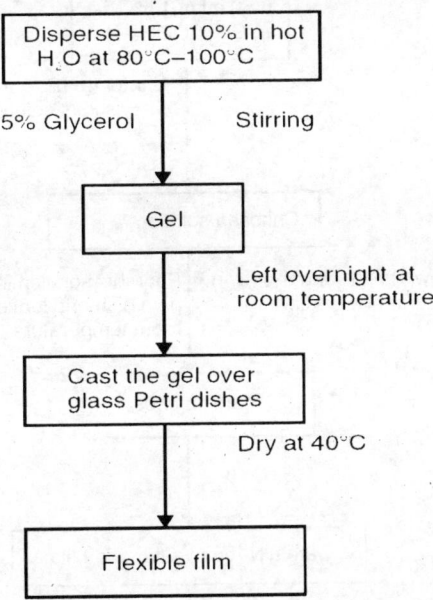

Scheme: 3.4 *Preparation of hydroxyethyl cellulose buccal patches*

Chitosan Buccal Patches

Dissolve 1.0 g chitosan in 50 ml of 1.5% v/v aqueous acetic acid under constant stirring using a magnetic stirrer for 48 h. Filter the resultant viscous solution through gauze. Leave the filtrate to stand until all air bubbles have disappeared.

- Pour the chitosan solution into a clean, dry, glass petri dish (10 mm in diameter) and leave to dry at room temperature. To improve elastic and film forming properties of the patches, add hydrophilic additives, i. e. 1% w/v PVP and 5% w/v gelatin may be added to the chitosan solution.
- Carefully remove the dried films (plain patches) from the petri dish, check for any imperfections or air bubbles.

- Cut the films into patches, 10 mm in diameter.
- Pack the sample films in aluminum foil and store in a glass container maintained at room temperature and 58% relative humidity this condition maintains the integrity and elasticity of the patches (Scheme 3.5).

Note: Patches containing drugs in all the methods as described above can also be prepared by dissolving the calculated amount of the drug in 20 ml distilled water. Then add this drug solution to the polymer gel under stirring. The films may be casted and then cut into patches, 10 mm in diameter, so that each patch contains 10 mg of the drug.

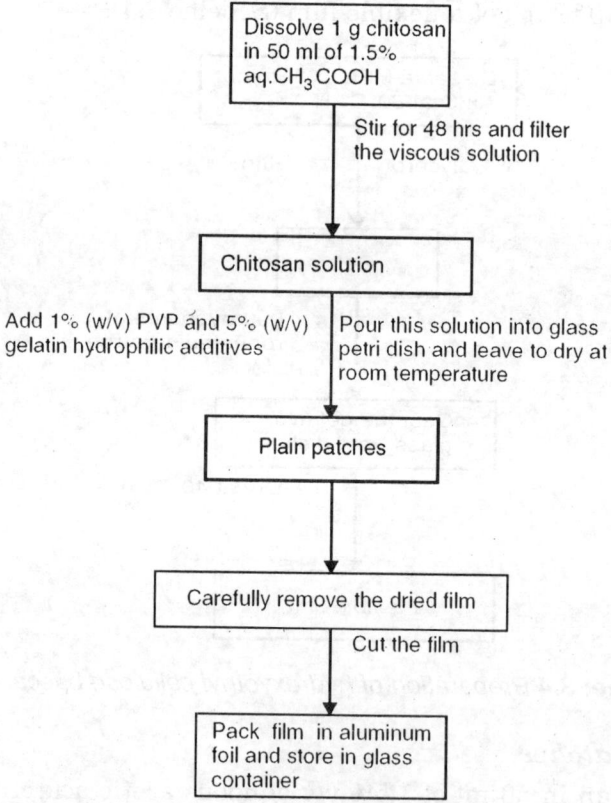

Scheme: 3.5 Preparation of chitosan buccal patches

Characterisation of Buccal Patches

Mass Uniformity and Patch Thickness

Determine the mass and thickness of small pieces of buccal patches individually of 10 patches selected randomly and report the mean and standard deviation.

Surface pH

Leave the prepared buccal patches to swell for 2 h on the surface of an agar plate prepared by dissolving 2% w/v agar in warmed isotonic phosphate buffer of pH 6.75 under stirring and then pour the solution into a petri dish till gelling at room temperature. Measure the surface pH by means of a pH paper placed on the surface of the swollen patch and record the mean of two readings.

Viscosity

Prepare the aqueous solutions containing both polymers and plasticiser in the same concentration as that of the patches. Use a model LVDV-II Brookfield viscometer attached to a helipath spindle number 4 to determine the viscosity of polymer solution with 20 rpm at room temperature.

Folding Endurance Test

The folding endurance of the prepared patches, is determined by repeatedly folding one patch at the same place till it breaks. Folding up to 300 times is considered satisfactory to reveal good film properties.

The number of times the film could be folded at the same place without breaking gives the value of the folding endurance.

Swelling

First determine the original patch diameter, allow the sample to swell on the surface of an agar plate kept in an incubator (hot air incubator) maintained at 37 °C. Measure the diameter of the swollen patch at one-hour intervals for 5 h. Perform the experiments in triplicate and calculate the radial swelling from the following equation:

$$S_D\,(\%) = [(D_t - D_0)/D_0 \times 100]$$

Where $S_D\,(\%)$ is the per cent swelling obtained by the diameter method, D_t is the diameter of the swollen patch after time t, D_0 is the original patch diameter at time zero.

In vitro Residence time

- Modified USP disintegration apparatus can be used for the determination of the *in vitro* residence time.
- Prepare the disintegration medium of 800 ml isotonic phosphate buffer of pH 6.75 (IPB) maintained at 37°C. Glue a segment of rabbit intestinal mucosa (3 cm long) to the surface of a glass slab and attach vertically to the apparatus.
- Hydrate the mucoadhesive patch from one surface using 15 µL IPB and then contact the hydrated surface with the mucosal membrane.
- Fix the glass slab vertically to the apparatus and allow to move up and down so that the patch may be completely immersed in the buffer solution at the lowest point and out at the highest point.

- Record the time taken for complete erosion or detachment of the patch from the mucosal surface (mean of triplicate determinations).

Bioadhesion Force

- The tensile strength required to detach the bioadhesive patch from the mucosal surface is used as a measure of the bioadhesive performance. The apparatus can be locally assembled.

- The device is mainly composed of a two-arm balance. Replace the left arm of the balance by a small platinum lamina vertically suspended through a wire on the same side, maintain a movable platform in the bottom in order to fix the model mucosal membrane.

- For determination of the bioadhesion force, fix the mucoadhesive patch to the platinum lamina using cyanoacrylate adhesive. A piece of rabbit intestinal mucosa (3 cm long) is glued to the platform as well.

- Moisten the exposed patch surface with 15 μL of IPB and leave for 30s for initial hydration and swelling. Raise the platform upward until the hydrated patch comes in contact with the mucosal surface.

- Place a preload of 20 g over the platinum lamina for 3 min as initial pressure. Add a constant weight of 5 g at 2 min intervals on the right pan. The total weight required for complete detachment of the patch is calculated and the bioadhesion forces are calculated per unit area of the patch as follows:

$$F = (W_W - g)/A$$

Where F is the bioadhesion force (kg m^{-1} s^{-2}), W_W is the mass applied (g), g is the acceleration due to gravity (cm s^{-2}), A is the surface area of the patch (cm^2).

Content Uniformity

Allow the medicated patch to dissolve in 100 ml isotonic phosphate buffer, pH 6.75 and the amount of drug in the solution may be determined spectrophotometrically.

In vitro Release Study

- To determine the *in vitro* release rate from the medicated buccal patch USP 24 dissolution apparatus type 1 (six-station dissolution apparatus) can be used with slight modification in order to overcome the small volume of the dissolution medium.

- Fill the dissolution medium with 50 ml IPB, pH 6.75, maintain at 37 ± 0.5 °C and keep it in a glass beaker fixed inside the USP dissolution flask.

- Fix the prepared patch to the central axis, which rotates at 50 rpm. Collect the samples at different time interval and filter the samples (2 ml). After collection of the samples fill the fresh medium containing an equal volume of IPB kept at the same temperature.

- Estimate the amount of drug in the medium spectrophotometrically at appropriate absorption maxima after suitable dilution with the dissolution medium as and when necessary. The same experiment should be carried out in triplicates.

Ageing/Accelerated Stability Studies

Accelerated stability testing is perfomed, to assess the effect of storage on the medicated buccal patches. Pack the prepared patches in glass petri dishes lined with aluminum foil and keep them in an incubator maintained at $37 \pm 0.5 \, °C$ and $75 \pm 5\%$ RH for 6 months. Changes in the appearance, residence time, release behaviour and drug content of the stored bioadhesive patches may be investigated and recorded after 1, 2, 3, 4, 5, and 6 months.

PROTOCOL: 3.6
Mucoadhesive Carbapol-cysteine Conjugates

Materials

Polyacrylic acid

Carbopol 974P (neutralised with NaOH)

1-ethyl-3- (3-dimethylaminopropyl) carbodiimide hydrochloride (EDAC)

L-cysteine hydrochloride monohydrate

Microcrystalline cellulose

Procedure

Synthesis of the Polyacrylic Acid Conjugates

- First hydrate the 250 mg of the sodium salt of polyacrylic acid in 62.5 ml of demineralised water for 1 h.

- Then activate the carboxylic acid moieties of the polymer for 45 min with EDAC in a final concentration of 50 mM.

- Thereafter, add the 125 ml of L-cysteine hydrochloride monohydrate to the reaction mixture and adjust the pH to 5 by adding 1 M NaOH or 1 M HCl, respectively.

- Then incubate the reaction mixture for 3 h at room temperature.

- Isolate the resulting conjugates by dialysing at $10 \, °C$ in the dark against 0.2 mM HCl at pH 3.0, two-times against the same medium but containing 1% NaCl and two times exhaustively against 1 mM HCl.

- Adjust the pH-value of the dialysed polymer-cysteine conjugates to 4.5 with 1 M NaOH and lyophilise in a lyophiliser.

- Store the polymer-cysteine conjugates at $4 \, °C$ until further use (Scheme 3.6).

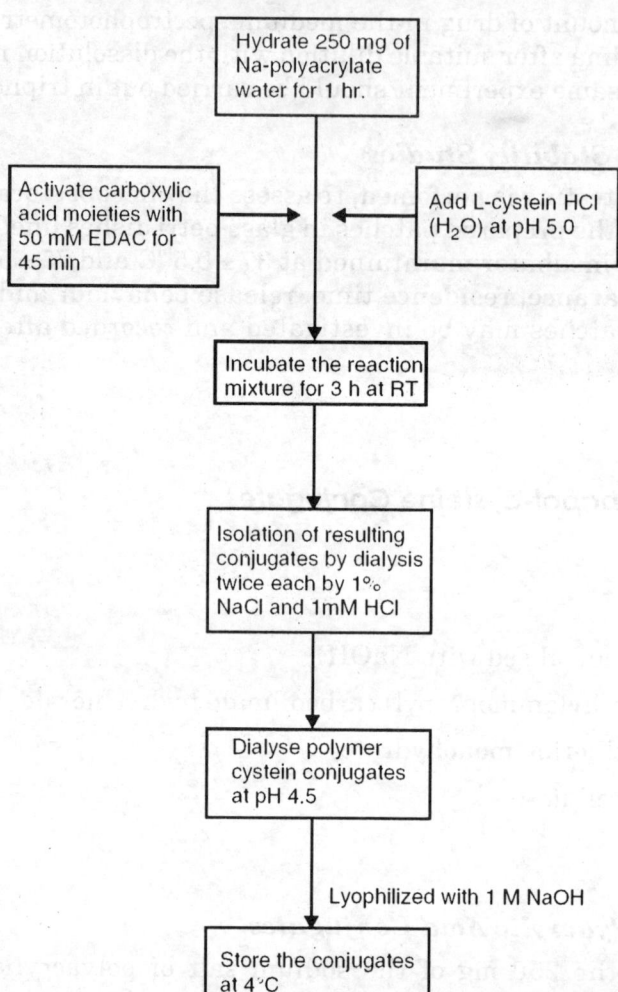

Scheme: 3.6 *Mucoadhesive carbapol-cysteine conjugates preparation*

SUGGESTED READINGS

- Alpar H.O., Somavarapu S., Atuah K.N., Bramwell V.W.(2005) Advanced Drug Delivery Reviews 3: 411.
- Andreas Bernkop-Schnürch Reprinted from Journal of Controlled Release 77 (2001) 323.
- Bernkop-Schnwich and Steininger, 2000.
- Blanco-Fluente et, al, 1996.
- Charlton S.T., Davis S.S., IIIum L.(2007) Journal of controlled release. 2: 225.

- Chen and Cyr., 1970.
- Chickering and Mathiowitz, 1995.
- Chickering D .E., Jacob J .S., Mathowitz E. (1995) Reactive Polymers 25 189.
- Chickering et. al, 1997.
- Dave B.S., Amin A.F., Patel M.M. (2004) AAPS Pharm Sci Tech 5 (2) 34.
- Guo L.Y., Zhao Y.P.,(2006) Journal of Adhesion Science and Technology. 20 (12): 1281.
- Huntsberger J.R. (1967) Treatise on adhesion and adhesives, (Ed. R Patrick), Vol. 1, New York: Marcel Dekker Inc.
- Ishida et., al. 1983.
- Jaiswal J., Gupta S.K., Kreuter J.(2004) Journal of controlled Release. 96 (1): 169.
- Jasti B., Li X., Cleary G. Drug Delivery Polymer (A report).
- Kakaulider 1998.
- Kast CE, Valenta C, Leopold M, Bernkop-Schnürch A.(2002) J Control Release. 81 (3): 347.
- Kaul G., Amiji M.(2004), J Drug Target. 12 (9–10): 585.
- Kobayashi A., Takano S., Kubono T.,(1996) Int. Con. Elect. Cont. 16–20: 331.
- Lee W.F., Lin W.J. (2001),Journal of Polymer Research. 9 (1): 23.
- Lenaerts V., Gurny R.(1990) Bioadhesive Drug Delivery Systems, CRC Press. 25.
- Lopez C.R., Portero A., Vila-Jato J.L., Alonso J.M. (1998) Journal of controlled release. 55 (2–3): 143.
- Luciano M., Freitas D., Osvaldo.(2005), Drug Development and Industrial Pharmacy, 3: 293.
- Madan et. al, 1999.
- Mathiowitz 1999.
- Mikos A.G., Peppas N.A. (1989) Int. J. Pharm. 53,1.
- Nafee N.A., Boraie N.A., Ismail F.A., Mortada L.M. (2003) Int. Jour. Pharm. 264 (1–2): 1.
- Nafee N.A., Boraie N.A., Ismail F.A., Mortada L.M.(2003) Acta Pharm. 53 199.
- Park and Robinson 1984.
- Peppas et. al, 1994.
- Perioli L., Ambrogi V., Giovagnoli S., Ricci M., Blasi P., Rossi1 C.(2007) AAPS Pharm. Sci. Tech 8 (3).
- Rao and Chary, 1998.
- Rhodis et al, 1994
- Rossin R., Pan D., Kai Qi., Turner J.L., Sun X., Wooley K.L., Welch M.J.(2005) J Nucl Med. 46:1210.
- Sakuma et. al, 1999.
- Santos et. al, 1999.
- Sharma G., Jain S., Tiwary A.K., Kaur K.,(2006) Acta Pharm. 56: 337.
- Shojaei H.A.(1998) J Pharm Pharmaceut Sci. 1 (1): 15 .
- Shrinivasa Rao et. al, 2003.

- Smart et. al, 1984.
- Sudhakar Y., Kuotsu K., Bandyopadhyay A.K.(2006) Journal of Controlled Release 1: 15.
- Valenta C., Kast E.C., Harich I., Bernkop-Schnürch A.(2001) Journal of controlled release. 77 (3): 323–332 .
- Vasir JK, Tambwekar K, Garg S.(2003) Int J Pharma 14:13.
- Vishnu M. P., Prajapati B.G., Patel M.M.(2007) Acta Pharm. 57: 61.

4

Multiple Emulsion

The emulsion can be defined as the dispersion of one immiscible liquid in another, stabilised by a third component called the emulsifying agent. Two main classes can be identified: the dispersion of water droplets in oil (W/O) and the reverse systems, the dispersion of oil droplets in water (O/W). Emulsion systems have been used in medical practices since the earliest time for the administration of oils and fats. Today they find use as drug-delivery systems, for nutritional and diagnostic applications, and as blood substitutes. Emulsion can be administered by injection by different route for variety of reasons. For example W/O emulsions given by intramuscular (IM) injection are known for their sustained release properties and adjuvant effects in immunology. Oil in water emulsions are normally given by the intravenous route as carriers of lipid-soluble compounds including anticancer agents.

More complex types of emulsion can be produced in which the dispersed droplets themselves contain smaller dispersed droplets. These systems known as multiple emulsions are easily prepared by the re-emulsification of simple primary O/W or W/O system to provide O/W/O or W/O/W systems (Fig 4.1). These systems can then be re-emulsified further to produce even more complicated systems.

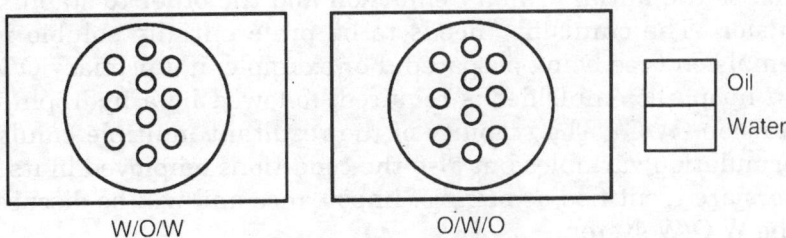

Fig. 4.1: Multiple emulsions

Emulsion can be administered by injection of different route for a variety of reasons-

- Sustained release.
- Adjuvant effects in immunology.

Sustained drugs release from the multiple emulsion systems can be explained on the basis of three possible mechanisms (i) diffusion of unionised drug through the oil layer,

(ii) diffusion of unionised and/or ionised drug through oil-water lamellae (liquid membrane) (iii) coalescences of the internal aqueous phase and rupture of the oil droplet. A combination of all three mechanisms may be possible *in vivo*.

The potential of multiple emulsions as drug delivery vehicle and drug targeting depends on successful formulation using oils and emulsifier that provide good stability characteristics and have low toxicity.

FORMULATION ASPECTS OF MULTIPLE EMULSIONS

Florence and Whitehill described three different types of multiple emulsions, which they termed A, B and C (Fig. 4.2). Type A multiple emulsions were those in which only one large internal drop was contained into the secondary emulsion droplet. In type B emulsions, there were several small internal droplets contained in the secondary emulsion droplet, and type C emulsions were those with a large number of internal droplets present. Only the type C systems have application in drug delivery and drug targeting.

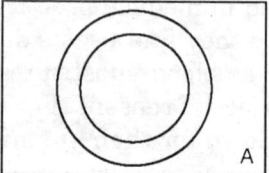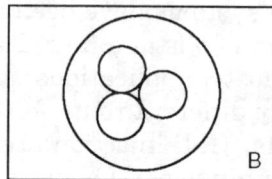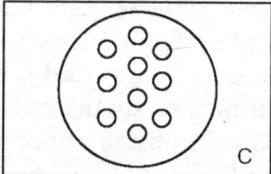

Fig. 4.2: Types of multiple emulsions

Multiple emulsions can be formed by the deliberate re-emulsification of primary emulsion, or they can occur when an emulsion inverts from one type to another, for example W/O to O/W. Thus for experimental studies, multiple emulsions are best prepared by the re-emulsification of a primary emulsion employing at least two surfactants one of which is used to stabilise the initial primary emulsion and the other to stabilise the secondary multiple emulsion. The emulsifier needs to be preferentially soluble in the dispersed phase of the emulsion type being prepared. For example, if a primary O/W emulsion is to be prepared, a lipophilic emulsifier is required, followed by a hydrophilic emulsifier for secondary emulsion (W/O). The stability of the resultant multiple emulsion will depend on not only formulation variables but also the conditions employed in its production. The following factors are identified as being of importance and will be discussed in turn with reference to the W/O/W system:

- Emulsification equipment
- Nature of the oil phase
- Volumes of the two dispersed phase
- Nature and quantity of the emulsifying agents
- Nature of entrapped materials including the drug substances
- Added stabilising components.

GENERAL METHODS OF PREPARATION

Two-Step Emulsification (Double Emulsification)

Two-step emulsification methods involve re-emulsification of primary W/O or O/W emulsion using a suitable emulsifier agent. The first step involves obtaining an ordinary W/O or O/W primary emulsion wherein an appropriate emulsifier system is utilised. In the second step, the freshly prepared W/O or O/W primary emulsion is re-emulsified with an excess of aqueous phase or oil phase. The finally prepared emulsion could be W/O/W or O/W/O respectively. The method is schematically illustrated in Fig. 4.3.

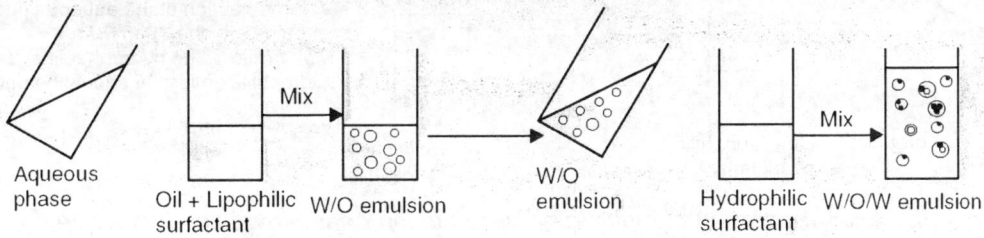

Fig. 4.3: Two-step preparation of a W/O/W multiple emulsion

In two step emulsification it was observed that on scale of acceptability, the physicochemical characteristics of multiple emulsion systems were directly related to the ratio of the amount of Span 80 to that of a series of the hydrophilic emulsifiers existing in the entire system (Matsumoto *et al.,* 1976; Matsumoto *et al.,* 1977a; Matsumoto *et al.,* 1977b). It was observed that twice or less Span 80 than Tween 80 is necessary for obtaining higher yields of O/W/O emulsions in contrast to the amount and ratio recommended for W/O/W emulsion (Kang and Matsumoto, 1988).

Recently, Okochi and Nakano, 2000 reported a modified two-step emulsification technique for the preparation of W/O/W emulsion. This method is different from the conventional two-step technique in two points: Firstly, sonication and stirring are used to obtain fine, homogenous and stable W/O emulsion. Secondly, a continuous phase is poured into a dispersed phase for preparing W/O/W emulsion (in contrast to conventional method in which a dispersed phase is poured into a continuous phase). Moreover, the composition of internal aqueous phase-oily phase-external phase is fixed at 1:4:5, which produces most stable formulation as reported for most of W/O/W emulsions.

PHASE INVERSION TECHNIQUE (ONE STEP TECHNIQUE)

Matsumoto and co-workers first reported the development of W/O/W system during the phase inversion of the concentrated W/O emulsion (Matsumoto, 1983; Matsumoto *et al.,* 1985a,b). An increase in volume concentration of dispersed phase may cause an increase in the phase volume ratio, which subsequently leads to the formation of multiple emulsions. The method typically involves the addition of an aqueous phase containing the hydrophilic emulsifier [Tween 80/sodium dodecyl sulphate (SDS) or Cetyl trimethyl ammonium salt (CTAB)] to an oil phase consisted of liquid paraffin and containing lipophilic emulsifier

(Span 80). A well-defined volume of oil phase is placed in a vessel of pin mixer. An aqueous solution of emulsifier is then introduced successively to the oil phase in the vessel at a rate of 5 ml/min, while the pin mixer rotates steadily at 88 rpm at room temperature. When volume fraction of the aqueous solution of hydrophilic emulsifier exceeds 0.7, the continuous oil phase is substituted by the aqueous phase containing a number of the vesicular globules among the simple oil droplets, leading to phase inversion and formation of W/O/W multiple emulsion (Fig. 4.4).

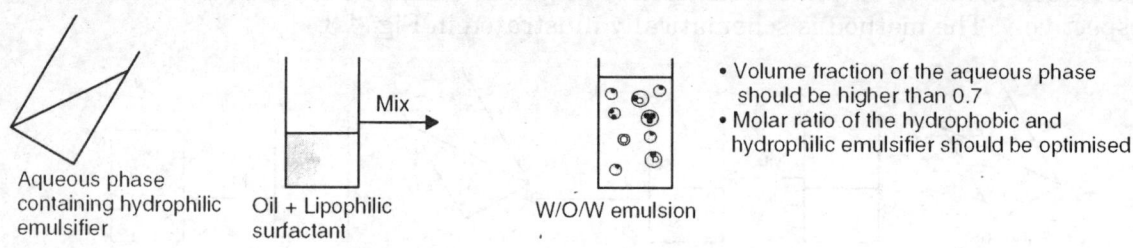

Aqueous phase containing hydrophilic emulsifier
Oil + Lipophilic surfactant
W/O/W emulsion

• Volume fraction of the aqueous phase should be higher than 0.7
• Molar ratio of the hydrophobic and hydrophilic emulsifier should be optimised

Fig. 4.4: Preparation of multiple emulsion using phase inversion technique

MEMBRANE EMULSIFICATION TECHNIQUE

In this method, a W/O emulsion (a dispersed phase) is extruded into an external aqueous phase (a continuous phase) with a constant pressure through a Porous Glass Membrane, which should have controlled and homogenous pores (Higashi *et al.*, 1995; 1999). The particle size of the resulting emulsion can be controlled with proper selection of Porous Glass Membrane as the droplet size depends upon the pore size of the membrane.

Multiple Emulsions Using Micro-channel Emulsification

Monodispersed multiple emulsions are useful for both industrial applications and basic studies. Rheology, appearance, chemical reactivity, and physical properties are influenced by both the average size and size distribution, and drug-release properties from multiple emulsions depend on their size (Fig. 4.5). Monodispersed emulsions can be obtained by fractionation from polydispersed emulsion, but repeated operations are required. Several research groups are investigating how to produce quasi-monodisperse W/O/W emulsions. Membrane emulsification, in which the pressurised dispersed phase permeates a microporous membrane and forms emulsion droplets, enables us to produce monodispersed emulsions with a coefficient of variation of approximately 10%. This technique has been applied to W/O/W emulsions. However, it is not clear how internal water droplets penetrate through the membrane pore.

Recently, novel microfabricated channel emulsification methods has been developed for making monodisperse emulsion droplets. This emulsification technique is called microchannel (MC) emulsification. Oil-in-water emulsions with a coefficient of variation of less than 5% and a droplet size of 3 to 100 μm have been successfully prepared using this technique. MC emulsification exploits the interfacial tension, the dominating force on a micrometer scale, as the driving force for droplet formation. During the droplet formation,

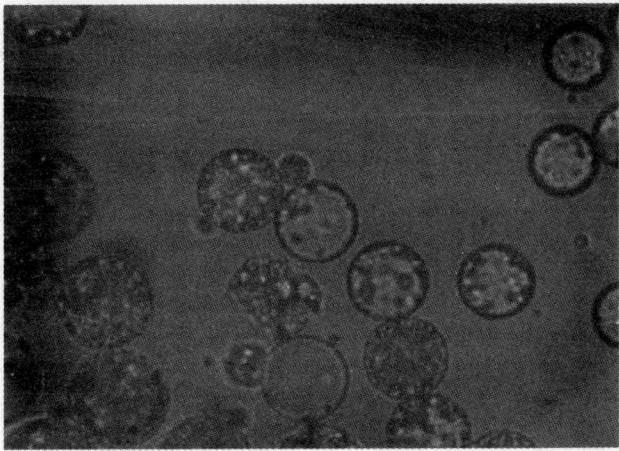

Fig 4.5: Photomicrograph of multiple emulsion droplets

the distorted dispersed phase is spontaneously transformed into spherical droplets by interfacial tension. The dispersed phase is forced into a distorted (elongated) disk-like shape in the MC. This distorted disk-like shape is the essential point for spontaneous transformation since the disk-like shape has a higher interface area than a spherical shape, resulting in instability from the viewpoint of interface free energy. The dispersed phase with disk-like shape spontaneously transforms into spherical droplets. Therefore, the droplets are formed without shear by continuous phase flow, and the required energy input is very low compared with conventional emulsification techniques. The mechanism is similar to the breakup of cylindrical flow at the point where transformation is caused by interfacial tension. The droplet size is controlled by MC geometry. An advantage of this technique is direct observation of emulsification through a microscope. Microchannel (MC) emulsification can be applied to prepare several types of oil-in-water emulsions, water-in-oil emulsions, lipid microparticles, and polymer microparticles. A disadvantage is its low production rate. Usually, less than 1 ml/h of dispersed phase can be emulsified.

CHARACTERISATION OF MULTIPLE EMULSIONS

Average Globule Size, Size Distribution and Yield of Multiple Emulsion

The optical microscopy method using calibrated ocular and stage micrometer can be utilised for globule size determinations of both multiple emulsion droplets and droplets of internal dispersed phase as well as yield. Florence and Whitehill (1982) used inverted phase contrast microscope and a high-speed camera. With the help of this technique, they classified multiple emulsions as coarse (>3μm diameter), fine (1–3 μm diameter) and micro-multiple emulsion (<1 μm diameter). The droplet size distribution of freshly made emulsion can be measured by light scattering using a Malvern Mastersizer and surface mean droplet diameter and the specific surface area (or SSA: area per unit mass of emulsion) can also be derived. Brightfield micrographs equipped with differential interference contrast optics have been used to characterise the internal droplet of multiple emulsions. Various other techniques used to characterise colloidal carriers like Coulter counter, freeze-fracture electron microscopy and scanning electron microscopy are also used to determine average globule size and size distribution of multiple emulsions.

Area of interfaces

The average globules diameter determined can be used in the calculation of the total area of interface using the formula:

S = 6/D

S = Total area of interface (sq.cm)

D = Diameter of globules (cm)

Number of globules

Number of globules per cubic mm can be measured following the method reported by Levius and Drommond (1953) using the hemocytometer cell. The emulsion is appropriately diluted; a countable number of globules are observed in each small square of the cell and counted. The globules in five groups of 16 small squares (total 80 small squares) are counted and the total number of globules per cubic mm is calculated using the formula (Chatterjee, 1977):

$$\text{No. of globules/mm}^3 = \frac{\text{No. of globules} \times \text{Dilution} \times 4000}{\text{No. of small squares}}$$

Rheological Evaluation

The rheology of multiple emulsion is an important parameter as it relates to emulsion stability and clinical performance. The viscosity and interfacial elasticity are two major parameters, which relate to product rheology. The viscosity of the multiple emulsions can be measured by Brookfield rotational viscometer. Samples are sheared for one minute at 100 rpm, using an appropriate spindle and readings are taken after equilibrium of the indicator dial. Oil phase viscosity can be measured by stress viscometry using a Bohlin controlled rheometer. Three different geometries stant (5 µL) were used according to the viscosity of the samples: double-gap DG 40/50, cone-plate 4/40, and concentric cylinder C25. The shear rates were varied between 0.5 and 200 s^{-1} depending on viscosity of the sample and geometry of the measuring head. The resulting viscosity was taken as the mean viscosity over the shear rate range. Interfacial film strength can be evaluated by interfacial rheology measurements, i.e. elasticity of (W/O) and (O/W) components of (W/O/W) multiple emulsions and these data may relate to emulsion stability. Interfacial rheology (i.e. interfacial elasticity at the oil-aqueous interface) can be investigated at the mineral oil/water interface using an Oscillatory Surface Rheometer. The effect of adding hydrophilic surfactant, Tween and Spans on interfacial elasticity can also be investigated and this may provide an insight on interfacial interactions that occur at the secondary O/W interface.

Zeta Potential

The zeta potential measurements are pivotal in the designing of surface modified or ligand anchored multiple emulsion systems. The zeta potential and surface charge can be calculated using Smoluchowski's equation from the mobility and electrophoretic velocity of dispersed globules using the Zeta-potentiometer. Nakhare and Vyas (1997) used a cylindrically bored micro-electrophoresis cell equipped with platinum-iridium electrodes to measure the electrophoretic mobility of the diluted W/O/W emulsion and using the following equation, zeta potential was calculated.

$$\zeta = \frac{4\pi\eta}{\varepsilon E} \times 10^3$$

Where,

ζ = Zeta potential (mV)

η = Viscosity of the dispersion medium (poise)

μ = Migration velocity (cm/s)

ε = Dielectric constant of the dispersion medium

E = Potential gradient (Voltage applied/ Distance between electrodes).

Per cent Drug Entrapment

Per cent entrapment of drug or active moiety in the multiple emulsion is generally determined using dialysis, centrifugation, filtration and conductivity measurements. However, recently an internal tracer/marker is used to evaluate the entrapment of an impermeable marker molecule contained in the inner aqueous phase of W/O/W emulsion. The unentrapped marker is calculated and the amount entrapped can be thus calculated by deducting unentrapped amount from the initially added amount. The % drug entrapment in the inner aqueous phase of W/O/W emulsion can be determined by using the dialysis method as reported by Nakhare and Vyas (1995, 1996). The % entrapment can be calculated using the following equation:

$$C = 100/[1 - n_1 V_0/n_{10} - n_1)V_1]$$

$$V = V_2 + \frac{V_d}{V_s}$$

Where,

n_{10} = Initial concentration of drug in inner aqueous phase

n_1 = Concentration of drug in dialysate

V_1, V_2 and V_0 represent the volume of inner and outer aqueous and middle oil phase respectively, and V_s and V_d represent volume of dialysing media and dialysed emulsion respectively.

In vitro Drug Release

The drug released from the aqueous inner phase of a W/O/W emulsion can be estimated using the conventional dialysis technique. Nakhare and Vyas (1995) investigated the release of drug from W/O/W emulsion employing the dialysis method using cellophane tubing (Fig. 4.6). The W/O/W emulsion was placed in the dialysis bag and dialysed against 200 ml of phosphate saline buffer (PBS, pH 7.4) at $37 \pm 1°C$ and a sink condition was maintained while sink contents were stirred continuously using a magnetic stirrer. Aliquots were withdrawn at different time intervals and estimated using standard procedure and the data were used to calculate cumulative drug release profile.

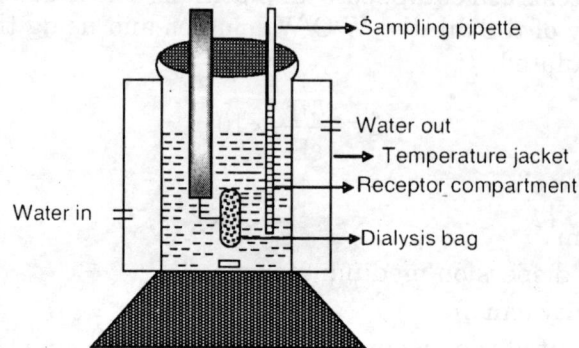

Fig. 4.6: Assembly used for in vitro drug release assay

In vitro stability studies

Emulsion stability is determined by phase separation on storage of W/O/W emulsions. Freshly prepared multiple emulsion allowed to stand for one week at room temperature and the volume of aqueous phase separated (Vsep) is measured at suitable time intervals and percent phase separation is calculated using following formula (*Nakhare* and *Vyas,* 1996):

$$B(\%) = 100 \ (V_{sep}/20) \ / \ [(V_1+V_2) \ (V_1+V_2+V_3)]$$

Where, V_1, V_2 and V_3 are the volumes of internal, external aqueous phase and middle oil phase respectively.

Photomicrography, difference in release of model drug and analysis of mean droplet diameters of the multiple emulsion systems as a function of time could be followed and used to study stability of W/O/W emulsions. However, to test flocculation in multiple emulsion, 5 and 100 drops of SDS (10%) are added immediately after the measurement and the emulsion is stirred gently. Then the droplet size distribution measurement is repeated and the degree of flocculation is microscopically assessed. Change in the stability of multiple emulsions can be assessed by measuring the number and size of multiple droplets over a period of time or by studying changes in rheological properties.

Nakhare and Vyas (1996) characterized *in vitro* stability to establish the suitability of W/O/W emulsion as suitable injectable drug carrier. Osmotic fragility and turbulence shock tests were performed in addition to assess *in vitro* stability.

PROTOCOL: 4.1

Preparation of Multiple Emulsion by Double Emulsification Method
Principle

Two separate steps of emulsification technique considered to be one of the reproducible and reliable method for multiple emulsion preparation. In first step, the W/O emulsion is prepared by a drop-wise addition of the water phase (W_1) containing NaCl as marker to the oil phase containing lipophilic emulsifiers. The second step involves the drop wise addition of primary W/O emulsion to an equal volume of aqueous phase W_2 containing the second emulsifier.

Materials and Composition

Formula I (Primary Emulsion)
Water
Sesame oil
Emulsifiers
Emulsifiers Span 85: Tween 80 (75:25), HLB 5.1
Formula II (Multiple Emulsion)
Primary emulsion
Water
Emulsifiers
Emulsifiers Span 80: Tween 80 50:50, HLB 9.6

Procedure

Preparation of Primary Emulsion

- Solubilise emulsifier of Formula I in sesame oil.
- Add water drop wise to oily phase and emulsify with sonication.
- Sonicate for 10 minutes.
- W/O type primary emulsion will be obtained.

Preparation of Multiple Emulsion

- Solubilise emulsifier of Formula II in given amount of water; a solution of hydrophilic emulsifiers will be obtained.
- To this solution add primary emulsion drop-wise with gentle stirring
- Stir for 1 minute and W/O/W multiple emulsions will be obtained (Scheme 4.1).

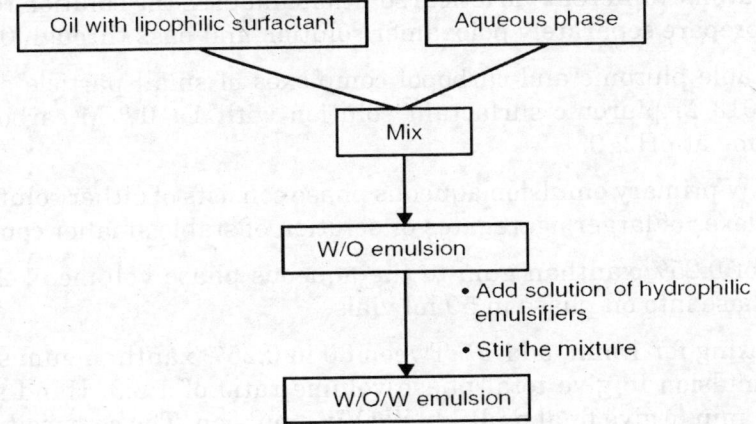

Scheme: 4.1 Preparation of multiple emulsion by double emulsification method

Process Variables

During First Step

Required HLB, emulsifier blend type, concentration of emulsifier blend, primary phase volume ration, emulsification equipment and emulsification time.

During Second Step

Required HLB, type of emulsifier, concentration, and secondary phase volume ratio emulsification equipment and emulsification time.

PROTOCOL: 4.2

W/O/W Multiple Emulsion Based on Pluronic and Polyarcylic Acid Complexes

Materials

Polyacrylic acid (carbapol 907)

Xanthan gum

Poloxamer surfactants (pluronics F68, P75, P85, P103, P104, P127)

Tween 80

Span 80

Isopropylmyristate (IPM)

Sesame oil

Procedure

- Prepare pluronic (different varieties) solution and pass the solution through 0.22 μm filter and prepare separately poloxamer solution and pass through 0.45 μm filter.
- Prepare stable pluronic and carbopol complexes of small particle size by reacting 0.0023−0.013 M pluronic surfactant solution with 1×10^{-6} M carbopol solution in equal volume at pH 2.0.
- Prepare O/W primary emulsion aqueous phase consists of either solution of Pluronic: PAA complexes of larger aggregates or solution of stable smaller complex particles.
- Add 50 μl of 0.25% xanthan gum to the aqueous phase volume of 2.5 ml. Add this aqueous phase into oil phase in 50 ml vials.
- After vortexing for 1 min, add 1% Tween 80 in 0.25% xanthan gum solution to each primary emulsion to give total phase volume ratio of 1:2:3. Hand shake the each phase for 1 min to give final multiple W/O/W emulsion. The compositions of multiple emulsions are given in Table 4.1.

Table: 4.1 summary of composition of various W/O/W multiple emulsions

Formula	Internal aqueous phase	Oil phase	External aqueous phase
A	Stable Pluronic F127: PAA complex pH 2	5% pluronic L101 in IPM	1% Tween 80 in 0.25% Xanthan gum
B	1×10^{-6} M PAA pH 2	5% Abuk WE 09 in miglycol	Same as above
C	Stable F127: PAA complex pH 2.0	7.5 Span 80 in sesame oil	Same as above
D	Stable F127: PAA	7.5 Span 80 in sesame oil	1% Pluronic P103 in 0.25 xanthan gum complex pH 2.0
E	Stable F127: PAA complex pH 2.0	7.5 Span 80 in sesame oil	1% Pluronic P123 in 0.25 xanthan gum

PROTOCOL: 4.3

Multiple Emulsion (W/O/W Type)

Principle

W/O/W emulsion is prepared by two-step emulsification method.

Materials

Drug rifampicin

Span-80 (sorbitan monooleate)

Polyvinyl alcohol

Polyvinylpyrrolidone

Soyalecithin

Liquid paraffin

Acacia and

Calcium stearate

Procedure

- Prepare the internal aqueous phase consisting of PBS (pH 7.4) containing rifampicin (10 mg/ml) and 2% of one of the macromolecules, polyvinyl alcohol, acacia, or polyvinyl pyrrolidone.
- Liquid paraffin, containing 30% w/w Span-80 is used as the oil phase.
- Carry out emulsification by stirring at 4000 rpm to produce the W/O primary emulsion. Prepare the W/O/W emulsion by subsequent emulsification of the primary W/O emulsion, with an equal part of phosphate buffered saline (pH 7.4) containing 0.5% Tween 80 as the secondary emulsifier using a whirl mixer. The final phase volume ratio is maintained at 1:1.
- Following the same method, prepare multiple W/O/W emulsion containing 2% W/V calcium stearate and soyalecithin in their organic phase.

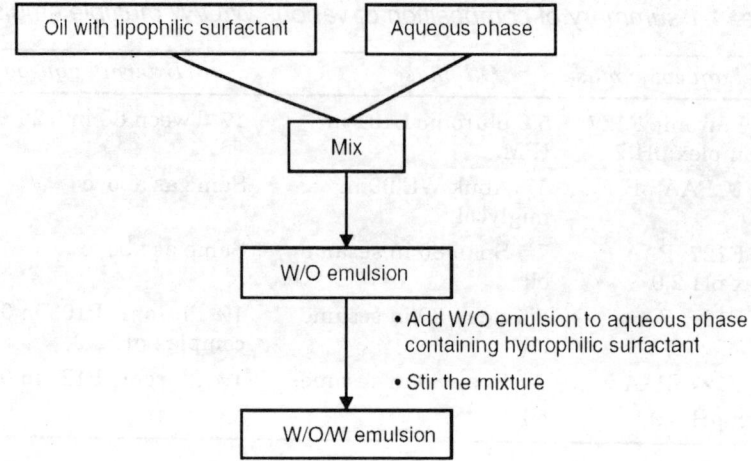

Scheme: 4.2. Preparation of multiple emulsions by two-step emulsification method

---

PROTOCOL: 4.4

Preparation of Polysaccharides Gel Based Multiple Emulsion by Two-step Emulsification Procedure

Principle

Two separate steps of emulsification technique is considered as one of the reproducible and reliable method for multiple emulsion preparation. In first step, the W/O emulsion is prepared by a drop-wise addition of the water phase (W1) containing NaCl as marker to the oil phase containing lipophilic emulsifiers. The second step involves the drop wise addition of primary W/O emulsion to an equal volume of aqueous phase W2 containing the second emulsifier (Scheme 4.2).

Materials and Composition

Formula I (Primary Emulsion)

NaCl (0.1 M)

Gelatin (5%)

Tryptophan (0.05 M)

Emulsifier polyglycerol polyricinoleate (PGPR, 75% tri- and tetraglycerol polyricinoleate)

Formula II (Multiple Emulsion)

Primary emulsion   40% w/w

Water   48% w/w

Medium chain fatty acid triglycerides (MCT, c_8-c_{10})

Neobee M5 Emulsifiers

Procedure

Preparation of Primary Emulsion

- Solubilise emulsifier of Formula I in oil.
- Add water drop-wise to oily phase and emulsify with sonication.
- Sonicate for 10 minutes.
- Pass through a high pressure homogeniser under high pressure (up to 3000 atms)
- W/O type primary emulsion is obtained.

Preparation of Multiple Emulsion

- Solubilise emulsifier of Formula II in given amount of water; a solution of hydrophilic emulsifiers will be obtained.
- To this solution add primary emulsion drop wise with gentle stirring
- Stir for 1 minute and pass through a high pressure homogeniser under high pressure (up to 1MPa)
- W/O/W multiple emulsions is obtained.

Process Variables

During First Step

Required HLB, Emulsifier blend type, concentration of emulsifier blend, primary phase volume ration, emulsification equipment and emulsification time.

During Second Step

Required HLB, type of emulsifier, concentration, and secondary phase volume ratio emulsification equipment and emulsification time.

PROTOCOL: 4.5

Preparation of Polysaccharides Stabilised Multiple Emulsion by Two-step Emulsification Procedure

W/O Primary Emulsion

H_2O

Glycerol

Glucose

Medium chain fatty acid triglycerides

Polyglycerol polyricinoleate

Monoglyceride oleate (MGO),

Dimodan MO-90

W/O/W Double Emulsion

W/O primary emulsion

H$_2$O

Whey protein isolate

Preparation of Primary Emulsion

- Drop wise addition of the aqueous phase containing glucose (marker), and glycerol to the oil phase that contains the hydrophobic surfactants.
- Sonicate for 10 minutes.
- Pass through a high pressure homogeniser under high pressure (up to 3000 atms)
- W/O type primary emulsion is obtained.

Preparation of Multiple Emulsion

- Solubilise emulsifier of Formula II in given amount of water; a solution of hydrophilic emulsifiers will be obtained.
- To this solution add primary emulsion drop wise with gentle stirring.
- Mix and pass through a high pressure homogeniser under high pressure (up to 600 atms).
- W/O/W multiple emulsions is obtained.

SUGGESTED REA DINGS

- Absolom, D. R. (1986). Methods Enzymol., 132 281.
- Adeyeye, C.M. and Proce, J.C. (1990). Drug Dev. Ind. Pharm., 16, 1055.
- Ali, A.A. and Mulley, B.A. (1978) J. Pharm. Pharmacol., 30, 205.
- Baker, R.W. and Lonsdale, H.K. (1974). Controlled release of biologically active agents (Tonquary, A.O. and Lceoy, R.E., Eds.), Plenum Press, New York, pp15.
- Benichou, A., Aserin, A., Garti, N., (2007). Colloids and Surfaces A: Physicochem. Eng. Aspects 294 ,20.
- Bhatnagar, S., Nakhare, S. and Vyas, S.P. (1995). J. Microencap., 12, 13.
- Boyd, J.V., Krog, N. and Sherman, P. (1976). The theory and practice of emulsion technology, Smith, A.L., Ed., Academic Press, London,123.
- Brodin, A.F., Kavaliunus, D.R. and Frank, S.G. (1978). Acta pharm. Suec., 15, 1.
- Burck, S.D. (1983). Controlled drug delivery, CRC press, Boca Raton, Vol. I, pp. 187.
- Chen, C.C., Tu, Y.Y. and Chang, H.M. (1999) J. Agric. Food Chem., 47, 407.
- Cole, M.L. and Whately, T.L. (1997) J. Control. Rel., 49, 51.
- Collings, A.J. (1971). British patent, 1, 235,667.
- Davis, S.S., Illum, L. and Walker, I.M. (1987). Int. J. Pharm., 38, 133.
- Dogru, S.T., Calis, S. and Oner, F. (2000). J. Clin. Pharm. Ther., 25, 435.

- Elson, C.O., Tomasi, M., Dertzbaugh, M.T., Thaggard, G., Hunter, R. and Weaver, C. (1996). Ann. N. Y. Acad. Sci., 778, 156.
- Fattal, E., Roques, B., Puisieux, F., Blanco-Prieto, M.J. and Couvreur, P. (1997). Adv. Drug Deliv. Rev., 28, 85.
- Fidler, I.J. (1980). Science, 208, 1469.
- Florence, A.T. and Whitehill, D. (1982) Int. J. Pharm., 11, 277.
- Florence, A.T. and Whitehill, D. (1982) J. Pharm. Pharmacol., 34, 687.
- Florence, A.T. and Whitehill, D. (1985) Macro- and Micro-Emulsions: Theory and Application, ACS Symposium Series, (Shar, D.O., Ed.), vol. 272, 1985, pp. 359.
- Florence, A.T., Al-Saden, A.A. and Whateley, T.L. (1980) Int. J. Pharm., 53, 17.
- Florence, A.T., Al-Saden, A.A. and Whateley, T.L. (1981) Colloids and Surfaces, 2, 49.
- Florence, A.T., Law, T.K. and Whateley, T.L. (1985) J. Colloid Interface. Sci., 79, 243.
- Frieberg, S. and Mandell, I. (1970) J. Pharm.Sci., 59, 1001.
- Fukushima, S., Juni, K. and Nakano, M. (1983) Chem. Pharm. Bull., 31, 4048.
- Fukushima, S., Nishida, M., Shibuta, T., Juni, K., Nakano, M., Uchara, N., Ohkuma, T., Yamishita, Y. and Takahashi, M. (1986), J. Pharmacobio-Dyn. 9, 18.
- Furuno, T., Ikeda, A., Iso, M., Omi, S. and Yokota, H. Zairyou Gijitsu, (1987) 5, 141.
- Gallarate, M., Carlotti, M.E., Trotta, M. and Bovo, S. (1999) Int. J. Pharm., 188, 233.
- Garti, N., Aserin, A. and Cohen, Y. (1993) J. Control. Rel., 29, 41–51.
- Garti, R.H., Frenkel, M. and Schwartz, R. (1983) J. Disperse Sci. Technol., 4, 237.
- Goldberg, E.P. (1983) Targeted drugs, John Wiley, New York, pp. 296.
- Gregoriadis, G. (1977) Nature, 265, 407.
- Hashida, M., Liao, M.H., Muranishi, S. and Sezaki, H. (1980) Chem. Pharm. Bull., 28, 1659.
- Hashida, M., Muranishi, S. and Sezaki, H. (1977) J. Pharmacokinetics and Biopharmaceutics, 5, 241.
- Hashida, M., Muranishi, S., Takahashi, Y. and Sezaki, H. (1977) J. Pharmacokin. Biopharm., 5, 241.
- Herbert, W.J. (1967) British Patent, 1, 080, 994.
- Higashi, H., Shimizu, M., Nakashima, T., Iwata, K., Uchiyama, F., Tateno, S. and Setoguchi, T. (1995) Cancer, 75, 1245.
- Higashi, H., Tabata, N., Kondo, K.H., Maeda, Y., Shimizu, M. and Nakashima, T. (1999) J. Pharmacol. Exp. Ther., 289, 816.
- Hino, T., Kawashima, Y. and Shimabayashi, S. (2000) Adv. Drug Deliv. Rev., 45, 27.
- Illum, L., Davis, S.S., Wilson, C.G., Thomas, N., Frier, M. and Hardy, J.G. (1982) Int. J. Pharm., 12, 135.
- Iso, M., Shirahase, T., Hanamura, S., Urushiyama, S. and Omi, S. (1989) J. Microencaps., 6, 165.
- Iwamoto, K., Kato, T., Kawahara, M., Koyama, N., Watanabe, S., Miyake, Y. and Sunamoto, J. (1991) J. Pharm. Sci., 80, 219.
- Iwata, M. and McGinity, J.W. (1992) J. Microencaps., 9, 201.
- Iwata, M., Nakamura, Y. and McGinity, J.W. (1999) J. Microencaps., 16, 49–58. J. Control. Rel., 52, 99.

- Kajita, M., Morishita, M., Takayama, K., Chiba, Y., Tokiwa, S. and Nagai, T. (2000) J. Pharm. Sci., 89, 1243.
- Kang, W.W. and Matsumoto, S. (1988) Int. Conf. Surface Colloid Sci., Kakone, Japan.
- Kanke, M., Simmons, G.H., Weiss, D.L., Bivins, B.A. and Deluca, P.P. (1980) J. Pharm. Sci., 69, 755.
- Kita, Y., Matsumoto, S. and Yonezawa, D. (1978) Nippon Kagaku Kaishi, 1, 11.
- Konno, T., maeda, H., Iwai, K., Tashiro, S., Maki, S., Morinaga, T., Mochinaga, M., Hiraoka, T. and Yokoyama, I. (1983), J Cancer Clin. Oncol., 19, 1053.
- Kramer, P.A. (1974) J. Pharm. Sci., 63, 1646.
- Lanier, J.G., Newman, M.J., Lee, E.M., Sette, A. and Ahmed, R. (1999) Vaccine, 18, 549.
- Laugel, C., Rafidison, P., Potard, G., Aguadisch, L. and Baillet, A. (2000) J. Control. Rel., 63, 7–17.
- Law, T.K., Florence, A.T. and Whateley, T.L. (1984) J. Pharm. Pharmacol., 36, 50.
- Law, T.K., Whateley, T.L. and Florence, A.T. (1986) J. Control. Rel. 3, 279.
- Leo, E., Pecquet, S., Rojas, J., Couvreur, P. and Fattal, E. (1998) J. Microencaps., 15, 421.
- Li, N.N. (1960) U.S. Patent, 3, 410.794.
- Lin, S.Y., Wu, W.H. and Lui, W.Y. (1992) Pharmazie, 47, 439.
- Makryalease, K., Scheper, T., Schugent, K. and Kurla, M.R. (1985) Germ. Chem. Eng., 6, 345.
- Matsumoto, S. (1983) J. Colloid Interface. Sci., 94, 362.
- Matsumoto, S. and Khoda, M. (1980) J. Colloid Interface. Sci., 73, 13.
- Matsumoto, S. and Sherman, P. (1981) J. Texture Studies, 12, 243.
- Matsumoto, S., Inoue, T., Khoda, M. and Ikura, K. (1980) J. Colloid Interface. Sci., 73, 555.
- Matsumoto, S., Khoda, M. and Murata, S. (1977a) J. Colloid Interface. Sci., 62, 149.
- Matsumoto, S., Kita, Y. and Yonezawa, D. (1976) J. Colloid Interface. Sci., 57, 353.
- Matsumoto, S., Kitayama, T. and Koh, Y. (1985a) J. Japan Oil Chemist's Soc., 34, 688.
- Matsumoto, S., Koh, Y., and Michiura, A. (1985b) J. Disp. Sci. Tech., 6, 507.
- Matsumoto, S., Ueda, Y., Kita, Y. and Yonezawa, D. (1977b) Agric. Biol. Chem., 42, 739.
- May, S.W. and Li, N.N. (1972) Biochim. Biophys. Res. Commun., 68, 786.
- McGinity, J.W. and O'Donnell, P.B. (1997) Adv. Drug Deliv. Rev., 28, 25.
- Mishra, B. and Pandit, J.K. (1989) Drug Dev. Ind. Pharm., 15, 1217.
- Miyakawa, T., Zhang, W., Uchida, T., Kim, N.S. and Goto, S. (1993) Biol. Pharm. Bull., 16, 268.
- Moghimi, S.M. and Patel, H.M. (1989) Biochim. Biophys. Acta, 984, 379.
- Mohan, R.R. and Li, N.N. (1974) Biotechmol. Bioenerg., 16, 513.
- Mohan, R.R. and Li, N.N. (1975) Biotechnol. Bioeng., 17, 1137.
- Morimoto, Y., Yamaguchi, Y. and Sugibayashi, K. (1982) Chem. Pharm. Bull., 30, 2980.
- Nakhare, S. and Vyas, S.P. (1995) J. Microencaps., 12, 409.
- Nakhare, S. and Vyas, S.P. (1996) J. Microencaps., 13, 281.
- Nakhare, S. and Vyas, S.P. (1997) Pharmazie, 52, 224.
- Nakhare, S., Vyas, S.P. and Jain, N.K. (1994) The Eastern Pharmacist, , 65.

- Oh, I., Kang, Y.G., Lee, Y.B., Shin, S.C. and Kim, C.K. (1998) Drug Dev. Ind. Pharm., 24, 889.
- Okochi, H. and Nakano, M. (2000) Adv. Drug Deliv. Rev., 45, 5.
- Omotosho, J.A. (1990) Int. J. Pharm., 62, 81.
- Omotosho, J.A., Whateley, T.L. and Florence, A.T. (1989) Biopharm. Drug Dispos., 10, 257.
- Omotosho, J.A., Whateley, T.L., Law, T.K. and Florence, A.T. (1986) J. Pharm. Pharmacol., 38, 865.
- Onuki, Y., Morishita, M., Takayama, K., Tokiwa, S., Chiba, Y., Isowa, K. and Nagai, T. (2000) Int. J. Pharm., 198, 147.
- Opaware, F.O. and Burgess, D.J. (1998) J. Pharm. Pharmacol., 50, 965.
- Oza, K.P. and Frank, S.G. (1989) J. Dispersion Sci. Technol., 10, 163.
- Pandit, J.K., Mishra, B., Krishnamurthy, Y. and Mishra, D.N. (1988) Ind. J. Pharm. Sci., 50, 274.
- Pavanetto, F., Perugini, P., Conti, B., Modena, T. and Genta, I. (1996) J. Microencaps., 13, 679.
- Rao, Y.M. and Bader, F. (1993) The Eastern Pharmacist, 36, 431.
- Rojas, J., Pinto-Alphandary, H., Leo, E., Pecquet, S., Couvreur, P. and Fattal, E. (1999) Int. J. Pharm., 183, 67.
- Scheper, T. (1990) Adv. Drug Deliv. Rev., 4, 210.
- Scheper, T., Halwachs, W. and Schugent, K. (1984) Chem. Eng., B-31, B-37.
- Shah, M.V., De Gennaro, M.D. and Suryakasuma, H. (1987) J. Microencaps., 4,223–228.
- Shimizu, M. and Nakane, Y. (1995) Biosci. Biotechnol. Biochem., 59, 492–496.
- Shinoda, K. and Friberge, S. (1986) Emulsion and solubilization, John Wiley and Sons, New York, pp. 33.
- Shively, M.L. (1997) Pharm. Biotechnol., 10, 199–211.
- Singh, S., Singh, R. and Vyas, S.P. (1995) J. Microencap., 12, 609–615.
- Su, J., Flanagan J., Singh, H, (2008) Food Hydrocolloids 22 ,112–120.
- Sugiura, S., Nakajima, M., Yamamoto K., Iwamoto S., Oda T., Satake M., and Seki M., (2004) Journal of Colloid and Interface Science, 270. 221.
- Suzuki, A., Morishita, M., Kajita, M., Takayama, K., Isowa, K., Chiba, Y., Tokiwa, S. and Nagai, T. (1998) J. Pharm. Sci., 87, 1196.
- Takahashi, T., Mizuno, M., Fujita, Y., Ueda, S., Nishioka, B. and Majima, S. Gann., (1973) 64, 345.
- Takahashi, T., Ueda, S., Kono, K. and Majima, S. (1976) Cancer, 38, 1507.
- Tomasi, M., Dertzbaugh, M.T., Hearn, T., Hunter, R.L. and Elson, C.O. (1997) Eur. J. Immunol., 27, 2720.
- Tomlinson, E., Burger, J.J., Mevie, J.G. and Hoefnagel, K. (1984) Recent advances in drug delivery systems (Anderson, J.H. and Kim, J.W., Eds.), Plenum Press, New York, pp. 199.
- Verma, R. and Jaiswal, T.N. (1997) Vaccine, 15, 1254.
- Weiss J., Scherze I., Muschiolik G., (2005) Food Hydrocolloids. 19, 605.
- Wisse, E. and De Leeuw, A.M. (1984) Microspheres and drug therapy: Pharmaceutical, immunological and medical aspects (Davis, S.S., Illum, L., Mevie, J.G. and Tomlinson, E., Eds.), Elsevier, Amsterdam, pp.1.

- Yashioka, T., Ikeuchi, K., Hashida, M., Muranishi, S. and Sezaki, H. (1982) Chem. Pharm. Bull., 38, 1408.
- Yazan, Y., Seiller, M. and Puisieux, F. (1993) Boll. Chim. Farm., 132, 187.
- Zheng, S., Zheng, Y., Beissinger, R.L., Wasan, D.T. and McCormick, D.L. (1993) Biochim. Biophys. Acta., 1158, 65.
- Zweitach, B.W. (1980) Adv. Microcir., 9, 206.
- Levius and Drommond (1953).
- Chatterjee, 1977.

5

Colon Specific Delivery

Enteric Coated Tablets, Pectin Based Systems

Colon has been extensively evaluated as a site for drug delivery, not only for local colonic pathologies but also for systemic drug delivery and for delivery of protein and peptide drugs. This site may also be useful in the treatment of diseases susceptible to diurnal rhythm such as asthma, arthritis, etc.

For a formulation to act as an effective colon specific drug delivery system, the primary condition is that a minimum amount of drug should be released in the environment of the upper gastrointestinal tract, i.e. in stomach and small intestine. The normal transit time in the stomach is 2 h (though this may vary), while in the small intestine it is relatively constant and is around 3 h. The usual colonic transit time varies from 20–30 h. Thus, for a dosage form to be effective as a colon drug delivery system, the drug release is required to be retarded in the upper GIT conditions. Thereafter, the drug release should be complete within the next 20–30 h. As a site for drug delivery, colon offers a near neutral pH, reduced digestive enzymatic activity, a long transit time and an increased responsiveness to absorption enhancers. This has led to the development of various systems for targeting drugs to the colon. These include pH- controlled release systems, enzyme-controlled delivery systems (including prodrugs and polysaccharide based delivery systems), time-controlled release systems and pressure/osmotically controlled release systems. However, the coated dosage forms, especially the enteric-coated dosage forms are most popular.

ENTERIC-COATED SYSTEMS

Enteric-coated systems are designed to provide protection to tablets and other version of novel drug delivery systems in the stomach. Application of a thicker coat causes a delay in drug release in the small intestine and slows down the drug release, which is both pH and time controlled. This time-controlled drug release may be retarded by 3–4 h. This ensures drug delivery to be colon specific. For the preparation of such tailor-made formulations, the selection of a polymer with a suitable coat level is crucial. Most of the commercially available systems for colon specific drug delivery utilise Eudragit (L-100/S-100) or cellulose acetate phthalate (CAP). Other coating polymers such as shellac (SH) and ethyl cellulose (EC) may provide an alternative polymer for the development of these systems. Eudragit S-100 (ES) is a methacrylic acid methylmethacrylate co-polymer, which is soluble at a pH of 7. Cellulose acetate phthalate is also an effective enteric film coating material as it dissolves at a pH of 6.0. As an enteric coating polymer, it is used at a concentration of 0.5–0.9%.

Shellac is a naturally occurring material obtained from lac, a resinous secretion of the insect *Laccifero lacca* Kerr. (*Coccidae*). It is an inexpensive and abundantly available polymer and is used for enteric coating of tablets and beads. Ethyl cellulose is a hydrophobic polymer used as a tablet coating material.

BIODEGRADABLE MATRIX AND HYDROGEL SYSTEMS (PECTIN BASED SYSTEMS)

The inability to digest certain plant polysaccharides by GIT enzymes is taken as an advantage to develop colon-specific drug delivery systems. The drug is embedded in the matrix core of the biodegradable polymer by compressing the blend of active drug, a degradable polymer and additives. Various polysaccharides such as pectin, guargum, chondroitine, etc. are being used for the purpose of colon targeting. The bacterial enzymes of colon degrade the carrier polymer in a defined way to release the contents for localised colonic delivery or systemic absorption through colon.

The gelling properties of pectin offer several advantages, including formation of viscous diffusional barriers and fermentability in the large intestine, which are useful attributes in colon-specific drug delivery systems (Fig. 5.1) (Sriamornsak *et al.,* 1997). Calcium pectinate is a lower water-soluble pectin salt used in colonic delivery systems. Calcium pectinate-indomethacin compressed tablets reportedly degraded by enzymes of aspergillus and colonic bacteria *Bacteroides ovatus*. Similarly, compression coated tablets comprised of natural pectin could protect the bio-susceptible core during GI transit.

Drug carriers made up of natural and modified polysaccharide hydrogels tend to swell following their hydration. The degree of swelling is an important property of the hydrogels. Initially, the swollen hydrated polymer creates a diffusional barrier on the surface and eventually, allows the penetration of colonic enzymes, which cause the degradation of polymer. The swelling property therefore, limits the use of hydrogels for poorly water-soluble drugs and in case of highly water-soluble drugs; an addition of compressed polymer layer is designed to delay the diffusion of drug for longer time.

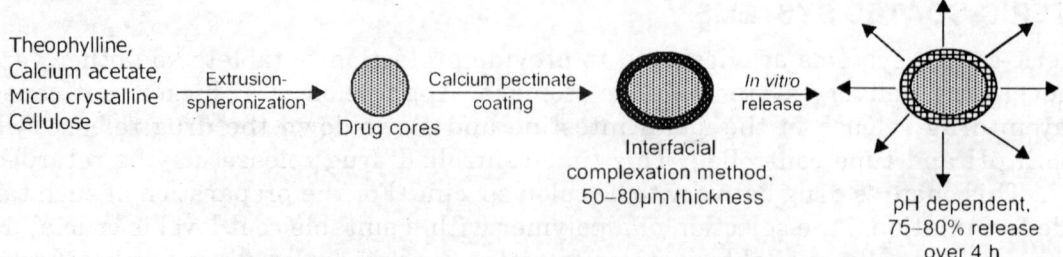

Fig. 5.1: *pH dependent theophylline release from pectin based biodegradable matrix system (Sriamornsak et al., 1997)*

Amidated pectins are more tolerant to pH variations and fluctuations in calcium levels as well as susceptible for enzymatic degradation (Figs. 5.2 and 5.3) (Wakerly *et al.*, 1996). Inclusion of calcium as a crosslinking agent increases the viscosity of amidated pectin gels while the amidation of pectin affects the release rate due to matrix erosion.

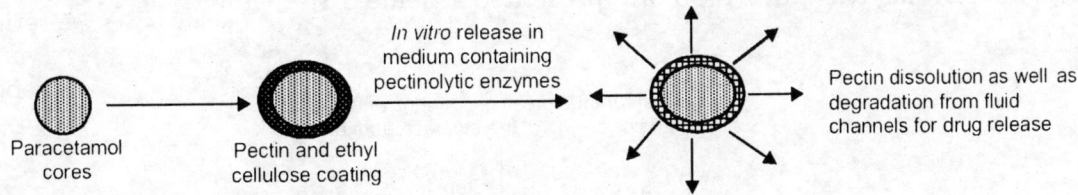

Fig. 5.2: *Working principle of system based on pectin-ethylcellulose combination (Wakerly et al., 1996)*

Chondroitin sulfate is a soluble mucopolysaccharide that is utilised as a substrate for bacteria (*Bacteroides thetaiotaomicron* and *B. ovatus*) in large intestine. Chondroitin breakdown occurs by the enzyme chondroitin sulfate lyase. Natural chondroitin sulfate is crosslinked, because of its higher water solubility. The hydrophilicity may be however altered by varying degree of crosslinking.

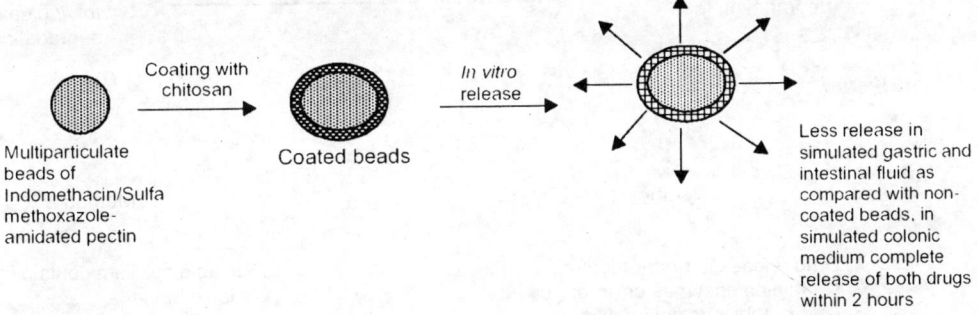

Fig. 5.3: *Working principle of multiparticulate system based on amidated pectin (Munjeri et al., 1997)*

PRECLINICAL EVALUATION AND ANIMAL MODELS

Colon-specific drug delivery systems significantly differ from other drug delivery systems by not releasing the drug in stomach and small intestine. They release the drug specifically in colon. Various *in vitro* and *in vivo* evaluation techniques have been developed and proposed to test the performance and stability of colon-specific drug delivery systems.

In Vitro Models

There is no standardised evaluation technique(s) available for evaluation of colon-specific drug delivery systems because an ideal *in vitro* model should possess the *in vitro* conditions of GIT such as pH, volume, stirring, bacteria, enzymes, and other components of food. Generally, these conditions are influenced by the diet and physical stress, and these factors make it difficult to design a standard *in vitro* model. Some *in vitro* models for drug release monitoring (Ashford *et al.,* 1993) and enzymatic degradation (Ashford *et al.,* 1994; Brondsted *et al.,* 1995) are presented scheme 5.1.

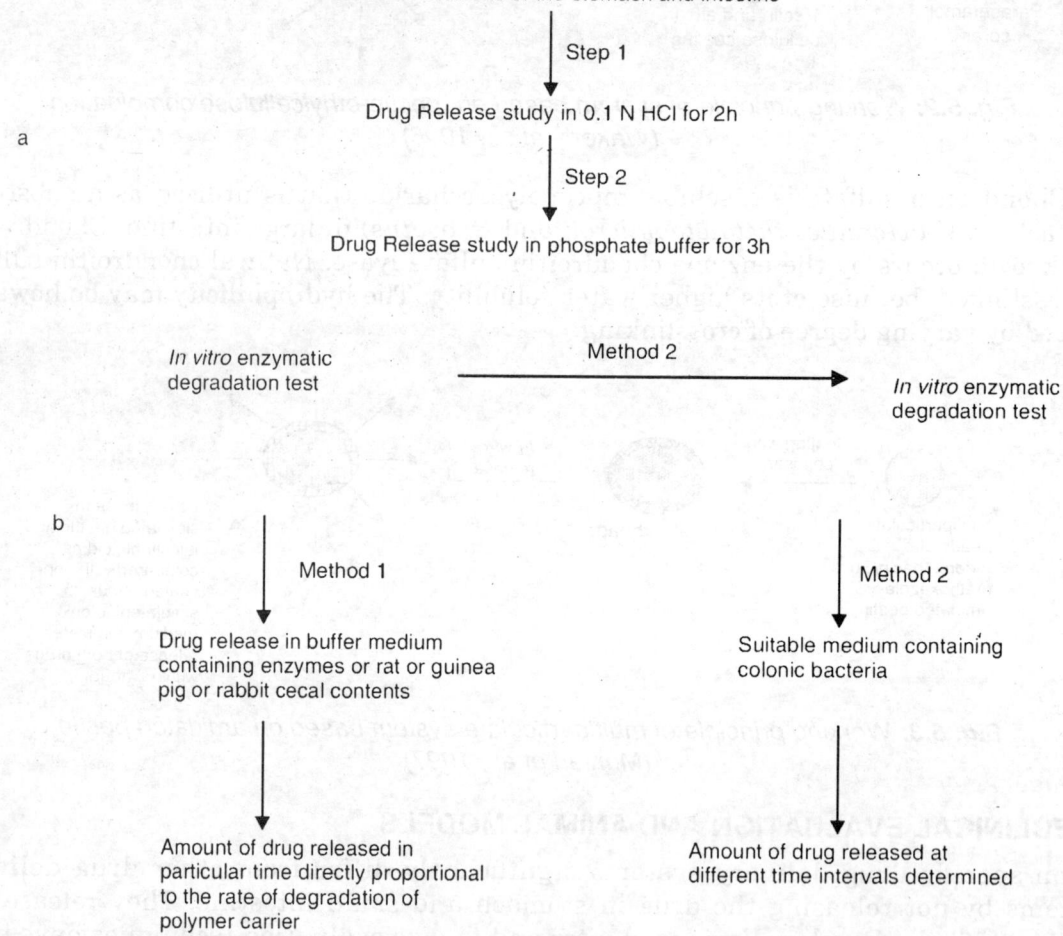

Scheme 5.1: *In vitro assessment of colon-specific drug delivery systems. (a) In vitro drug release test (b) In vitro enzymatic degradation tests*

In Vivo Animal Models

A number of animals have been used to evaluate the delivery of drug(s) to the large intestine of mammals. Various animals such as dogs, guinea pigs, rats and pigs are used because they resemble the anatomic and physiological conditions as well as the microflora of human GIT. While choosing a model for testing a colon drug delivery system, relative model for the colonic disease should also be considered. For example, guinea pigs are commonly used for experimental IBD model. To evaluate drug delivery and efficacy, particularly for treatment of IBD, the anatomy and physiology of all the potentially used animals differ considerably from those of human.

The primary difference in bacterial glycosidase activity between human and animals exists in the Proximal Small Intestine (PSI) and Distal Small Intestine (DSI). The relatively high levels of glycosidase activity in the PSI and DSI of laboratory animals may lead to hydrolysis of glycoside prodrugs in the small intestine. In contrast, glycosidase activity is more in human colon/cecum. This difference suggests that laboratory animals are not good models for the evaluation of glycoside prodrugs. However, rabbit and guinea pig show equal glycosidase activity in the large intestine when compared with humans. In contrast to the distribution of glycosidase activity, the distribution of azoreductase activity in the rat and rabbit GIT is fairly comparable to that in the human GIT (Renwick, 1982).

The GIT anatomy of rodents and humans is significantly different. Guinea pigs have a very large caecum (about 3 times the size of its stomach). In contrast, humans have a poorly defined caecal region continuous with the colon. Guinea pigs also possess a colonic furrow, which is a part of separation mechanism. Nitrogen and viable bacteria are transported in a retrograde manner from the colon into the cecum where the cecum uses the surplus of microorganisms by means of cecotrophy (Holtenius and Bjornhog, 1985). For slowly absorbed drugs, such transport may help to maintain the drug in the cecal area for longer time prior to excretion. The rats and mouse have total intestinal transit times similar to that of humans (20–30 hours) while beagle dogs show relatively shorter transit time (6–8 hours). The small intestinal transit time is about 3–4 hours, 1–2 hours (shorter) and 4–5 hours (longer) in humans, guinea pigs and rats, respectively (Pettersson *et al.,* 1976).

In fact, rodents are coprophagic and, hence, it is commonly observed that these animals have large quantities of feces and other substances in their stomach even under fasting conditions. The consumption of feces by rodents leads to a higher number of bacteria in their stomach and small intestine. The bacteria present in human food are killed by stomach acidity (Draser and Hill, 1974). In contrast, the stomach pH of many rodents is not sufficiently low to kill the bacterial load of their feed.

The eating behaviour, anatomy and physiology of GIT of guinea pigs are comparable to human. This makes guinea pigs most suitable animal for the evaluation of colon delivery systems (Kararli, 1995; Dressman and Yamada, 1991). Bacterial flora in colon and digestive properties of small intestine are also almost similar to human. They also possess an interdigestive, migrating myeloelectric complex, which is known to be a critical factor in gastric emptying of indigestible solids (Ruckbusch and Buene, 1976). The size of guinea pigs is comparatively larger than rats that make the possibility of oral ingestion and the data obtained can be extrapolated to human. To study the absorption properties of the systems, a fistula is generally created in the terminal ileum of guinea pigs (Gardner *et al.,* 1996). Rats are suitable for the initial screening of absorption properties and effect of absorption enhancers, on colon drug delivery (Van den Mooter *et al.,* 1995). The smaller size of rats, however make oral ingestion difficult. In some cases, the systems are surgically inserted directly into the desired region of absorption site in rats. The biodegradation studies of polymers can be carried out in rats because of the similarity of microflora of rats and human. Azobond prodrugs can be evaluated by using rabbits, which have azoreductase activity, comparable to human GIT. The *in vivo* drug release data can be compared, correlated and eventually standardised by adopting simulated human intestinal microbial system (Molly *et al.,* 1993). For rapid evaluation of colon specific drug delivery systems, a novel model has been proposed. In this model, the human foetal bowel is transplanted into a subcutaneous tunnel on the back of a thymic nude mice, which vascularises within 4 weeks, matures and becomes capable of developing a mucosal immune system from the host (Winter *et al.,* 1991).

PROTOCOL: 5.1
Preparation of Colon Specific Tablets
Material
[A] Tablets
Formula for Tablet Preparation

Model drug	2.5 g
Starch	0.45 g
Lactose	18 g
Starch paste	10% w/v
Magnesium stearate	1% w/w
Talc	1.5% w/w

[B] Coating Solution
Formula I

Eudragit S-100	12.5% w/v
PEG-400	1.25% *w/w*
Isopropyl alcohol	q. s.

Formula II

Cellulose acetate phthalate (CAP)	15% w/v
PEG-400	1.5% *w/w*
Acetone	q. s.

Formula III

Shellac	30% w/v
Isopropyl alcohol	q. s.

Formula IV

Ethyl cellulose	5% *w/v*
Ethyl alcohol	1.5% w/w
Acetone	q. s.

Procedure

Step 1. Tablet Preparation

- Prepare model drug containing tablets by wet granulation, using lactose as the main filler.
- For a batch of 100 tablets (25 mg dose), mix 2.5 g of active drug and 18 g of lactose. Add starch (0.45 g) as disintegrant. The prepared powder mix is granulated using starch paste (10% w/v).
- Pass the wet mass through a sieve with a nominal aperture size of 2 mm and dry in an oven at $45 \pm 2\,°C$ for 6 h. Sieve the dried granules again with a sieve of nominal aperture of 1 mm.
- Mix sieved granules with talc (1.5% w/w) and magnesium stearate (1% w/w) and blend. Prepare tablets weighing 225 mg and containing 25 mg of active drug individually on a single punch tableting machine.
- Evaluate tablets for thickness, mass and content uniformity, friability, disintegration, hardness test and dissolution test, etc.

Step 2. Tablet Coating

- Prepare coating solutions using the usual (10–12% w/v) concentrations of polymers used for coating. For Eudragit-S100, 12.5% w/v, Eudragit S-100 (ES) using isopropyl alcohol and PEG-400 (1.25% w/w) as plasticiser.
- In the case of cellulose acetate phthalate, use 15% w/v solution in acetone for coating and propylene glycol (1.5% w/w) as plasticiser.
- In the case of coating with shellac, use a 30% (w/v) solution in isopropyl alcohol.
- For ethyl cellulose, use a solution of 5% (w/v) in acetone and ethyl alcohol (1.5% w/w) as plasticiser.
- Coat the tablets with different polymers, at two or three different concentrations. Pour the desired volume of coating solution on the pre-warmed tablet (batch size 50 g) bed in a pan coater.
- Coat the tablets and dry with the help of inlet air (temperature 35–45 °C). Repeat the coating process till the desired level of coating is achieved.
- The per cent mass increase of the tablets upon coating indicates the coat thickness (Scheme 5.2).

Note

In the dissolution test, use USP 24 method (USP dissolution test apparatus, basket method, 75 rpm, $37 \pm 0.5°C$).

For the initial 2 h, conduct the study in 750 ml of 0.1 M HCl followed by dissolution at a pH of 6.8 (adjusted by addition of 250 ml of 0.2 M trisodium phosphate). Collect aliquots manually with the help of pipette at predetermined time intervals and analyse for active drug using a UV-visible spectrophotometer or HPLC.

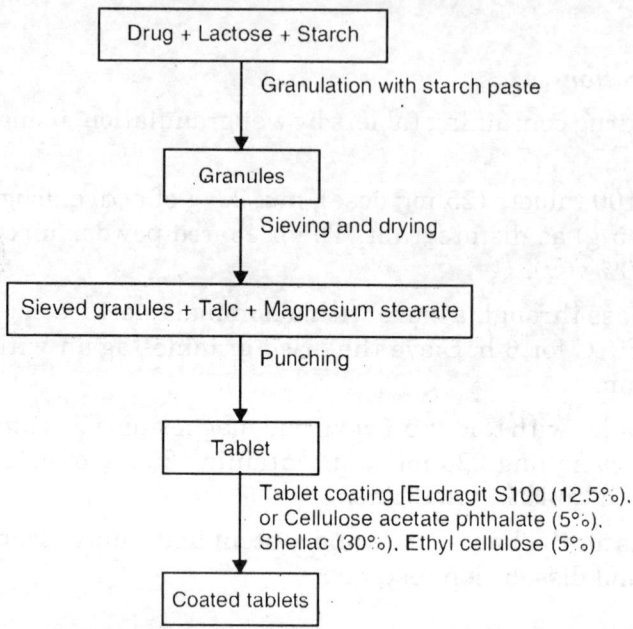

Scheme: 5.2 *Preparation of colon specific tablet*

PROTOCOL: 5.2
Colon Specific Tablets Using Guar Gum Matrix
Materials

Drug	200 mg
Guar gum (20%)	90.0 mg
Microcrystalline cellulose	101.5 mg
Starch paste	45 mg
Talc	9 mg
Magnesium stearate	4.5 mg

Procedure

- Prepare the matrix-containing drug and guar gum by the wet granulation method using 10%w/v starch paste. Use MCC as diluent and talc and magnesium stearate in 2:1 ratio as lubricant.
- Sieve guar gum (<250 μm) separately and mix with drug (<150 μm) and MCC (<250 μm). Blend the powder and granulate with starch paste (10% w/v).
- Pass the wet mass through a mesh (1680 μm) and dry so obtained granules at 50 °C for 2 h.
- Pass these dried granules through mesh (10/12 μm) and mix with the talc and magnesium stearate in 2:1 ratio.
- Compress the lubricated granules with the single station tableting machine using round flat and plain punches.

- Test the compressed tablets for thickness, mass and content uniformity, friability, disintegration, hardness test, drug release studies and dissolution test, etc.

PROTOCOL: 5.3
Ethylcellulose Enteric Coated Tablets

Principle
Granule preparation by wet granulation method.

Materials
[A] Formula for Granulation

Ingredients	Composition ratio
Drug	60
Lactose (diluent) adjust the quantity according to the die cavity of tablet machine	
Calcium phosphate	20
Succinic acid (adjust the pH of their microenvironments)	10
Tartaric acid (adjust the pH of their microenvironments)	-
Citric acid (pH-regulating additive)	-
Eudragit™ S-100 (enteric polymer)	10

[B] Coating Materials

Eudragit S
Eudragit L
Hydroxypropyl methylcellulose acetate succinates,
Cellulose acetate phthalate

The enteric polymers of coating material dissolve around or below pH 7, cellulose acetate phthalate at pH 6.2, Eudragit L at pH 6 and Eudragit S at pH 7.

Incorporate Triethylcitrate (Ph. Eur.), diethylphthalate (Ph. Eur.), talc, magnesium stearate and polysorbate 80 (Ph. Eur.) in the coating solution, which is to be prepared in demineralised water.

Procedure
Step 1 Preparation of Matrix Granules

- Prepare 20% solution methacrylate polymer (Eudragit™ S-100) in ethanol slowly with continuous stirring for 2 hr. Sieve the dry substances through a 1.18 mm sieve.
- Weigh accurately different ingredients. Mix the drug with the diluents and other components. Moist the powder masses (each weighing approximately 200 g) with binder solution in a mortar and sieve manually through a 2.0 mm sieve.
- Dry the granules overnight at room temperature and separate the fraction 1.18–1.68 mm by sieving.

Step 2 Enteric Coating of Matrix Granules

- Prepare coating solution with the 10% polymer as film former, 3.5% triethylcitrate as plasticiser, 3% magnesium stearate as lubricant and 83.5% demineralised water.

- Coat the enteric matrix granules by the fluidised-bed coater.
- Add triethylcitrate in the cold water and stir the solution using a magnetic stirrer for half an hour. Then mix magnesium stearate.
- Pass the coating solution through a 0.3 mm sieve, and keep in an ice bath.
- Heat the granules for 5 minutes at an outlet temperature of 40 °C ± 5 °C and an airflow rate of 40 m^3/h (coating parameters: airflow rate 70 m^3/h, outlet temperature 40 °C ± 5 °C, spraying pressure 1 bar, spraying rate 5 g/min)
- Continue the coating until a theoretical weight gain is 20%.
- Dry the granules after coating at the same temperature for 5 minutes, and then overnight at room temperature (Scheme 5.3).

Note: Add triethylcitrate to cold water and the solution was stirred magnetically for half an hour.

Step 3. Prepare tablets using microcrystalline cellulose (Emcocel™ LP200) magnesium stearate, talc as lubricants using single station tableting machine.

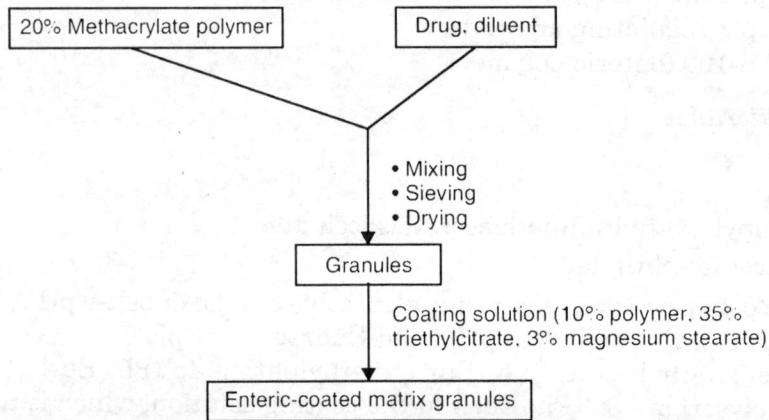

Scheme: 5.3 Preparation of enteric-coated matrix granules

PROTOCOL: 5.4

Pectin and Ethyl Cellulose Coated Tablet

Principle: By direct compression method

Materials

[A] Composition of Tablets

Drug	5–7.5%
Emdex	> 90%

(direct compressible materials composed of dextrose and maltodextrin)

Magnesium stearate   1%

[B] Coating Solution

Pectin solution— (2% w/v solution of pectinex in deionised water)

Ethylcellulose

Procedure

- Weigh accurately ingredients including drugs, emdex and lubricants and mix well using blender.
- After uniform mixing compress powder mass using single station tableting machine.
- Mix 2% w/v solution of pectin and ethyl cellulose in 50:50 ratio
- Coat the prepared tablet with the coating solution using a fluidised bed spray drier (coating conditions: outlet temperature— 75°C, spray nozzle diameter 1.1 mm, spray rate 2 g/min.)
- Check the samples of coated tablets periodically to confirm the uniform thickness.
- Evaluate the prepared tablets for drug content, content uniformity, weight variation, thickness, hardness, drug release behaviour, friability and disintegration time, etc.
- Store the prepared tablets in plastic sealed pack at room temperature for longer time.

PROTOCOL: 5.5
Pactin Based Microspheres Systems
Materials

Formula–I

Model drug (lipophilic)	33.3
Pectin (PEC),	66.7
Sodium fluorescein (NaFlu)	-

Formula–II

Model drug (lipophilic)	20
Pectin (PEC),	80
Sodium fluorescein (NaFlu)	-

Formula–III

Model drug (lipophilic)	31.25
Pectin (PEC),	62.50
Sodium fluorescein (NaFlu)	6.25

Formula–IV

Model drug (lipophilic)	-
Pectin (PEC),	100
Sodium fluorescein (NaFlu)	-

Procedure

- Prepare 1% w/v solutions of pectin in distilled water and 1% w/v drug solution in acetone separately at room temperature. Mix both the solutions in different ratios, depending on the intended composition of the microspheres.
- Dry the mixture by spray-drying.
- Prepare the microspheres containing sodium fluorescein by dissolving the appropriate amount of sodium fluorescein in the pectin solution, then mix the drug solution and proceed as described above.
- Collect the drug-free microspheres by spray-drying the aqueous solution of PEC.
- The process conditions, to obtain the highest production yields are— inlet air temperature $128-129 \pm 2\,°C$; outlet air temperature $62–63 \pm 2\,°C$; spray flow rate of the solution, about 10 ml/min.
- Keep the microspheres, harvested in the final collector vessel, at room temperature in vacuum for 48 h.

PROTOCOL: 5.6

Calcium Pectinate Beads for Colonic Delivery

Materials

Amidated LM pectin with DE of 36% and DA of 14%
Model drug
Zinc acetate
Calcium chloride

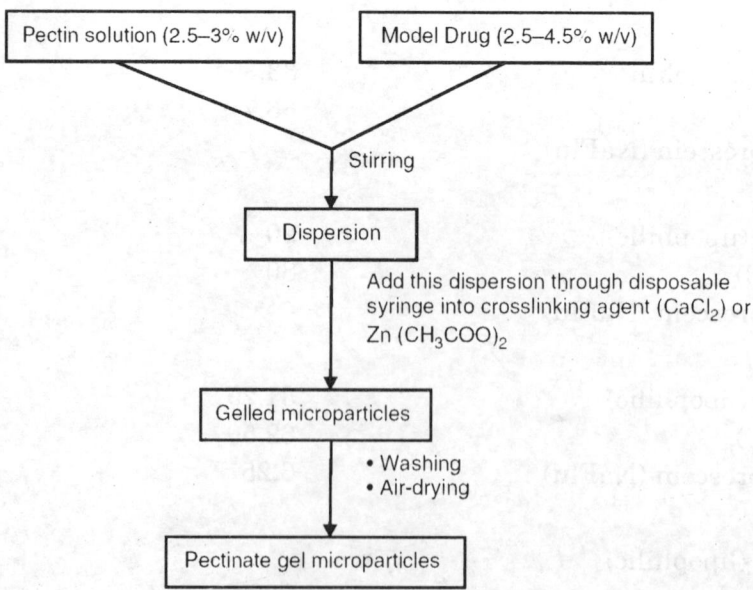

Scheme: 5.4 Preparation of pectinate beads for colonic delivery

Preparation of Pectinate Gel Microparticles (2.5–3% w/v)

- Prepare pectin solution at a concentration of 2.5–3% w/v initially. Disperse appropriate amount of the model drug (2.5–4.5% w/v) in this stirred solution until a uniform dispersion was obtained.

- Finally, add the homogenous, bubble-free slurry drop wise, at an average rate of 1 ml/min from falling distance of 5 cm through a disposable syringe (a nozzle of 1 mm inner diameter) into 20 ml of a gently agitated solution of the crosslinking agent [$CaCl_2$ or $Zn\,(CH_3COO)_2$].

- Allow the gelled microparticles thus formed to stand in the crosslinking solution, unless otherwise noted, to be cured for 24 h (Scheme 5.4).

SUGGESTED READINGS

- Ashford, M., Fell, J., Attwoods, D., Sharma, H., and Woodhead, P. (1993) J. Control. Rel., 26, 213.
- Ashford, M., Fell, J., Attwoods, D., Sharma, H., and Woodhead, P.(1994) J. Control. Rel., 30, 225.
- Brondsted H., Hovgaard L., and Simonsen L., (1995) STP Pharm Sci., 5, 60.
- Draser B.S. and Hill M.J. (1974) Human Intestinal Flora, Academic Press, London, 26.
- Dressman J. B. and Yamada K., (1991) In: Pharmaceutical bio-equivalence, Welling P.G., Tse F.L.S. and Dighe S.V. (Eds.), Vol 48, Marcel Dekker, New York, 727.
- Gardner N., Haresign W., and Spiller R. (1996) J. Pharm. Pharmacol., 48, 689.
- Holtenius K. and Bjornhog G. (1985) Comp. Biochem. Physiol., 82A, 537.
- Ibrahim El. Gibaly (2001) INt. J. pharma, 232 (1–2), 199.
- Kararli T.T., (1995) Biopharm. Drug Dispos., 16, 351.
- Molly K., Vande Woestyne M. and Verstraete W., (1993) Appl. Microbiol. Biotechnol. 39, 254.
- Pettersson G., Ahlman H., and Kewenter J. (1976) Acta. Chir. Scand., 142, 537.
- Renwick A.G., (1982) In Clinical Pharmacology and Therapeutics (Vol. 1), George C.F., Shand G. and Renwick A.G. (Eds.) Butterworth, London, 3.
- Ruckbusch Y. and Buene L., (1976) Br. J. Nutr., 35, 397.
- Van den Mooter G., Samyn C., and Kinget R., (1995) Pharm Res. 12, 244.
- Winter H.S., Hendren R.B., and Fox C.H. (1991) Gastroenterology 100, 89.

6

Transdermal Delivery Systems

TRANSDERMAL DRUG DELIVERY SYSTEMS

In contemporary therapeutics the oral route has been most preferred route of drug administration. The rise to prominence of modern therapeutics based on so many existing medicinal agents and the drug of future; due to their poor oral availability has generated need of focusing the attention on non-oral route for routine and effective drug administration. Para or non-oral routes which include nasal, rectal, buccal, vaginal and transdermal are considered as due to first pass metabolism drug availability is poor or administered moles are poor permeant to gastrointestinal barrier. Due to frequent pricking, need of constant medical supervision and lack in patient compliance associated with parenteral the transdermal route has been introduced as an alternative to bolus system. The skin is also identified to pose a barrier to permeating molecules and could selectively metabolise some drugs. The loss on this account could be compensated by providing better trans skin flux to drug permeant molecules via incorporation of penetration enhancers chipping of skin sonophoresis, electrophoresis, and pro-drug approach.

Basic Component of Transdermal Device(s)

The component of device include (i) The polymer matrix or matrices that regulate the release of drug (ii) The drug absorption/permeation enhancer (iii) Excipients and (iv) Adhesives.

Polymer Matrix

The polymer that is used in the preparation of various compounds of transdermal drug delivery systems should fulfill the following requirement.

- Molecular weight, physical characteristics and chemical functionality of the polymer must allow the diffusion of the drug substances.
- The functionality of the polymer should be chemically non-reactive.
- The polymer and its degradation products must be nontoxic.
- The polymer must not decompose on storage or during the life of the device.

- The polymer must be easy to manufacture and fabricate into the desired product. It should allow incorporation of large amounts of active agent.
- The cost of the polymer should not be excessively high.

Drugs

The important drug properties that affect its diffusion from the device as well as across the skin include molecular weight, chemical functionality, physical properties and effect of drug structure on skin including molecular weight, chemical functionality, physical properties and effect of drug structure on skin penetration. Although, diffusion of the drug in an adequate amount to produce a satisfactory therapeutic effect is of paramount importance. Other parameter such as skin irritation and clinical need should also be considered before drug is selected as a candidate for transdermal delivery. The drug should be non-irritating and non-allergic to the human skin.

Enhancers and Excipients

Skin permeability enhancers and other excipients, which promote skin permeation have to be considered as an integral part of the most of transdermal formulations because of the barrier properties of the stratum corneum. The penetration enhancers have been classified into three categories, i.e. lipophilic solvents, surface-active agents and two component systems.

Lipophilic solvents have been found to increase permeation of lipophilic drugs. Dimethyl sulfoxide has been found to increase permeation of lipophilic drugs, possibly by affecting the continuous lipophilic pathway of the skin. Surface-active agents also have been found to enhance the skin permeation especially of hydrophilic drugs. However their use is limited because of their skin irritating property. Two component systems have been found to be very effective permeation promoters. Systems are composed of oleic acid and propylene glycol. The system affects the multilaminate hydrophilic, lipophilic layers as well as the continuous path.

Adhesive and Packaging

The adhesion of all transdermal devices to the skin has so far been affected using a pressure sensitive adhesive. The adhesive system however should possess the following requisites.

- It should not cause an irritation, sensitisation or imbalance in the normal skin flora.
- It should adhere to the skin strongly during the dosing interval and should be resistant to the normal routine disturbances such as— bathing, clothing, abrasion, and exercise.
- It should easily be removable without leaving any unwashable remains.
- It should have intimate contact with the skin at both macroscopic and microscopic levels.

The pressure sensitive adhesive can be positioned on the face of the delivery (face adhesion systems) and such devices has to fulfill the additional requirement that include—

- It should be physically compatible with the drug and other dosage form excipients.
- It should not interfere with the permeation characteristics of the drug.
- It should allow the delivery of simple or blended percutaneous absorption enhancers.
- The adhesive properties should not deteriorate on ageing or on delivery of dosage form active components.

Based on the component used for the preparations of these delivery systems, they could essentially be classified as

1. Membrane moderated
2. Adhesion-diffusion controlled
3. Matrix dispersion type
4. Micro reservoir type

MEMBRANE MODERATED TDDS (Reservoir Type Device)

In membrane moderated systems the drug reservoir is encapsulated in a shallow compartment molded from a drug impermeable metallic plastic lamination whilst the drug delivery side is covered by a controlling polymeric membrane. The drug molecules are allowed to be released only through the controlling membrane. In the drug reservoir compartment the drug solids are dispersed in a solid polymer matrix or suspended in an unleachable viscous fluid that forms a paste like suspension. On the external surface a thin layer of drug compatible adhesive polymer may be applied for an intimate delivery face to skin contact. The rate of drug release from this type of transdermal drug delivery system can be tailored by varying the polymer composition permeability coefficient and thickness of the rate limiting membrane. Several transdermal therapeutic systems have been successfully developed using this technology, i.e. Transderm Scop® for three day protection of motion sickness and Transderm nitro® for once a day medication of angina pectoris.

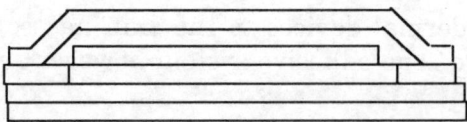

Fig. 6.1: *Cross sectional view of membrane moderated transdermal drug delivery system*

This approach has also been used for the development of transdermal therapeutic system for the controlled percutaneous absorption of oestradiol, clonidine and prostaglandin.

Adhesion Diffusion Controlled TDDS

This type of delivery systems is a simplified form of the membrane moderated drug delivery system. Instead of completely encapsulating the drug reservoir in a compartment the drug reservoir is prepared by direct dispensing the drug in an adhesive polymer and then spreading the medicative adhesive by solvent film casting method over a flat sheet of drug impermeable metallic plastic backing membrane to form a thin drug reservoir layer. The drug reservoir layer is covered by a non-medicated rate controlling adhesive polymer of constant thickness to produce an adhesive diffusion controlled drug delivery system.

MATRIX DISPERSION TYPE TRANSDERMAL DRUG DELIVERY SYSTEM

The matrix dispersion type transdermal systems are formed by homogeneous dispersing the drug in a hydrophilic-lipophilic mix polymer matrix and the polymer matrix is then moulded into form of a medicated disc of defined surface area and thickness. The drug reservoir containing polymer disc is then glued over an occlusive base plate consisted of compartment fabricated using an impermeable plastic backing. Instead of spreading the adhesive polymer onto the surface of the medicated disc, the polymer is applied along the circumference to form an adhesive rim around the medicated disc. This type of polymeric device is exemplified by developing Nitro Dur® system, which is used for one day medication of angina pectoris. The delivery system can also be used for transdermal administration of oestradiol diacetate and verapamil.

MICRORESERVOIR TYPE TRANSDERMAL DRUG DELIVERY SYSTEMS

This type of delivery systems has some essential features of both, i.e. reservoir and matrix dispersion type drug delivery systems. In this approach the drug reservoir is formed by suspending the drug solid in an aqueous solution of water-soluble liquid dispersion, by high shear mechanical agitation to form thousand of unleachable microspheres of the drug. This thermodynamically unstable dispersion is stabilised by immediately crosslinking of the polymer chains *in situ*. This technology has been utilised in the development of Nitro Dur® for one day treatment of angina pectoris.

Characterisation of Transdermal Drug Delivery Systems

Evaluation of Pressure-sensitive Adhesives

The pressure-sensitive adhesives are evaluated for general adhesive properties as well as for dermal toxicity and human wear.

Adhesive Properties

For evaluation of adhesive properties, adhesive laminates are prepared, consisting of a backing sheet or membrane, an adhesive film and a release liner. For the preparation of test laminate in laboratory transfer coating process is used. Pressure-sensitive adhesive can be evaluated on the basis of their three basic properties: peel adhesion, tack and shear strength (Chein, 1987).

Peel Adhesion Properties

The force required to remove an adhesive coating from a test substrate is referred to as peel adhesion. Molecular weight of adhesive polymer, the type and amount of additives, *i.e.* tackifiers and polymer composition are the variables that determine the peel adhesion properties. Adequate adhesion to skin and nontraumatic removal of TDD systems from skin depend on the peel adhesion properties.

A single tape is applied to a stainless steel plate or a backing membrane of choice and then tape is pulled from the substrate at a 180° angle, and the force required for tape removed is measured. The force is expressed in ounces (or grams) per inch width of tape, with higher values indicating greater bond strength. If the pulled tape does not leave any residue on the plate, it indicates "adhesive failure", which is desirable for most of the applications, especially for TDD system. If some residue is left behind, it suggests "cohesive failure", which often signifies a lack of cohesive strength.

Tack Properties

Tack is the ability of a polymer to adhere to a substrate with little contact pressure. Molecular weight, composition of polymer and tackifying resins affect the tack properties of TDD systems. In the case of TDD systems, which are applied with finger pressure, tack is an important property. There are four generally used tests for tack determination namely thumb, rolling ball, quick-stick (peel-tack), and probe tack test.

Thumb Tack Test

It is a qualitative test applied for tack property determination of adhesive. In this test, the thumb is simply pressed on the adhesive and the relative tack property is detected. By experience one can differentiate between relative degree of tack.

Rolling Ball Tack Test

This test measures the softness of a polymer that relates to tack. In this test, a stainless steel ball of 7/16 inches in diameter is released on an inclined track so that it rolls down and comes into contact with horizontal, upward-facing adhesive. The distance the ball travels along the adhesive provides the measurement of tack, which is usually expressed in inch. The less tacky the adhesive, the farther the ball will travel.

Quick-stick (peel-tack) Test

In this test, the tape is pulled away from the substrate at 90°C at a speed of 12 inches/min. The peel force required to break the bond between adhesive and substrate is measured and recorded as tack value, which is expressed in ounces (or grams) per inch width. The higher values of force required indicates the higher degree of tack.

Probe Tack Test

In this test probe tack tester is used. The tip of a clean probe with a defined surface roughness is brought into contact with adhesive, and when a bond is formed between probe and adhesive. The subsequent removal of the probe mechanically breaks it. The force required to pull the probe away from the adhesive at fixed rate is recorded as tack (expressed in grams).

Shear Strength Properties

Shear strength is the measurement of the cohesive strength of an adhesive polymer. If transdermal device has adequate cohesive strength, it will not slip after application and will leave no residue upon removal. It can be influenced by the molecular weight, the degree of crosslinking and the composition of polymer, as well as by the type and the amount of tackifier added. In this particular test, adhesive-coated tape is applied onto a stainless steel plate. A specified weight is hung from the tape, to affect its pulling in a direction parallel to the plate. Shear strength is determined by measuring the time it takes to pull the tape off the plate. The longer the time taken for removal, greater is the shear strength.

In vitro Release Kinetics

Controlled release kinetics of drug from technologically-different transdermal therapeutic systems can be evaluted and compared by using Franz diffusion cell assembly. For example in the case of nitroglycerine TDD systems, the release of nitroglycerine from Transderm-Nitro® (a membrane-moderated transdermal system) and Deponit® (an adhesive diffusion controlled system) can be compared by plotting the data for cumulative amount of drug released from these systems as a function of time (Q *vs.* t). Keshery *et al.*, 1985 found that the release of nitroglycerin from the Transderm-Nitro is almost three times greater than that from the Deponit® system. They suggested that the rate-controlling adhesive layers in Deponit system play a greater rate-controlling role for release of nitroglycerin than does the rate-controlling membrane in the case of Transderm-Nitro® system. Similarly, the release flux of nitroglycerine from the Nitro-Dur® system (a matrix dispersion type TDD system) is about two folds greater than the Nitrodisc® system (a microreservoir type TDD system) (Huang, 1987 Keshary and Chein, 1994, Robinson and Lee, 1987).

IN VITRO SKIN PERMEATION KINETICS

Animal Model and Human Cadaver

In vitro permeation kinetics studies can be performed on hairless mouse skin or human cadaver skin by using either Franz diffusion cell or two-reservoir diffusion cell (Valia-Chien permeation cell). In two-reservoir diffusion cells, sink conditions can be maintained. The permeation of nitroglycerine across human cadaver and hairless mouse skin from different TDD therapeutic systems was compared for their kinetics. It was noted that the rates of skin permeation generated from the excised skins of hairless mouse agree fairly with the data obtained from human cadaver skin, suggesting that hairless mouse skin could be an acceptable animal model for human skin permeation kinetics studies (Chien et al, 1986; Chein and Vallia, 1985).

Transdermal Delivery: New Approaches

Several new techniques have recently been developed which reduce the barrier properties of the stratum corneum and as a result significantly enhance the skin permeation of drugs. Potential approaches used in overcoming the skin barrier properties are as follows.

Physical Approaches

1. Iontophoresis

2. Ultrasound
3. Thermal energy
4. Stripping of stratum corneum
5. Hydration of stratum corneum

Chemical Approaches

1. Delipidisation of stratum corneum
2. Synthesis of lipophilic analog
3. Co-administration of cutaneous enzyme inhibitor

Biochemical Approach

1. Synthesis of bioconvertible prodrugs
2. Co-administration of cutaneous enzyme inhibitors.

PROTOCOL: 6.1

Prodrugs for Dermal Delivery

The prodrugs approach is used to enhance bioavailability, passage through various biological barriers, and duration of pharmacological effects. Increased site specificity reduces the toxicity and adverse action associated with drug molecules. Improved organoleptic properties can also be achieved thereby improving an overall stability and phycochemical properties associated with drug molecule.

PROTOCOL: 6.2

Preparation of Esters of Testosterone for Dermal Application

Testesterone Cysteine Ester

- Add 2.0 ml thionyl chloride to 0.727 g of cysteine and reflux the mixture for 2 h at 60 °C. Remove the excess of thionyl chloride under reduced pressure.
- After removing thionyl chloride, add 10 ml pyridine followed by 1.730 g of testesterone. Reflux the mixture with constant stirring at 100 °C for 4 h. Remove the pyridine in vacuum and add 5 ml methanol water mixture (80:20) to the residue.
- Then, cool the mixture and solid crystals will be obtained. Recrystalise the crystals using methanol-acetone mixtures (Scheme 6.1).

Testesterone Cysteine Ester

- Add 2.0 ml thionyl chloride to 1.2 g of cystine and reflux the reaction mixture for 4 h at 60 °C temperature. Remove the excessive thionyl chloride under reduced pressure.

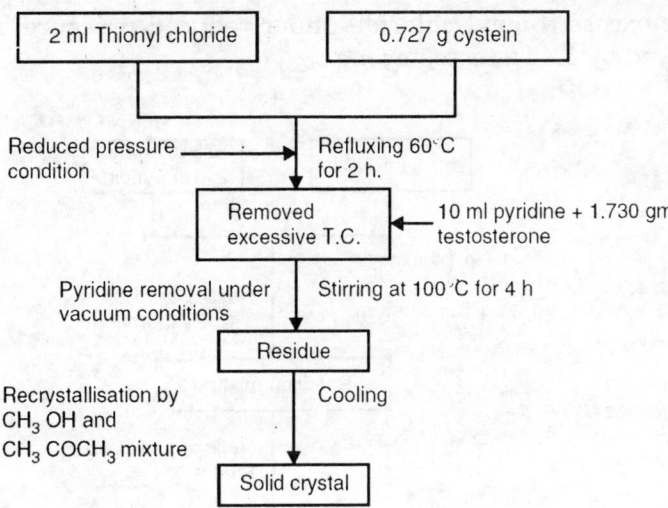

Scheme 6.1: *Preparation of esters of testosterone for dermal application*

- Add the pyridine (10 ml) to the mixture followed by testesterone, reflux the mixture with continuous stirring at 100°C for 4 h.
- Remove the pyridine and wash the residue with ether. Dissolve the residue in methanol-ethanol mixture (60:40) and recrystallise. Further purify the crystals using the same solvent system (Scheme 6.2).

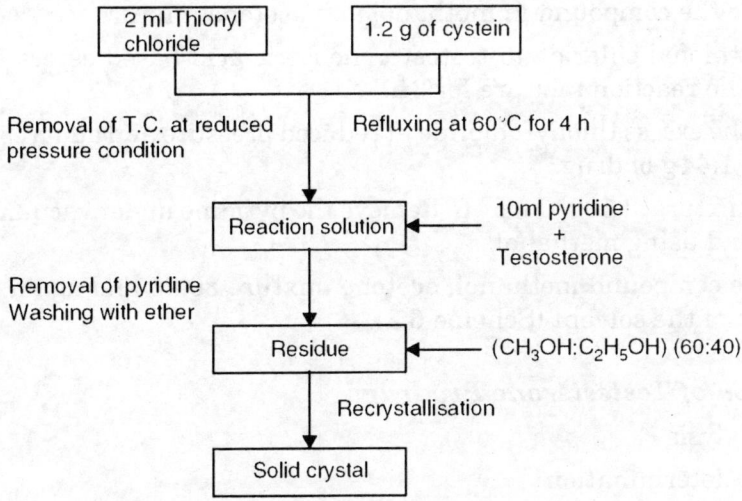

Scheme 6.2: *Preparation of testosterone cystein ester*

Hydroxy Acid Based Prodrugs of Testosterone
Testosterone Tartaric Acid Based Esters

- Add 0.5 ml thionyl chloride to the 0.75 g of tartaric acid in pyridine and reflux the mixture for 3 h.

- Evaporate the excess thionyl chloride under reduced pressure. Add fresh 10 ml of pyridine followed by 1.44 g testosterone.

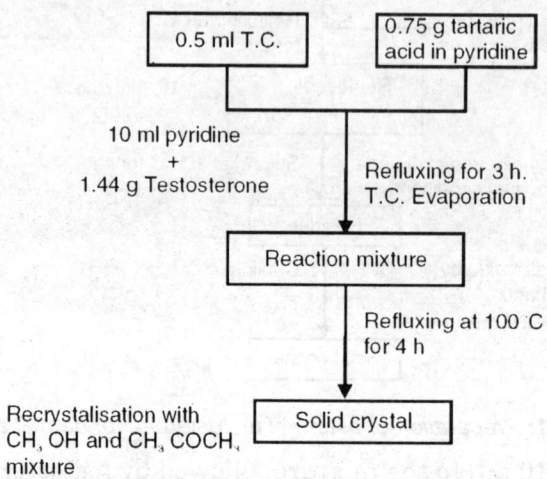

Scheme 6.3: *Preparation of testosterone tartaric acid based esters*

- Reflux the mixture at 100°C for 4 h. Remove the pyridine under vacuum and recrystallise the compound in methanol and acetone mixture.
- Add 0.6 ml thionyl chloride to testosterone citric acid based esters acid in pyridine and reflux the reaction mixture for 3 h.
- Evaporate the excess thionyl chloride at reduced pressure and add fresh 10ml pyridine followed by 1.44 g of drug.
- Reflux the mixture at 100°C for 4 h. Remove the pyridine under vacuum and crystallise the compound using methanol.
- Dissolve the compound methanol: acetone mixture 80:20 and again recrystallise by evaporation of the solvent (Scheme 6.3).

Characterisation of Testesterone Prodrugs

Elemental analysis

Melting point determination

Chromatographic method (TLC)

Solubility measurement

Critical micellar concentration (CMC) determination

Structural confirmation methods

IR, FT-IR, ^{1}H-NMR, ^{13}C-NMR, Mass- spectroscopy

PROTOCOL: 6.3

Preparation of Monolithic Controlled Transdermal Drug Delivery System (Matrix Diffusion Controlled T. D. D. S.)

Principle

The low temperature drying method is utilised for the film preparation. Dimension of film was controlled with the help of glass rings of defined diameter.

Procedure

- Prepare 10% w/v solution of polymer in solvent (according to Table 6.1 and 6.2) at room temperature then add 2% w/v drug and 5% w/v Glycerol (based on total weight) to this polymer solution.
- Pour this drug containing polymer solution into the glass ring placed over the mercury substrate previously cold with the ice. Keep the frozen film of polymer at –20°C for drying (freeze dryer).
- Keep the films for 48 h at room temperature in a desiccator. Store the product at 40% RH at room temperature.
- The rate of evaporation of the polymer solvent can be kept consistently slow and controlled, by covering the mercury substrate by an inverted glass funnel of appropriate diameter. The inverted glass funnel also avoids the dew formation on mercury substrate during substrate pre-cooling for the preparation of films at low temperature.
- Prepare backing membrane using 10 % w/w polystyrene solution containing 5% dibutyl phthalate (based on polymer weight). Mount the prepared polymeric backing film, which is relatively oversized on it and pressed with one of the premoist surface of drug reservoir. The solvent of the polymer in the form of spray is used for moistening the reservoir surface.
- Complete the sealing accomplished by applying a moderate pressure. Sealing is checked by the air entrapment method.
- Polystyrene films, because of low permeation of water act as an occlusive type of backing membrane. When the non-occlusive type of backing membrane is needed waterproof band-aid (Johnson and Johnson) may also be used as backing membrane.
- Coat the dosage form with release liner to protect its adhesive ring.
- Solubilise drug in the solvent systems used for the preparation of reservoir.

Table 6.1. Polymeric composition of monolithic controlled transdermal drug delivery system

S. No.	Product composition (Type)	Polymeric composition / concentration
1.	**Hydrophilic and hydrophobic polymers blend**	
	Eudragit RL(EuRL)-Polyvinyl Pyrrolidone system	EuRL-100 : PVP (different ratio)

Table 6.1. *Polymeric composition of monolithic controlled transdermal drug delivery system*

Cond...

S. No.	Product composition (Type)	Polymeric composition / concentration	
	Polyethylene (PE)-Polyvinyl Pyrrolidone (PVP)	PE-PVP in different ratio	
	Poly Methyl Methacrylate-Polyethylene glycol (PMMA-PEG)	PMMA-PEG 4000 in different ratio	
2.	**Copolymer Blend type systems**		
	Ethylene-Vinyl acetate (EVAc) type copolymer system	E:VAc in different ratio (60:40, 75:25, and 82:18)	
3.	**Swellable polymers**		
	Poly Hydroxy Ethylmethyl Acrylate (PHEMA)		6 % w/v
	Hydroxy propyl methyl cellulose (HPMC)		6 % w/v
	Methyl vinyl ether maleic anhydride (MVEMA copolymer)		6 % w/v
4.	**Swelling controlled systems**		
	MVEMA-PMMA copolymer	MVEMA-PMMA (5:0.5, 5:0.75, 5:1.0, 5:1.5 ratio of polymers)	
5.	**Swelling controlled polymer Ca^{++} compositions**		
	MVEMA:PMMA:CaCl$_2$	5:1:0.5	
	MVEMA:PMMA:CaCl$_2$	5: 1 :1.5	

Table 6.2. *Polymer and solvent used for the preparation of polymeric drug solution*

Polymer	Solvent system used
Eudragit RL-100	Methanol
Polymethyl Methacrylate	Ethyl Methyl Ketone
Polyvinyl Pyrrolidone	Methanol
PEG-4000	Methanol
Ethylene vinyl acetate copolymer	Dichloromethane
Hydroxypropyl methyl cellulose	Methanol + Methylene chloride (10:90)
Methyl vinyl ether maleic anhydride copolymer	Ethyl Methyl Ketone
Polyhydroxy ethyl methacrylate	Methanol

PROTOCOL: 6.4

Preparation of Aqueous Dispersion Based Controlled Transdermal Monolithic System

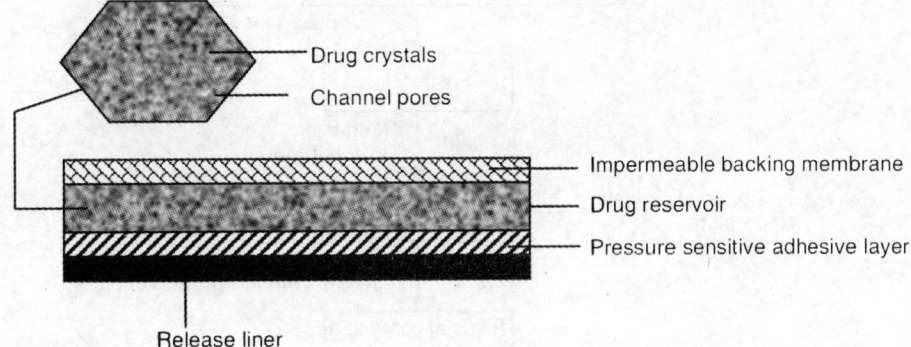

Scheme 6.4: Preparation of aqueous dispersion based controlled transdermal monolithic system.

Procedure

- Mix 10% w/v aqueous portion in low volume (1–2ml) with polymeric solution (Table 6.3) containing 2% w/v drug and vortexed in a glass vial for 5 minutes to prepare a suspension.
- Then, pour the mixture into the glass ring over a mercury substrate previously cooled using dry ice for 5–10 min, during pre-cooling to avoid frost formation on mercury substrate an inverted funnel as a cover is used.
- Keep the films after cooling at drug ice kept at –20°C (Lyophiliser) under vacuum.
- Equilibrate the films further at ambient temperature in a vacuum desiccator (Scheme 6.4).
- To avoid the effect of atmospheric moisture and to check the effect of rate of evaporation during whole drying process films should be covered with inverted funnels.
- Store the films at controlled humidity (RH 40% at room temperature).
- Then after prepare the delivery device in the same way as discussed earlier in the preparation of transdermal monolithic system (Protocol 6.3) (Scheme 6.5).

Table 6.3 Formulation composition of aqueous dispersion based TDDS

Formulation	Polymers	Polymer Concentration (%w/v)	Water content
1	EVAc18 Copolymer	10%	0.0 ml
2.	EVAc18 Copolymer	10%	0.5 ml
3.	EVAc18 Copolymer	10%	1.0 ml
4.	EVAc18 Copolymer	10%	1.5 ml
5.	EVAc18 Copolymer	10%	2.0 ml

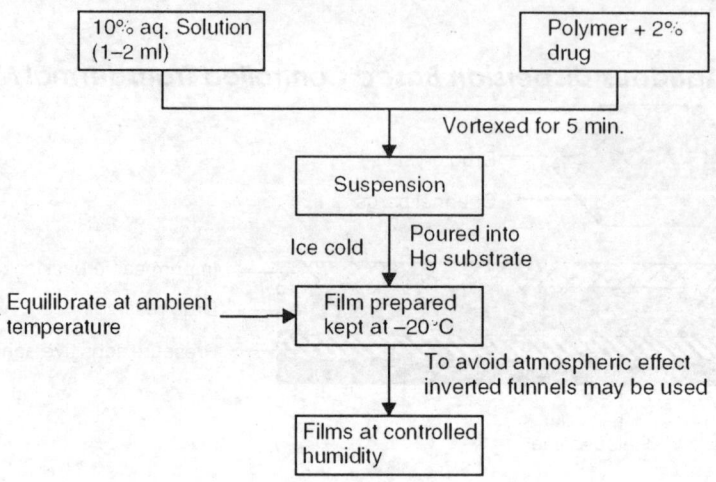

Scheme 6.5: *Preparation of transdermal monolithic systems*

PHYSIOCHEMICAL CHARACTERISATION OF DRUG MATRIX FOR TDDS
Thickness Measurement

Any suitable scale can be used.

Water Vapour Transmission

A modified method of the American Standard Test Method (ASTM test)

- Wash and dry the film in an oven.
- Take the fused calcium chloride in the cells and apply a thin layer of an adhesive over the brims, allow to dry in air for 5 min. Weigh the cells accurately and keep in the humidity chamber maintaining at 60% relative humidity. Weigh the cells again after 24 h. the differences in the weights is considered as the moisture transmitted through the film.
- Calculate water vapour transmission by Kanning and Goodman formula in g/h/cm^2.

$$\text{Water vapour transmission} = \frac{\text{Amount of moisture transmitted}}{\text{Area (cm}^2) \times \text{time (h)}}$$

Equilibrium Water Content

- Cut the drug reservoirs in to strips of definite size and place in an oven (50°) until constant weight is obtained.
- Equilibrate the films in the water for 12 h. the equilibrium water content is calculated by using formula reported by Zenter *et al,* 1978.

$$\text{Equilibrium water content} = \frac{(\text{Weight of exposed films} - \text{weight of swelled film})}{\text{Weight of swelled films} \times 100}$$

Water Uptake Studies

- Swellable polymers used in drug matrix should be studied for water uptake studies.
- Soak the drug reservoir in the distilled water and after films attain equilibrium at 24 h weigh them and calculate the per cent water uptake by using following formula

$$\% \text{ water uptake} = \frac{\text{Weight of film} \times 100}{\text{Weight of the swelled film}}$$

Drug Content Determination

- Dissolve accurately weighed 5 g drug reservoir in their corresponding solvents. Centrifuge the solvent at $3000 \times g$ for 10 min. Transfer the supernatant to 10 ml volumetric flasks. Dry the solution by vacuum drying and redissolve in methanol. After appropriate dilution estimate the drug concentration spectrophotometrically.
- *In vitro* diffusion across cellophane membrane

Preparation of Skin

- Remove the dermal fat and other subcutaneous fat from the skin of abdomen region of human cadaver.
- Store it at 4 °C in the surgical gauze saturated with the medium (PBS 7.4) containing 0.1mg/ml gentamycin.

Preparation of Elution Solution

75% PEG-400 in the medium enhances the aqueous solubility of testosterone and maintain perfect skin condions with regard to the biological sink.

Mounting Skin

Mount the skin on the donor cell after clamping the skin by horse clamp. The epidermal side was exposed to ambient laboratory conditions and application of delivery devices while dermal side was bathed with isotonic solution in the receptor compartment. Because of high metabolism and low permeability of drug across the skin the receptor compartment is not attached to the jar as done in the previous experiment to avoid impairment in the drug estimation.

Permeation Studies

After placing the different delivery devices on the epidermal sides of skin, the studies are run. Maintain the temperature of the cell at 37°C. Stir the contents of receptors compartment using Teflon coated magnetic bar (80 rpm) the constant flow is maintained by peristaltic pump.

PROTOCOL: 6.5

Skin Irritation and Sensitisation Testing of Transdermal Drug Products

Principle

To fully evaluate the equivalence of transdermal products, skin irritation and sensitisation should be assessed because the condition of the skin may affect the absorption of a drug from a transdermal system. More severe skin irritation may affect the efficacy or safety of the product. Transdermal products have properties that may lead to skin irritation and/or sensitisation. The delivery system, or the system in conjunction with the drug substance, may cause these reactions. In the development of transdermal products, dermatologic adverse effects are evaluated. Separate skin irritation and skin sensitisation studies also are used for this purpose. These studies are designed to detect irritation and sensitisation under conditions of maximal stress and may be used during the assessment of transdermal drug products.

Procedure

Recommended designs for skin irritation and skin sensitisation studies for the comparative evaluation of transdermal drug products are delineated below.

Cumulative Skin Irritation Study

- *Sample size:* 30 subjects
- *Exclusion criteria:* Dermatologic disease that might interfere with the evaluation of test site reaction
- *Duration of study:* 22 days
- *Study design:* A randomised, controlled, repeat patch test study that compares the test patch to the innovator patch. Placebo patches (transdermal patch without active drug substance) and/or high- and low-irritancy controls (e.g. sodium lauryl sulphate 0.1% and 0.9% saline) can be included as additional test arms.
- *Patch application:* Each subject applies one of each of the patches to be tested. Test sites should be randomised among patients. Patches should be applied for 23 ± 1 h daily for 21 days to the same skin site. At each patch removal, the site should be evaluated for reaction and then patch is reapplied. Application of a test patch should be discontinued at a site if predefined serious reactions occur at the site of repeated applications. Application at a different site may subsequently be initiated.
- *Evaluations:* Scoring of skin reactions and patch adherence should be performed by a trained and blinded observer at each patch removal using an appropriate scale.

I. *Dermal response:*

0 = no evidence of irritation

1 = minimal erythema, barely perceptible

2 = definite erythema, readily visible; minimal oedema or minimal papular response

3 = erythema and papules

4 = definite oedema

5 = erythema, oedema, and papules

6 = vesicular eruption

7 = strong reaction spreading beyond test site

II. *Other effects:*

A = slight glazed appearance

B = marked glazing

C = glazing with peeling and cracking

F = glazing with fissures

G = film of dried serous exudate covering all or part of the patch site

H = small petechial erosions and/or scabs

Dermal reactions should be scored on a scale that describes the amount of erythema, oedema, and other features defining irritations.

- *Data presentation and analysis:* Individual daily observations should be provided, as well as a tabulation that presents the percentage of subjects with each grade of skin reaction and degree of patch adherence on each study day. The mean cumulative irritation score, the total cumulative irritation score, and the number of days until sufficient irritation occurs to preclude patch application for all the study subjects should be calculated for each test product, and a statistical analysis of the comparative results should be performed.

Skin Sensitization Study (Modified Draize Test)

- *Sample size:* 200 subjects
- *Exclusion criteria:*
  - Dermatologic disease that might interfere with the evaluation of the test site reactions.
  - Use of systemic or topical analgesics or antihistamines within 72 h of study enrollment or systemic or topical corticosteroids within 3 weeks of study enrollment.
- *Duration of study:* 6 weeks
- *Study design:* A randomized, controlled study on three test products: the test transdermal patch, the innovator patch, and the placebo patch (transdermal patch without the active drug substance).
- *Patch application:* Test sites should be randomized among patients. The study is divided into three sequential periods:
  - *Induction Phase:* Applications of the test materials should be made to the same skin sites 3 times weekly for 3 weeks, for a total of 9 applications. The patches should remain in place for 48 h on weekdays and for 72 h on weekends. Scoring of

skin reactions and patch adherence should be performed by a trained and blinded observer at each patch removal, using an appropriate scale. Dermal reactions should be scored on a scale that describes the amount of erythema, edema, and other features relating to irritation.

— *Rest Phase:* The induction phase is followed by a rest phase of 2 weeks, during which no applications are made.

— *Challenge Phase:* The patches should be applied to new skin sites for 48 h. Evaluation of skin reactions should be made by a trained blinded observer at 30 min and at 24, 48, and 72 h after patch removal.

• *Data Presentation and Analysis:* The individual daily observations should be made, as well as a tabulation of the percentage of subjects with each grade of skin reaction and degree of patch adherence on each study day. The mean cumulative irritation score and the total cumulative irritation score for all the subjects should be calculated for each test product, and a statistical analysis of the comparative results should be performed. A narrative description of each reaction in the challenge phase should be provided, together with the opinion of the investigator as to whether such reactions are felt to be indicative of contact sensitisation.

SUGGESTED READINGS

• Bodor, N. and Loftsson, T. (1989) US Patent 4,885,174.
• Chein, *et al.* 1987,
• Chein, Y.W. and Valia, KH. (1985) Drug Dev Ind. Pharm. 11, 1195.
• Guy RH (1996) Pharm. Res. 13, 1765.
• Huang, 1987,
• Keshary P.R., Y.C. Huang, and Y.W. Chien. 1985. Mechanism of Transdermal Controlled Nitroglycerin Administration (III) Control of Skin Permeation Rate and Optimization. Drug Development and Industrial Pharmacy II: 1213–1253.
• Keshary, P.R. and Chein, Y.W. (1994) Drug Dev Ind. Pharm. 10, 883.
• Keshery, *et al.* 1985,
• Misra, N. and Rao, V.U. (1996) Ind. J. Expt. Bio. 34(2), 171.
• Okabe. H., Suzuki. E., Saitoh. T. Takayama, K. and Nagai, T. (1994) J. Control. Rel., 32, 243.
• Okomoto, H., Hasida, M. and Sezaki, H. (1990) Pharm. Res. 7(1), 64.
• Patil, S., Singh, P., Szolar-Platzer, C. and Maibach, H. (1996) J. Pharm. Sci., 85(3), 249.
• Robinson, J.R. and Lee, V.H.L. (1987) Controlled Drug Delivery: Fundamentals and Applications, Marcel Dekker, New York, 523.
• Sanders, H.F., Cheng, Y.L., Enscore, D.J. and Libcki, S. S.B. (1989) US Patent. 4,764,379.
• Sanders, H.F., Cheng, Y.L., Enscore, D.J. and Libicki, S. S.B. (1989) US Patent. 4,820,720.
• Scheuplein, J. (1965) J. Invest. Dermatol. 45, 334.
• Scheuplein, J. (1965) J. Invest. Dermatol. 48, 334.
• Scheuplein, J. (1965) J. Invest. Dermatol. 48, 79.

- Shah, H.S., Genier, S., Yu, C.D. and Patel, B (1993) US Patent 5,219,877.
- Sharata, H.H. and Burnette, R.R. (1988) J. Pharm. Sci. 77(1), 27.
- Wert, P.W. and Downing, D.T. (1982) Science 217, 1261.
- Williams, C. and Barry, B.W. (1992) Crit. Rev. Ther. Drug Syst 9 (3–4), 305.
- Xiong, G.L., Quan, D., Maibach, H.I. (1996) J. Control. Rel. 42, 289.
- Zenter, *et al.* 1978,

7

Spherical Crystallisation

The spherical crystallisation technique also involves the use of a bridging liquid that improves compressibility by acting as granulating fluid. Thus, spherical crystallisation is a method that helps to achieve good flowability and compressibility. Spherical crystallisation can be achieved by various methods such as simple spherical crystallisation, emulsion solvent diffusion, ammonia diffusion, and neutralisation (Paradkar *et al*, 1998; Kawashima *et al*, 1989). In the pharmaceutical industry, the crystal size growth and the formation of the spherical crystal agglomerates are very important for preparing the solid dosage forms (e.g. capsules, tablets, etc.). The particle size of the agglomerates produced by the spherical crystallisation techniques is 300–500 mm in diameter and

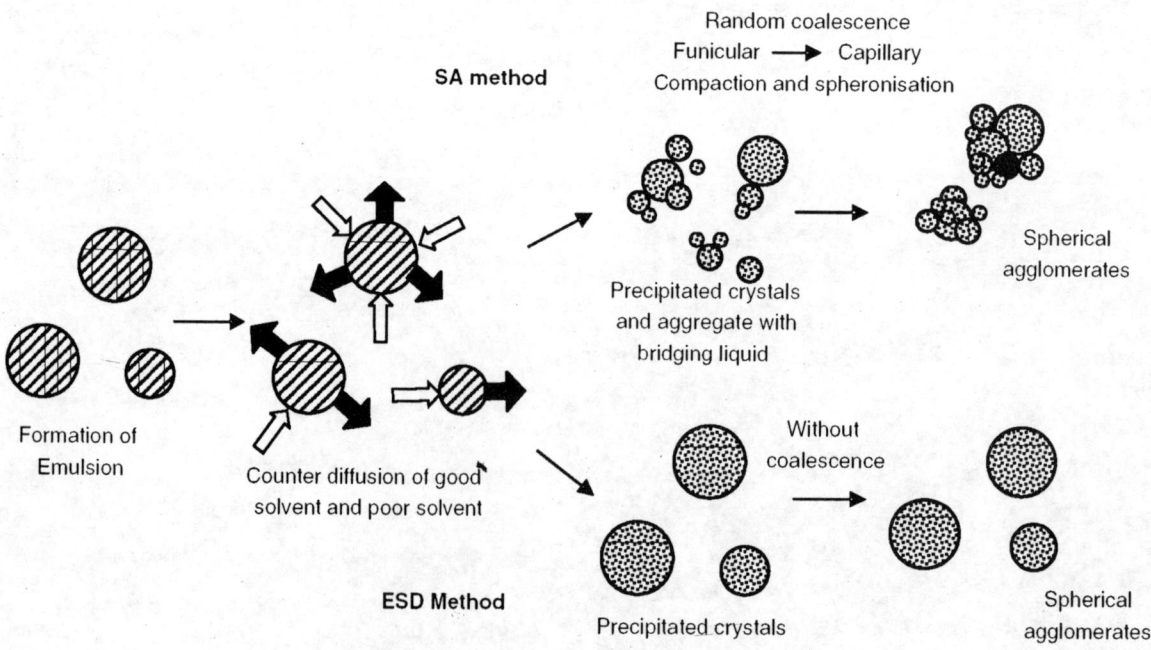

Fig.7.1. *Mechanism of spherical crystallisation*

their form is more or less spherical. The agglomerates have very good flow property, high bulk density and compressibility values. They can be used directly for capsule-filling (without excipients) and direct tablet making (without granulation, drying, etc.). The drug materials produced by the spherical crystallisation technique result in the economical process in the development of the solid dosage forms. The typical spherical crystallisation technique employs three solvents: one is the substance dissolution medium, another is a medium which partially dissolves the substance, and the third is the wetting solvent for the substance. The traditional crystallisation processes (salting-out precipitation, cooling crystallisation, crystallisation from the melting, etc.) (Fig. 7.1) can also be used to produce spherical crystal agglomerates (Kallies *et al*, 1993). It may be called a non-typical spherical crystallisation process.

PROTOCOL: 7.1

Spherical Magnesium Aspartate (MASP) Crystals by the Non-typical and Typical Spherical Crystallisation Process

Development of spherical magnesium aspartate (MASP) crystals by the non-typical spherical Crystallisation process (MASP developed)

- The agglomeration of magnesium aspartate is carried out by salting-out combined with cooling.
- The formation of salt precedes the crystallisation process.
- Perform the experiments in a mechanically stirred tank with a volume of 1000 ml.
- Use a Julabo thermostat with computer control (Julabo Labortechnik, Seelbach, Germany) for the cooling process.
- Place a total of 500 ml of 20 % (wt/wt) magnesium aspartate in the crystalliser tank. The good solvent for MASP is water and the poor solvent is methanol (10–50%, in relation to the measured solution).
- The other parameters of the crystallisation are as follows: stirring rate: 50–100 rpm, feeding rate of methanol: 0.36 l/h, temperature interval: 90–101°C and cooling rate: 0.71 °C/min.

Development of spherical acetylsalicylic acid (ASA) crystals by the typical spherical crystallisation process (ASA developed)

- The experiments are carried out in a mechanically stirred tank with a volume of 500 ml. A thermostat with computer control is used for the cooling process.
- Dissolve 121.6 g of ASA in 225 ml of ethanol (20–40% v/v) at 40–70°C, and add carbon tetrachloride–water mixture (1–5% w/v) to the solution, followed by cooling at 61 °C/min to 20°C with stirring (200 rpm).
- Use commercial magnesium aspartate (MASP control) and acetylsalicylic acid (ASA control) products as controls.

PROTOCOL: 7.2

Spherically Agglomerated Crystals of Ascorbic Acid for Direct Tableting

Materials

Raw ascorbic acid crystals (sieved at 100 mesh, average diameter <18.8 mm)

Procedure

- Dissolve ascorbic acid in purified water (good solvent) at 50°C to make saturated solution (0.4 g/ml).
- Pour the required amount of the resultant solution into 300 ml ethyl acetate (poor solvent), thermally controlled at 5°C under agitation with a propeller type agitator with four blades at rotation of 300 or 800 rpm for 20 min. The apparatus used for spherical crystallisation system is shown in Fig. 7.2.

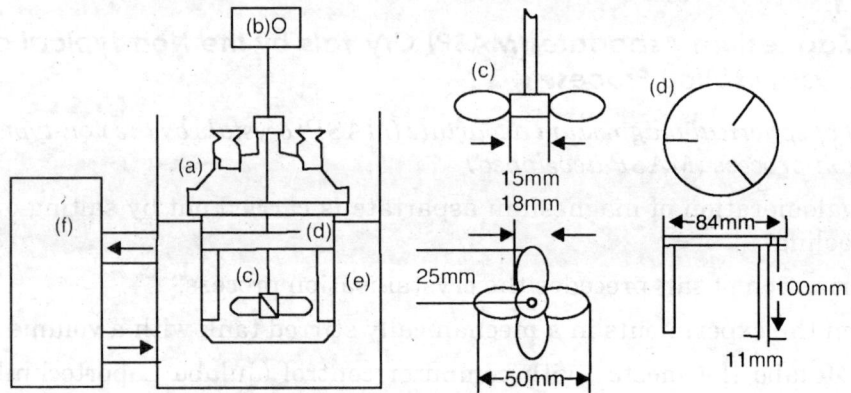

Fig. 7.2 *Apparatus for spherical Crystallisation (a) vessel (500 ml), (b) motor, (c) propeller type agitator, (d) baffle, (e) water bath, (f) thermoregulator vessel, agitator and baffles are coated with teflon .*

- Depending on the volume ratio of aqueous drug solution to ethyl acetate being 1:100 or 4:150, the spherically agglomerated crystals can be prepared in different processes. (At volume ratio = 1:100, the agglomeration and crystallisation of drug occurs in the quasi-emulsion (without) droplets form even in the miscible solvent system.
- At volume ratio = 4:150, both solvents are immiscible and form the emulsion droplets after mixing in which crystallisation occurs, followed by further agglomeration of the precipitated crystals with liberated water phase.
- Filter the agglomerated crystals, wash with a small amount of methanol and dry in vacuum.
- Fractionate the dried agglomerated crystals into 125–500 µm range.

Characterisation of the Spherical Crystals

Particle Size and Particle Roundness

For the determination of the particle size (length, breadth and roundness) use light microscope fitted with image processing and analysis system. Roundness is a shape factor that provides information about the circularity of particles. It is calculated by software according to the following formula:

Roundness = perimeter^2/ $4\pi\times$ area × 1.064

The perimeter is calculated from the horizontal and vertical projections, with an allowance for the number of corners. An adjustment factor of 1.064 corrects the perimeter for the effect of the corners produced by digitisation of the image. When roundness value is close to one, the particles are close to spherical.

Drug Loading

The drug loading efficiency of crystals is determined by dissolving 100 mg of crystals in 100 ml of methanol, followed by measuring the absorbance of appropriately diluted solution spectrophotometrically (PharmaSpec UV-1700, UV-Vis Spectrophotometer, Shimadzu) at 253.5 nm.

Solubility Studies

Mix some quantity of crystals (about 100 mg (w/v)) and shake with 10 ml of distilled water or a solution of sodium lauryl sulphate (SLS) (2%, m/v) in a shaking water bath (100 agitations per min) for 24 h at room temperature, pass the solution through a 0.45 µm membrane filter and analyse the amount of the drug dissolved spectrophotometrically.

Morphological Study

Examine the morphology of the crystals by scanning electron microscopy (SEM). A Polaron sputter coating apparatus is used to induce electric conductivity on the surfaces of the samples. The air pressure applied is in between 1.3–13 mPa.

Study of Flow Time, Bulk Density and Carr Index
- Measure the flow time (s/100 ml) with an ASTMD 329–38 equipment.
- Determine the bulk densities (poured and tapped densities) with a Stampf volumeter 2003. The Carr index (carr R.L, 1965) is calculated from the densities:

$$\text{Carr index } (\%) = \frac{\text{Tapped volume} - \text{Poured density}}{\text{Tapped density}}$$

The Carr index reflects the compactibility of the powders, and there is a correlation between the Carr index and the flowability of the crystals (Wells, J.I.1988).
- Calculate the porosities of the spherical crystals from their bulk and true densities. Calculate the porosity of the tablets from apparent density of the tablets using the following equation:

Porosity ($\dot{\epsilon}$) =(apparent density/true density)

Compactibility and Cohesivity

The Stampf volumeter measurements allow calculation of the compactibility and cohesivity values via the modified Kawakita equation.

$$\frac{N}{C} = \frac{1}{a}N + \frac{1}{ab}$$

Where N is the number of taps, C is the degree of volume reduction, and a and b are constants: 1/a describes the degree of volume reduction at the limit of tapping and is called the compactibility; 1/b is considered to be a constant related to cohesion and is called the cohesiveness. C is calculated via the following equation, and graphs of N/C vs. N are plotted:

$$C = \frac{V_0 - V}{V_0}$$

The compactibility 1/a and cohesivity 1/b are obtained from the slope 1/a and the intercept 1/ab of the plot of the modified Kawakita equation.

In vitro Dissolution Studies

Carry out the *in vitro* dissolution studies using an eight-station USP 23 dissolution testing apparatus (Electrolab, India) (Babu *et al,* 2002). The dissolution medium used may be 900 ml of distilled water or 2%, (*m/v*) SLS. Weigh the agglomerates and fill into a hard gelatin capsule. Introduce the capsule into the dissolution medium and stir the medium at 75 rpm using a paddle at 37 ± 0.5 °C. Collect the samples and analyse spectrophotometrically.

BET and BJH Methods

For the determination of specific surfaces and micropore volumes of samples use Micromeritics ASA 2000 equipment from data (20 points each) of nitrogen adsorption and desorption isotherms at the boiling point of liquid nitrogen under atmospheric pressure. The specific surface is calculated in the validity range of the BET isotherm (Brunauer *et al,* 1938), from the slope and intercept of a line characterised by 5 measuring points. The micropore volume is calculated via the BJH method (Barrett *et al,* 1951).

Compaction Behaviour of Agglomerated Crystals

The compaction behaviour of agglomerated crystals is analysed by applying Heckel equation (Heckel R.W., 1961; Heckel R.W., 1961)

$$\text{In } [1/1–D] = KP + A$$

Where D is relative density of tablet to true density of powder, 1/K is average yield pressure (p). At lower compression pressure, the data of agglomerated crystals may deviate from the linear relation.

$$A = \text{In } [1/1–D_0] + B$$

Where D_0 is relative density of powder bed at P=0.

$$D_A = 1 – e^{-A}$$

$$D_B = D_B - D_0$$

The purity of spherical crystallisation can be determined by IR spectrum analysis (Perkin Elmer IR spectrometer) and melting point determination (Toshniwall apparatus).

SUGGESTED READINGS

- Babu, G. V. M., Shankar, V. G., Sankar, K. H., Seshasayana, A., Kumar, N. K. and Murthy, K. V. R. (2002) Indian J. Pharm. Sci., 6, 588–590.
- Barrett, E.P., Joyner, L.G., Halenda P.P. (1951) J. Am. Chem.Soc., 73, 373.
- Brunauer, S., Emmett, P.H., Teller, E. (1938) J. Am. Chem. Soc., 60, 309.
- Carr, R.L. (1965) Chem. Eng., 72, 69.
- Heckel, R.W. (1961a) Trans. Metall. Soc., AIME 221, 1001.
- Heckel, R.W. (1961b) Trans. Metall. Soc., AIME 221, 671.
- K. Kawakita, K.H. Ludde, (1971) Powder Technol., 4, 61.
- Kallies, A., Konig, J., Ulrich (1993) Solidification by crystallisation in drops, International Workshop for Industrial Crystallisation, Bremen, Germany, p-138.
- Kawashima Y. *et al.* (1989) J. Soc. Powder Technol. Japan, 26, 659.
- Paradkar, A.R., Mahadik, K.R. and Pawar, A.P. (1998) Indian Drugs 31, 6, 283.
- Wells, J.I. (1988) Pharmaceutical preformulation, in: M.M. Rubinstein (Ed.), The physicochemical Properties of Drug Substances, Ellis Horwood Limited, Chinchester, UK, pp. 209.
- Yamashiro, M., Yuasa, Y., Kawakita, K. (1983) Powder Technol., 34, 225.

8

Microemulsion

Microemulsion can be defined in general as thermodynamically stable isotropically clear dispersion of two immiscible liquids, consisting of microdomains of one or both liquids stabilised by interfacial films of surface active molecules (Gennes *et al*, 1982; Leung *et al*, 1981). Schulman and coworkers (1959) introduced the term microemulsion to describe the clear, fluid systems obtained by titration to the point of clarity of an ordinary milky emulsion (macroemulsion) by the addition of a medium chain alcohol such as pentanol or hexanol. Thus over the year the terms thermodynamically stable emulsions, transparent emulsion, micellar emulsions, swollen micelles and reverse micelles have been used in the literature to describe precisely the same systems that were called microemulsion by Schulman.

STRUCTURE OF MICROEMULSION

Microemulsions can be classified into three types (Fig.8.1): water-in-oil (water/oil), bicontinuous, and oil-in-water (oil/water).

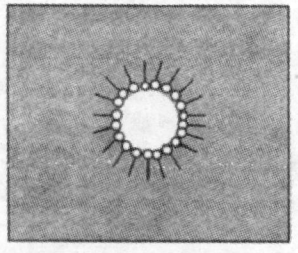
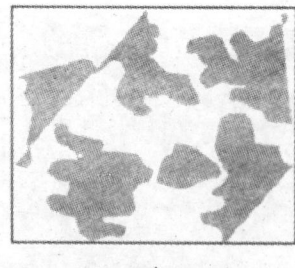
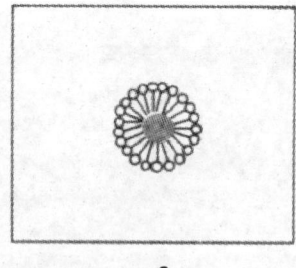

a.   b.   c.

Fig: 8.1 *Schematic representation of different types of microemulsion system:*
(a). W/O Microemulsion; (b). Bicontinous Microemulsion; (c). O\W Microemulsion

Two types of phases are thus shown to be associated with microemulsions

• Droplet phases
• Bicontinuous phases

Droplet Phases

At higher water concentration microemulsion consists of small oil droplets dispersed in water, i.e. O/W microemulsion, where as at lower water concentration the situation is reversed and the system consists of water droplets dispersed in oil, i.e. W/O microemulsion. In each phase the oil and water are separated by surfactant rich film.

The oil droplets in O/W microemulsions are surrounded by the electrical double layers, which can extend into the external phase for a considerable distance (up to 100 nm), depending on the electrolyte concentration. Thus the hard sphere volume of the droplet is generally considerably greater than of the oil core volume, which creates a strong osmotic (repulsive) force at relatively low disperse phase concentrations.

In contrast W/O systems are stabilised primarily by steric interactions between the absorbed film in such a way that the hard sphere volume of the droplets is only slightly greater than that of the water pools. The droplet interaction can take place at relatively short distances of separation where the tail of the hydrocarbon chains can interpenetrate with each other. This allows a great increase in droplet number concentration before a strong osmotic force is felt.

Bicontinuous Phases or Middle Phase Microemulsions

In many cases it is possible to effect a gradual transition from O/W to W/O microemulsion simply by changing the volume fraction of oil and water. The intermediate region, which contains approximately equal volumes of oil and water is composed of lamellar or bicontinuous structures. In this region both the oil and the water domains extend over macroscopic distances and the surfactant forms an interface of rapidly fluctuating curvature, but in which the net curvature is near zero.

THEORETICAL BASIS OF MICROEMULSIFICATION

When oil water and surfactants are mixed, microemulsions are only one of a number of association structures (including ordinary emulsions, micellar and mesomorphic phases of various construction such as lamellar hexagonal cubic and various gels and oily dispersions) that can form depending on the chemical nature and concentration of each of the components, as well as prevailing temperature and pressure. When a surfactant is added to a mixture containing equal amounts of oil and water either W/O or O/W emulsion will form depending on the molecular interaction of the surfactant with both the oil and water. Different interaction strengths on both sides of the surfactant film induce a tension gradient across the surfactant membrane and consequently produce curvature. A geometrical model has been proposed to describe quantitatively the correlation between the structure of surfactant aggregates and the geometric packing of surfactants at the interface is a packing ratio or critical packing parameter (CPP). CPP defined as the ratio of cross sectional area of hydrocarbon chain to that of the polar head of the surfactant molecule at the interface, i.e.

$$V/a_0 Ic$$

Where V = volume of the hydrocarbon chain of surfactant

a_0 = optimal cross sectional area per polar head in a planar interface.

Ic   =   approximately 80–90% of the fully extended length of the surfactant chain.

A greater cross sectional area of the tail than that of the head ($V/a_0Ic>1$) would favour the formation of W/O droplets, whereas a smaller cross area of the tail than that of the head ($V/a_0Ic<1$) would favour the formation of O/W droplets. A planer interface dictates $V/a_0Ic = 1$, leading to the formation of lamellar structure.

Many approaches have been used to explore the mechanisms of microemulsion formation and stability. Some emphasise the formation of an interfacial film and the production of ultra-low interfacial tensions (mixed film theories); other emphasise the monophasic nature of many microemulsions (solubilisation theories). Thermodynamic theories consider the free energy of formation of microemulsions and the bending elasticity of the film. No one approach alone covers all aspects of microemulsion structure and stability and all have a place in the overall understanding of microemulsions.

Formulation of Microemulsion

In the microemulsification, the film curvature and interfacial tension are crucial factors in the formation of microemulsions. Thus the key to microemulsion preparation lies in decreasing the interfacial tension and increasing the free energy of the newly created surfaces. In this respect, a relatively large amount of surfactant along with co-surfactant such as a short chain alcohol is required to lower the interfacial tension in formulating conventional microemulsion. Thus the formulation of microemulsion usually involves a combination of three to five components.

An oil phase, an aqueous phase, a primary surfactant and in many case secondary surfactant (co-surfactant), and sometimes an electrolyte. The formation of microemulsion is highly specific process involving spontaneous interactions among the constituent molecules. The type of association structure formed from these components at a particular temperature depends not only on the chemical nature of each component but also on their relative concentrations. Thus it is essential for a systematic study of microemulsion composition to establish phase diagrams for the system under investigation.

Oil

In the microemulsion formulations, usually aliphatic and aromatic oils are employed together with synthetic or natural amphiphiles to homogenise water forming isotropic transparent and stable dispersion of either water-in-oil or oil-in-water for various industrial purposes. Table 8.1 shows a list of oils that have been for the preparation of microemulsions.

Solubilisation of a single-chain oil (ethyl ester of fatty acid oil) is easier than the three-chain (triglycerides) oil and within the same series of oil; the oil with shorter alkyl chain length is solubilized to greater extent than the longer chain length oils. Thus as expected, the structure and in part the molecular volume of the oils used influences the amount of oil incorporated within the microemulsion. Within the triglyceride series of oils, tributyrin, the smallest molecular volume oil could be incorporated up to 3% (W/W) at a surfactant concentration of 35% w/w, while the larger molecular volume oils could only be solubilised to 2 and 1 % (W/W) at approximately 30% (W/W) and 10–35% (W/W) surfactant for Miglycol

812 and soyabean oil respectively. Similarly for the ethyl esters, the smallest molecular volume of ethyl butyrate was solubilised to the greatest extent, namely 16% (W/W) at a surfactant concentration of 30% (W/W), whereas the larger molecular volume oils, ethyl caprylate and ethyl oleate were incorporate at levels of 7% and 3% (W/W) respectively, at surfactant concentration of 25% (W/W). Surprisingly, however this trend was reversed in O/W microemulsions produced using a longer unsaturated alkyl chain surfactant, where the largest molecular volume were solubilised to the greatest extent.

Table 8.1 *Lists of oil phase in microemulsion preparation*

Hexane	Mineral oil	Cotton seed oil
Benzene	squalene	Corn oil
Toluene	Oleic acid	Sesame oil
n-Octane	eutanol G	Olive oil
Decane	Cetearyl octanoate	Ricebran oil
Dodecane	Isopropyl myristate (IPM)	Saffola oil
Hexadecane	IPM-Decanol	Clove oil
Isooctane	IPM octanoic acid	Linseed oil
n-tetradecane	Isopropyl palmitate	Palm oil
n-hexadecane	Tributyrin	
n-heptane	Miglycol	
xylene		

Surfactants

In the preparation of microemulsion a crucial step lies in the choice of surfactant (if necessary) and co-surfactant for the particular oil. The chosen surfactant must—

- Lower the interfacial tension to a very small value to aid dispersion processes during the preparation of the microemulsion.
- Provide a flexible film that can readily deform round small droplets,
- Be of an appropriate hydrophilic-lipophilic character to provide the correct curvature at the interfacial region for the desired microemulsion type, O/W, W/O, or bicontinuous.

These conditions have been achieved in several ways. For example by using a combination of an anionic or cationic surfactant of high HLB with a co-surfactant of lower HLB; a double chained surfactant of the appropriate molecular composition; or a single chained nonionic surfactant of the polyethylene glycol alkyl ether type at appropriate temperature.

In order to reduce the interfacial tension, it is necessary to maximise the interfacial adsorption of surfactant. A surfactant with a balanced hydrophilic and lipophilic property is desirable, meaning that a surfactant with equal solubility in both water and oil is most likely to be preferentially adsorbed at the oil-water interface. The relative sizes of the hydrophilic and hydrophobic groups of the surfactant molecules, that is, their HLB must be correctly balanced for a given oil and aqueous solution to produce a microemulsion. The HLB scheme, though originally defined for oil and water emulsions stabilised by nonionic surfactants, can be extended to microemulsion formulation and many ionic emulsifiers.

Recently much attention has been paid to utilisation of the phospholipids in formulating pharmaceutically acceptable microemulsions. Their non-toxicity makes them an ideal choice. Attempts to use lecithin as an amphiphile for the preparation of efficient microemulsions must take into consideration the characteristic solution properties of lecithin, which are as follows:

- Very strong hydrophobicity due to two long hydrocarbon chains
- A strong lipophilicity due to the Zwitter ionic polar head groups, which have dipole moments and are strongly hydrated.
- A close balance between hydrophilic and lipophilic properties although slightly displaced toward the lipophilic side.
- A strong tendency to form liquid crystals notably of lamellar structure.

PROTOCOL: 8.1
PREPARATION OF MICROEMULSION

Materials

Isopropyl myristate

Soyabean lecithin

Castor oil

Olive oil

Lecithin

Tween 80

Tween 20

Propylene glycol

Magnetic stirrer

pH meter

The following formulas are selected for the final microemulsion preparation:
Formula I

Isopropyl myristate	1 g
Soybean lecithin	0.05 g
Tween 80	0.25 g
Drug (Flurbiprofen)	0.05 g
Phosphate buffer pH 5.5	q.s. to 10 g

Formula II

Isopropyl myristate	1 g
Soybean lecithin	0.05 g
Tween 80	1 g
Drug (Flurbiprofen)	0.05 g
Phosphate buffer pH 5.5	q.s. to 10 g

Formula III

Isopropyl myristate	0.75 g
Propylene glycol	1.13 g
Tween 80	3.43 g
Drug (Flurbiprofen)	0.05 g
Phosphate buffer pH 5.5	q.s. to 4.63 g

Procedure

- Disperse soybean lecithin well in oil phase by keeping it at 50°C in an oven and add the co-surfactant (Tween 80 in formula I and II and propylene glycol in formula III) to the aqueous or oily phase depending upon their solubility in respective phase.

- Heat the oily and aqueous phase separately to 50°C and then add the aqueous phase to the oil phase. The homogeneous and stable lipid emulsion forms spontaneously.

- Drug incorporation depends upon the solubility of drug in oily or aqueous phase; drug is added into that particular phase before mixing of these two different phases (Scheme 8.1).

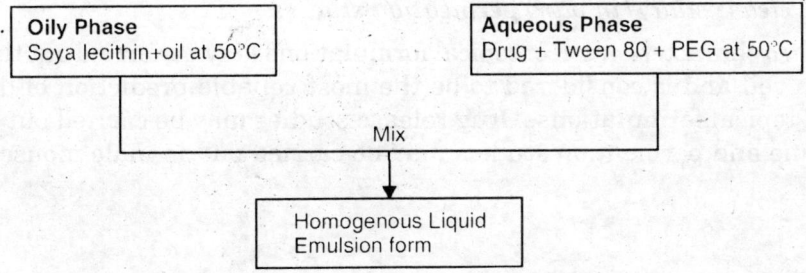

Scheme: 8.1 Preparation of Microemulsion

Characterisation of Lipid Microemulsion

1. *Size Shape and Size Distribution Measurements*

    Determine morphology and structure of oil globules with the transmission electron microscopy (TEM) by using negative staining with phosphotungstic acid.

    Determine size of the droplets for the formulations with the mastersizer (Malvern Instruments Ltd. UK) using laser light scattering technique.

2. *Rheology of the Microemulsion*

The prepared microemulsion system may be studied for its rheological behaviour using Brookfield viscometer. Viscosity can determine at various shear rates by subjecting the system at different torque values. Maintain the temperature constant at 25.2°C throughout experiment.

The spreadibility of formulation may be determined with the parallel-plate method. The spreadibility assembly consisted of two glass plates (lower stationary and upper moveable) designed to slide over each other, place approximately 0.5g formulations over defined area of the lower plate.

Cover with an upper moveable plate. Allow upper plates to slide over the lower one with gel in between at a rate of 1mm/sec for a total distance of 50 mm and record the force Vs distance graph construct spreadibility curve.

3. *Stability Studies*

Phase separation studies may be conducted by storing the formulation at different temperature conditions.

- Store three batches of same formulations in sealed glass containers at room temperature (25±5°C), in refrigerator (4°C) and at higher temperature (40±5°C) for 45 days.

- Evaluate the formulation in each time intervals for per cent oil separated (phase separation).

- The formulation can also be studied by applying shear rate by repeated centrifugation of the formulation at 10000 rpm and calculating the oil phase remaining after centrifugation treatment.

4. *In vitro release study / in vitro permeation studies*

The *in vitro* characterisation of topical formulations may be carried out through Franz's diffusion cell and is considered to be the most reliable prediction of drug transport through topical formulations. Drug release studies may be carried out using dialysis membrane and permeation studies may be carried out on male mouse skin.

PROTOCOL 8.2

PREPARATION OF EUCALYPTUS OIL MICROEMULSION FOR TRANSDERMAL DELIVERY OF HYDROCORTISONE

Materials

Hydrocortisone

Tween 80

Eucalyptus oil

Isopropanol

Methanol (HPLC grade)

Acetonitrile (HPLC grade)
Ethanol (96%)
Propylene glycol
Propylparaben

Construction of Pseudo-ternary Phase Diagrams

Eucalyptus oil may be selected as oily phase as it has been successfully used in transdermal delivery of steroidal drugs similar to hydrocortisone from microemulsion.

Tween 80 may be selected as the surfactant in this study as it is readily miscible with the eucalyptus oil. In the case of cosurfactants if needed the surfactant/cosurfactant ratio should be 1:1 (W/W) used. This ratio is selected on the basis that this ratio solubilises the greatest amount of water on titration compared to various surfactant/cosurfactant ratios when mixed with the oil at 1:1 weight ratios.

The pseudo-ternary phase diagrams may be constructed using water titration method at ambient temperature.

- Prepare mixtures of oil and surfactant or surfactant cosurfactant at weight ratios of 0.5:9.5, 1:9, 1.5:8.5, 2:8, 2.5:7.5, 3:7, 3.5:6.5, 4:6, 5:5, 6:4, 7:3, 8:2 and 9:1. Titrate the mixtures dropwise with water under gentile magnetic stirring.

- After being equilibrated observe the systems and select transparent fluid systems as microemulsion and highly viscous systems that did not show a change in the meniscus after being tilted to an angle of 90° as gel.

Preparation of Microemulsions

Microemulsion formulations selected from the constructed phase diagrams may be prepared according to the composition presented in Table 8.2.

- Select the formulation so that the concentrations of oil and water comes to be the same. The variables may be the presence or absence of cosurfactants and the type of cosurfactant.

Table 8.2: The composition of the microemulsion formulations

Material	TW ME	TW ETH ME	TW ISO ME	TW PG ME
Eucalyptus oil	20	20	20	20
Tween 80	60	30	30	30
Ethanol	–	30	–	–
Isopropanol	–	–	30	–
Propylene glycol	–	–	–	30
Water	20	20	20	20

- Prepare the microemulsions by mixing the oil with the surfactant or surfactant/ cosurfactant mixture before adding the required amount of water under magnetic stirring.

- Add the excess drug to prepare saturated drug solutions with excess crystals to maintain saturation. Equilibrate under continuous mixing in a water bath maintained at 32 °C for 72 h before application to the skin.

- Evaluate the formulations for transdermal drug delivery potential comparing with saturated aqueous drug solution with excess drug crystals as the control.

PROTOCOL 8.3

Competitive Solubilisation of Cholesterol and Phytosterols in Nonionic Microemulsions

Materials

Tween 60 [polyoxyethylene-(20)-sorbitan monostearate]

R-(+)-limonene (98%)

Ethanol (EtOH 99.8%)

Propylene glycol (PG, 99.5%)

Phytosterols (composed of 40–58% β-sitosterol, 20–30% campesterol, 14–22% stigmasterol, and 0–6% brassicasterol)

Cholesterol (98% purity)

Tri-distilled Water

Phase diagrams

The five-component systems may be prepared as reported elsewhere on pseudoternary phase diagrams.

Sterol Solubilisation in the Microemulsion System

- Solubilise sterols (PS, CH, or mixtures) in R-(+)-limonene, ethanol and Tween 60 solution (in 1:1:4.67 weight ratio) at 90 °C for 2–5 min in sealed Viton-corked tubes (preventing ethanol evaporation) to form a transparent, solution like system, termed as "concentrate."

- Cool the concentrates to room temperature.

- Add the aqueous phase (water and PG at 1:1 weight ratio) after the concentrate has cooled to 25 °C.

- Store the concentrates, as well as the aqueous phase as diluted formulations, in a 25 °C circulation bath.

The solubilisation capacity may be visually determined as the maximum quantity of solubilised sterols (CH, PS or their mixtures) which could be loaded without any observable sterols precipitation after 3–4 days.

PROTOCOL 8.4

Linker-based Lecithin Microemulsions for Transdermal Delivery of Lidocaine

Materials

Sorbitan monooleate (Span® 80)

Sodium caprylate

Caprylic acid

Isopropyl myristate

Sodium chloride

1-pentanol

Dulbecco's phosphate buffered saline (PBS)

Lidocaine powder (base form)

Laboratory grade soybean lecithin

Sodium phosphate monobasic, monohydrate (ACS grade)

Acetonitrile (HPLC grade)

Anhydrous ethyl alcohol

Microemulsion Preparation

Phase behaviour studies may be performed using equal volumes of aqueous solution and oil (5 ml of each) in flat bottom test tubes. To obtain a phase transition of Winsor Type II–Type III or IV–Type I, the concentration of sodium caprylate is gradually increased (using a separate test tube for each concentration increment) while maintaining the temperature ($23\pm1°C$ room temperature, unless stated otherwise), electrolyte concentration (0.9% NaCl in the aqueous solution) and pressure (1 atm) constant. This procedure will be referred to as a hydrophilic linker (sodium caprylate) scan.

- Introduce all the ingredients, vortex the test tubes thoroughly, then vortex once a day for 3 days, and leave to equilibrate for 2 weeks.

- After these systems reach equilibrium, calculate the microemulsion volume fraction by measuring the volume of the microemulsion and excess phase(s) (if any) in the test tube. Leave the selected systems to equilibrate in a water bath at 37°C with an objective of determining the phase behaviour at body temperature.

- Adjust pH of all microemulsions systems to 5.5 ± 0.5. Sorbitan monooleate to lecithin weight ratios of 1:1, 2:1 and 3:1 may be investigated.

- Note sorbitan monooleate to lecithin ratio of 1:1, microemulsions are rarely formed; instead, highly viscous liquid crystalline phases result. Tables 8.3a and b present a summary of the formulations which can be considered in this experiment.

- Lidocaine can be introduced in the formulations by predissolving this drug in IPM to a concentration of 10%.

Table 8.3 (a): *Microemulsion series used in phase behaviour studies (%w/w)*

Series	%LE	%SM	%CA	%SC	%NaCl	%Water	%IPM
A	4.0	8.0	–	0.5~7.0	0.9	45.1-%SC	42.0
B	4.0	12.0	–	0.5~7.0	0.9	45.1-%SC	38.0
	0.4	1.2	0.3	0.5~7.0	0.9	48.4-%SC	48.8
	0.8	2.4	0.6	0.5~7.0	0.9	47.7-%SC	47.6
	1.2	3.6	0.9	0.5~7.0	0.9	47.0-%SC	46.4
	1.6	4.8	1.2	0.5~7.0	0.9	46.3-%SC	45.2
	2.0	6.0	1.5	0.5~7.0	0.9	45.6-%SC	44.0
L	2.4	7.2	1.8	0.5~7.0	0.9	44.9-%SC	42.8
	2.8	8.4	2.1	0.5~7.0	0.9	44.2-%SC	41.6
	3.2	9.8	2.4	0.5~7.0	0.9	43.5-%SC	40.2
	3.6	10.8	2.7	0.5~7.0	0.9	42.8-%SC	39.2
	4.0	12.0	3.0	0.5~7.0	0.9	42.1-%SC	38.0

Table 8.3 (b): *Microemulsion formulations used in transdermal delivery studies*

Formulation	% LE	%SM	%CA	%SC	%NaCl	%Water	%IPM
L-Type II	4.0	12.0	3.0	1.0	0.9	41.1	38.0
L-Type IV	4.0	12.0	3.0	4.0	0.9	38.1	38.0
L-Type I	4.0	12.0	3.0	7.0	0.9	35.1	38.0
% Pentanol							
p-Type II	4.0	12.0	8.0		0.9	37.1	38.3

LE , Lecithin; SM, sorbitan monooleate; CA, Caprylic acid; SC, Sodium caprylate

SUGGESTED READINGS

* Acosta, E.J., Nguyen, T., Witthayapanyanon, A., Harwell, J.H., Sabatini, D.A. 2005. Environ. Sci. Technol. 39, 1275.

* Alany, R.G., Rades, T., Agatonovic-Kustrin, S., Davies, N.M., Tucker, I.G. 2000. Int. J. Pharm. 196, 141.

* Benita, S., In: microencapsulation and industrial applications, Marcel Dekker, New york, 411,1997.

* Biruss, B., Kahlig, H., Valenta, C., 2007. Int. J. Pharm. 328, 142.

* Chen, H., Chang, X., Weng, T., Zhao, X., Gao, Z., Yang, Y., Xu, H., Yang, X., 2004. J. Control. Rel. 98, 427.

* De Gennes, P. G., Taupin, C. (1982) J. Phys. Chem., 86, 2294.

- El Maghraby G M. Int J Pharm 355 (2008) 285.
- Gasco, M. R., Gallarate, M. and Pattarino, F. (1991) Int. J. Pharm., 69, 193.
- Kunieda, H and Ishikawa, N (1985) J. Colloid Interface Sci., 107, 122.
- Kunieda, H. and Shinoda K. (1980) J. Colliod Interface Sci., 75, 601.
- Kurihara, K., Kizling, J., Stenius, P., Fendler, J. H. (1983) J. Am. Chem. SOC., 105. 2574.
- Lawrence M. J., Rees G.D. (2000) Adv Drug Delivery Rev., 45:89,121.
- Lawrence, M. J. (1994) Eur. J. Drug Metab. Pharmacokinet., 3, 257.
- Leung, R., Hou, M. J., Manohar, C., Shah, D. O., Chun, P. W., Shah, D. O., Ed.; American Chemical Society: Washington DC, 325,1981.
- Lovell, M. W., Johnson, H. W., Hui, H. W., Cannon, J. B., Gupta, P. K. and Hsu C. C. (1994) Int. J. Pharm,. 109, 45.
- Paul B. K., Moulik S. P., (1997) J Disp Sci Technol., 18, 301.
- Ross S. and Morrison I. D. In: Colloidal System and Interfaces, Wiley, New York, 176 (1988).
- Rozner S, Aserin A, Garti N J Colloid Interface Sci 321 (2008) 418.
- Schulman J.H., Stockenius, W., and Prince, L.M. (1959) J. Phy. Chem., 63, 1677.
- Tarr B. and Yalkosky S. H. (1989) Pharm. Res., 6, 40.
- Yuan J. S., Ansari M, Samaan M, Acosta E J. Int J Pharm 349 (2008) 130.
- Zhu W, Yu A, Wang W, Dong R, Wu J, Zhai G Int J Pharm (In Press).

9

Implants and Inserts

Implantable drug delivery devices are devoid of aforementioned limitations associated with oral, intravenous topical drug administration vis-à-vis subcutaneously implantable drug delivery devices offer one unique advantage of a retrievable mechanism. This feature enables a readily reversible termination of drug administration whenever required. Some desirable properties of effective subcutaneous controlled release drug delivery systems are:

- It should improve patient compliance by reducing the frequency of drug administration over the entire period of treatment.
- It should be free from any major surgical procedure and ideally should be readily administered.
- It should release the drug in a rate-controlled manner, which leads to enhanced effectiveness and reduction in side effects.
- It should be readily retrievable by medical personnel to terminate medication.
- It should be easy to sterilise.
- It should be devoid of any potential medical complication.
- It should be easy to manufacture and relatively inexpensive.
- It should be stable and safe, and should have good mechanical strength.

CLASSIFICATION

- Transdermal implantable systems
- Subdermal implantable systems
- Implantable polymeric matrix

Subdermal implants of various types, namely pellets, rods and fibres of biodegradable and non-biodegradable polymers have been developed. They provide a means to avoid the first pass metabolism and to deliver sustained release of drugs in relatively smaller and safer quantities. A subdermal delivery system can provide constant and efficacious blood levels of drugs for a desired period with little likelihood of either drug insufficiency or accumulation due to lack of congruency between drug availability and depletion. Such a system would be easily administered, would eliminate patient intervention and increase patient compliance and would be effective for extended periods. Biologically compatible polymers are used in fabrication of subdermal implants for delivering drugs at an optimum rate and concentration.

Implantable Devices

Implantable infusion pumps

Vapour-pressure powered devices

Peristaltic pumps

Solenoid pumps

Electronic pumps

Implantable mini-osmotic pump (Alzet[@])

Ocular implantable system

Vaginal implants

Intra-arterial catheter infusion drug delivery systems

Needle injection catheter

Microcatheter

Helical catheter

Porous balloon catheters

Implantable drug delivery pump

CLASSIFICATION BASED ON MECHANISMS OF DRUG RELEASE FROM IMPLANTS

Diffusion Controlled

Reservoir

This type of system consists of a core of drug surrounded by a polymer and diffusion of the drug across the polymer layer is the rate-limiting step. Zero-order release kinetic can easily be obtained from reservoir systems by slight modifications. These systems are generally non-biodegradable therefore must be surgically removed. They are relatively expensive and can leak the contents, which lead to toxic manifestations.

Matrix

These systems rarely provide zero-order release rate, which can be achieved by compensating for the increase diffusional distance with an increasing area of the drug. Applications of these systems include cases of drugs, which are distributed uniformly in the matrix or chemically bound to a polymer backbone chain. It has been reported (Hopfenberg and Hsu, 1978) that if the kinetics of the biodegradation of polymer is known, a zero-order release can be generated by geometry where the surface area did not change with time. The most frequently used biodegradable polymer is polylactic acid or lactic-glycolic acid copolymers.

Chemically Controlled

These systems resemble diffusion type delivery systems except that the drug is distributed uniformly throughout the bioerodible polymer, which erodes and decreases in geometry/dimension with time to allow the drug release. Degradation products of the polymer should not be toxic. A zero-order kinetics can be achieved if the surface area remains unchanged with time.

Three dissolution mechanisms discussed by Heller [1980] are:

- Water-soluble polymers insolubilised by degradable crosslinks,
- Water-insoluble polymers solubilised by hydrolysis, ionisation or protonation of the side groups, and
- Water-insoluble polymers solubilised by backbone chain cleavage to small water, soluble molecules.

Swelling Controlled

This type of a swelling-controlled polymeric system (Fig.9.1) the release rate is equal to the product of surface area and a rate constant corresponding to rate of advance of the boundary separating the outer shell from central core. The release rate is constant if the absorption rate of the environmental fluid is constant.

In this system the rate-limiting step depends on ingression of an external agent and not on the diffusive or physicochemical properties of the incorporated drug.

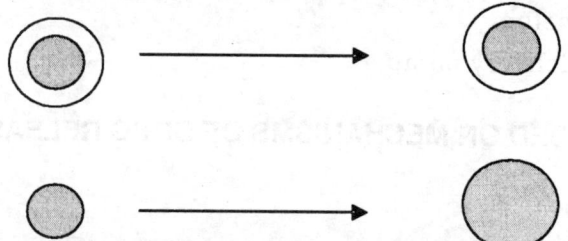

Fig. 9.1: *Swelling controlled delivery system*

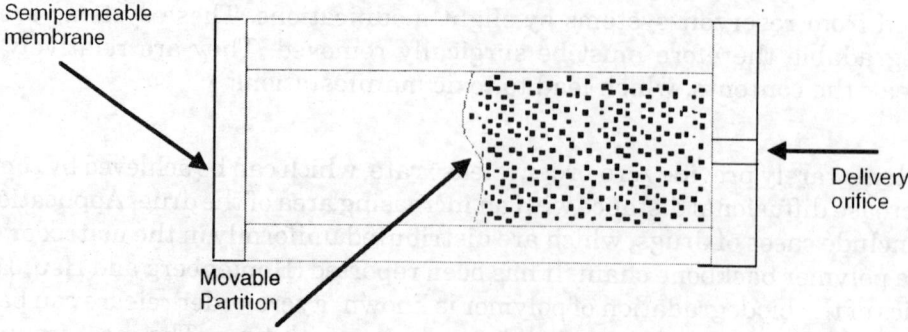

Fig. 9.2: *Schematic representation of osmotic pump*

Osmotically Controlled

This type of system utilises osmotic pressure as a driving force for delivery of drugs/bioactive. The systems in the form of matrix (Fig. 9.2) where the core is surrounded by a semipermeable film, zero-order release is difficult to achieve. However, if the system is fabricated in the form of a pump containing a laser-drilled hole at the outlet, zero-order release can be obtained. A typical example is the Alzet® osmotic minipump (Alza).

Magnetically Controlled

This type of system (Fig. 9.3) consists of the drug and small magnetic beads uniformly dispersed within a polymer matrix. In contact with aqueous media, the drug is released in a diffusion-controlled manner and the rate can be increased on exposure to a oscillating external magnetic field. A typical application of this type of system is when drug delivery is designed to correspond to the changes in steroid secretion during the menstrual cycle.

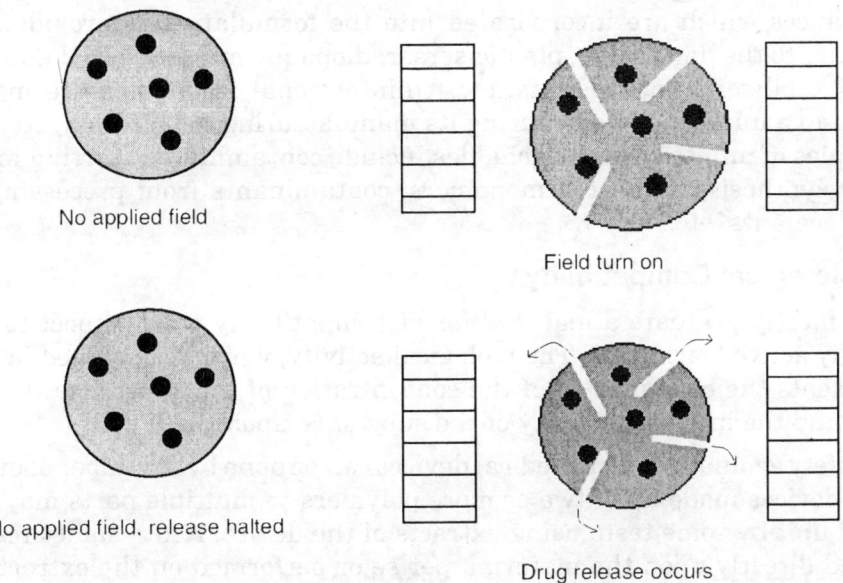

No applied field

Field turn on

No applied field, release halted

Drug release occurs

Fig. 9.3: Drug release from magnetically controlled delivery system

EVALUATION OF IMPLANTABLE POLYMERIC MATERIALS

Newer drug delivery devices and materials are being continually developed for various biomedical applications. Initially, the basis of selection of materials for biological applications was their physical properties while absence of any biological activity whereas biological acceptance (biocompatibility) of the material was not taken into account. Plastic containers were used frequently with a convention that these are quite inert against harsh acid and base treatments. However, studies indicated that plastics adversely affect the biological milieu. The adverse effects include thrombogenicity, cellular necrosis, carcinogenicity, etc. numerous clinical reports and continuous studies indicating adverse, reactions from plastic materials created concern as to whether or not the patient does better from use of the device than without use of the device. However, now-a-days emphasis is being laid on the fact that patient should receive maximum benefit from use of the device while being exposed to minimum risks from the device.

Acute Evaluations

Acute biological incompatibilities mostly arise due to presence of biologically active leachable substances in the medical material. The most common short-term response of the tissues to an implanted material is its encapsulation by fibrous tissue within few weeks.

A leachable is referred to a substance or component in the biomedical material or device, which may migrate from the material/device to the surrounding medium. The medium may be tissue fluids surrounding the implanted device, blood stored in a blood bag, therapeutic preparations with their solvent given by solution administration set, etc. Leachables may be divided into two categories, intentional or unintentional. Intentional additives include those substances which are incorporated into the formulation to provide some specific characteristics to the device like, plasticisers, radiopaque materials, UV absorbers, fillers, colourants, stabilisers, antioxidants, etc. Unintentional leachables are introduced into the material in a number of ways during its manufacturing, fabrication, sterilisation, etc. Some examples of unintentional leachables include contaminated starting materials used for polymer synthesis, unreacted monomers, contaminants from processing equipment, adhesive or sealants, etc.

Tests for Biological Compatibility

Acute tests mostly evaluate a material for biocompatibility with respect to the presence of biologically active leachables. The biological activity, which is observed in most of these tests, represents the combination of the concentration of the substance that reaches the target cells and the intrinsic activity of the substance upon these cells.

Acute safety evaluation of biomedical devices can be done by a number of biological tests. Biomedical devices made up of two or more polymers or multiple parts may be evaluated as an intact unit by some tests using extracts of the device. Acute safety tests can either be conducted directly upon the material, per se or performed on the extracts (eluates) of the material or device.

Rabbit Muscle Implant

This is a simple test conducted for short-term compatibility of a biomedical material with living tissues. The test, when supported by careful histopathologic examination of adjacent tissue, provides considerable information regarding biocompatibility of the material/device.

Healthy New Zealand albino rabbits of either sex are lightly anaesthetised by slowly injecting 25 mg/kg of pentobarbital sodium intravenously via the marginal ear vein. One negative control, one positive control and two test samples are inserted through the skin (at 90° to the surface) and into the paravertebral muscles to a sufficient depth. Seven days after implantation, the rabbit is sacrificed by an overdose of pentobarbital sodium intravenously and implant site along with adjacent tissues are examined and appropriately scored according to the severity of response. This test primarily detects histopathologic examination of the muscle tissue adjacent to the implanted sample and adds to the sensitivity of the test.

Agar Overlay Cell Culture

This is a relatively inexpensive and rapid test to detect the presence of leachable cytotoxic substance in a material/device. This test can be conducted to assess the cytotoxicity of almost any compound, which is capable of diffusing through the agar layer. In this test, a 24 h confluent monolayer of mouse fibroblast cells (L cells) is grown on Eagle's medium in petri dishes. The nutrient medium is replaced with agar composed of equal part of double strength Eagle's medium and 3% agar, cells are pink stained with a neutral red stain, and four samples, one negative control, one positive control and two test samples are placed on the agar. The petri dishes are incubated at 37°C for 24 h in an atmosphere of 5% CO_2 and 95% air. After 24 h each site is examined for cytotoxic activity. A clear zone with loss of pink colour produced by cytotoxic reaction around the "toxic" sample and "nontoxic" sample gives a pinkish, translucent appearance.

A semi-quantitative scoring system was developed for the primary acute toxicity screen in which size of the clear zone (zone index) and degree of lysis within the zone (lysis index) were observed and combined to get response index.

This basic test has shown good correlation with the rabbit muscle implant test, however the test is somewhat more sensitive compared to muscle implant test. In addition to these tests, many other tests are performed on extracts of materials like cell culture test, intradermal irritation, systemic toxicity, isolated perfused heart and sensitivity testing. However, whether the biological activity shown at the levels present would be toxic, beneficial or without appreciable effect to the patient is not answered directly by these tests. Nevertheless, positive test indicates the presence of toxicologically active substance, which should not present any effect, which they may exert upon the patient, should not be a part of the planned therapeutic regimen.

Chronic Evaluations

Biomaterials or devices may release leachables that elicit a mild, temporary effect or may produce irreversible damage to the organs or tissues and prolonged release may lead to progressive damage. This suggests that some acute subtle effects may become quite apparent in chronic studies. Polymeric material in contact with living tissues and biological fluids for long term may result in biodegradation. Long-term implantation of solid materials also raises another potential problems of carcinogenesis, which may or may not be associated with biodegradation.

Some investigators have suggested that biodegradation of a polymer produces free radical species which are carcinogens, however no data available indicating that the degradation products produce significant adverse effects in man and animals, except for those resulting from mechanical failure of the device.

Some studies in 1940s reported that local sarcomas formed when bakelite disks were implanted subcutaneously in rats. Tumours of this aetiology were called material induced cancers, solid-state cancers, foreign body cancers, and smooth-surface cancers. The risk of solid tumour formation can be reduced by selection of appropriate materials and /or devices. The true risk of material induced tumours is still unknown in case of human beings. Estimates made from published reports and from surveys of certain groups of patients indicated that the incidences of material associated tumours are quite small in human beings. Until, more accurate data are available for long term use of implants in human, it would be worthwhile to limit such implants to situation of decided therapeutic benefit.

MICROSEALED DRUG DELIVERY SYSTEMS

PROTOCOL: 9.1
Transdermal MDD device

- Thoroughly mix 11 parts of nitroglycerin-lactose triturate (10% w/w) with 7 parts of aqueous polyethylene glycol 400 solution (10% v/v) to form uniform paste.

- Add the drug dispersion compartment to 57 parts of silicone elastomer. Thoroughly mix the combination using a high torque mixer to form a homogeneous dispersion. A drug polymer microdispersion is produced.

- With continuing agitation, 13 parts of isopropyl palmitate, 6 parts of mineral oil and 6 parts of curing agent are added, in sequence, into the drug polymer microdispersion to form a pre-MDD formulation.

- Expose the well-mixed pre-MDD formulation to a vacuum of 71 cm, with continuing agitation, for at least 30 min or until all the entrapped air is removed.

- Pour an adequate amount of the deaerated pre-MDD formulation into disk type molds.

- Polymerise the pre-MDD formulation in the molds and glue them individually onto the occlusive baseplate at the centre of the adhesive foam pad. After covering with surlyn-laminated foil, a unit of Nitrodisc system is produced.

PROTOCOL: 9.2
Subdermal MDD implants

- Thoroughly mix 4 parts of finely milled norgestomer crystals with 6 parts of aqueous polyethylene glycol 400 solution (40% v/v) to form a uniform paste.

- Add the drug dispersion compartment of 82.5 parts of silastic elastomer 382. Thoroughly mix the combination using a high torque mixer to form a homogeneous dispersion. A drug polymer microdispersion is produced.

- With continuing agitation, 7.5 parts of Dow Corning medical fluid 360 and 15 drops of catalyst M (for every 100 g of mixture) are added, in sequence, into the drug polymer microdispersion to form a pre-MDD formulation.

- Expose the well-mixed pre-MDD formulation to a vacuum of 71cm with continuous agitation for 5 min or until all the entrapped air is released.
- Deliver the deaerated pre-MDD formulation into polymeric tubing, e.g. silastic tubings with a controlled membrane thickness, via a specially designed tube at 60°in an circulating air oven for 1 hr. MDD implants are thus formed (Scheme 9.1).
- Cut the MDD implants into section of 2–5 m in length. The subdermal MDD implants are thus produced.

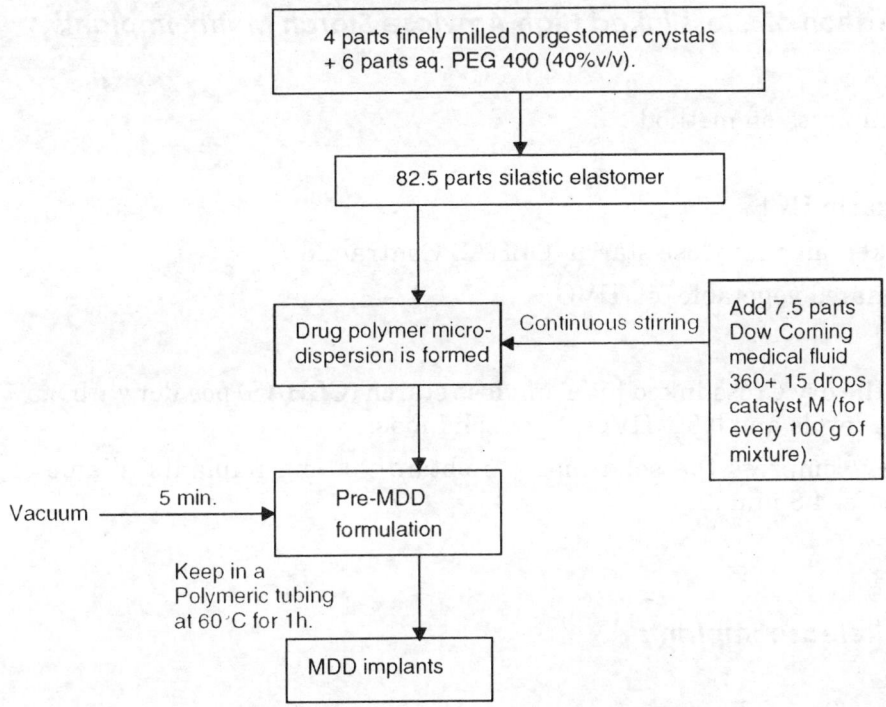

Scheme. 9.1: *Preparation of MDD implants*

PROTOCOL: 9.3
Vaginal MDD Rings

The procedure for the fabrication of vaginal MDD rings is similar to that outlined earlier for subdermal MDD implants except that in the final stage (step 7) the MDD implants are cut into 16 cm in length.

The ends of each section of MDD implant are then bound together to form a doughnut shaped vaginal ring by applying a thin layer of silastic Medical Adhesive and then inserting both ends into a small section (2 cm in length) of silastic (Medical grade) tubing, which has been swollen reversibly in diameter by an organic solvent.

Intrauterine Devices

The procedure for the fabrication of MDD –7 IUD is similar to that outlined earlier for sub dermal MDD implants, except that in the final stage the MDD implants are cut intersections of 2 cm in length. The implant is than bound to a unit of 7-shaped polypropylene frame by gluing the ends of each MDD implants to the vertical stem of the plastic frame.

PROTOCOL: 9.4

Characterisation of Crosslinked High Amylose Starch Matrix Implants

Principle

Direct compression method

Materials

Ciprofloxacin HCl

Crosslinked high amylose starch (CLHAS Contramid)

Hydrogenated vegetable oil (HVO)

Procedure

- Blend the dry Crosslinked high amylose starch (CLHAS) powder with 2.5% w/w CFX loading levels and 0.5% HVO to get solid mass.
- Directly compress the solid mass to obtain 200-mg implants (diameter, 7.1 mm; thickness, 4.8 mm).

PROTOCOL 9.5

Controlled Release Implants

Materials

Preparation of Type A Implants

- Mix the required quantity of Mannitol (15% w/v), sodium citrate (15% w/v), avidin and IL-1beta, mixed in Milli Q water and lyophilise.
- Mill the resulting powder to form fine and uniform particles and blend with silicone composed of a 1:1 ratio of part A, containing the catalyst, and part B, containing the crosslinking agent.
- Then press the mixture through an extruder with a 1.6 mm die, and cured at 37°C for 2–3 days.
- Prepare the Type A implants by cutting the extruded cores into 1 cm lengths.

Preparation of Type B Implants

- Fill a syringe with a kneaded mixture of the powder and silicone and another with silicone only, in a 1:1 ratio of part A and B.

- Co-extrude them under pressure through concentrically arranged nozzles (outer diameter: 1.9 mm), so that the avidin containing silicone formes the inner part and the avidin free silicone the outer.
- Cure the molding at 25–37 °C for 4–5 days and the implants cut into 1 cm lengths (Type B implant).

PROTOCOL 9.6

One-side-coated Insert

Tilisolol hydrochloride

Poly(2-hydroxypropyl methacrylate) (HPM)

Procedure

- Dissolve 5.0 μmol Tilisolol and HPM in methanol on petri dish and dry.
- Hollow out the thin polymer matrix as a disc (diameter: 6 mm, thickness: approximately 0.32 mm).
- Prepare one-side-coated insert by attaching a polypropylene tape on the one side of the disc.

Characterisation

Drug Release

- 'Place the inserts in a beaker containing 30 ml of pH 7.4 at 25 °C.
- Cover the insert with a wire net to prevent movement. Withdraw sample of the solution at periodic intervals.

SUGGESTED READINGS

- Ariel, I.M. (1965) Cancer 18, 1489.
- Baker, R.W. and Lonsdale, H.K. (1974) In: Controlled release of biologically Active Agents, AC Tanquary and RE Lacey (Eds), Pleum, New York, 15.
- Bawa, R. (1993) In: Ophthalmic Drug delivery Systems, AK Mitra (Ed.), Marcel Dekker, New York, 223.
- Clark BF (1973) J. Endocrinol. 58, 555.
- Desevaux C., Lenaerts V., Girard C., Dubreuil P., Journal of Controlled Release (2002) 82, 95.
- Duncan GW (1970) US Patent 3,545,439.
- Fang SM., Lin CS and Lyon V. (1977) J. Pharm. Sci. 66, 1744.
- Heller J (1980) Biomaterials 1, 51.
- Hitoshi Sasaki et al J. Controlled Release (2003) 92, 241.
- Hopfenberg, H. and Hsu, K.C. (1978) Polym. Eng. Sci. 18, 1186.
- Jackanicz, T.M., Nash H.A., Wise D.L. and Gregory, JB (1973) Contraception 8, 227.

- Kelly J., Molyneux, P.D., Smith, S.A. and Smith, S.E. (1989) Br. J. Ophthalmol.. 7, 360.
- Loewit, K. (1971) Contraception 3, 219.
- Maichuk, Y.F. (1976) In: Ocular Therapy, IH Leopold (Ed)., Wiley, New York,1.
- Markou, CP., Brown JE., Puresley MD and Hanson SP (1998) J. Control. Rel. 53,281.
- Tatum, H.J. (1970) US Patent 3,533,406.
- Zaffaroni, A. (1974) US Patent 3,854, 480.

10

Micellar Systems

INTRODUCTION

Colloidal carriers are frequently used to transport and deliver drugs through the body for the reason of protecting the drug against degradation and/or excretion, to prevent adverse side effects of toxic drugs, or to accomplish targeted drug delivery. Examples of such carriers are micro/nanospheres, polymer–drug conjugates, liposomes, and micelles. After micelles were first proposed as drug carriers by Ringsdorf in 1984, they have been emerging as a convenient carrier system (Bader *et al.,* 1984, Nostrum, 2004).

A notable feature of surfactant is their ability to self-associate to form micelles. Since micelles consist of surfactant molecules packing in a space-filling manner numerous parameters of the surfactant solution change at the critical micellisation concentration (CMC). The main driving force for micelle formation in aqueous solution is the effective interaction between the hydrophobic parts of the surfactant molecules, whereas interaction opposing micellisation may include electrostatic repulsive interaction between charged head groups of ionic surfactants, repulsive osmotic interactions between chainlike polar head groups, such as oligoethylene oxide chains, or steric interaction between bulky head groups. In aqueous solution, surfactants aggregate in different forms, such as spherical micelles, worm-like micelle, bilayer fragments, vesicles, or inverted structures (Kunitake, 1992). The way surfactant molecules aggregate is mainly determined by the attraction between the *hydrophobic* tails and electrostatic repulsions of the hydrophilic head groups, which are present in the surfactant molecules.

The type of aggregated surfactant can be determined by the packing parameter P as in the following equation (Israelachvili, *et al.,* 1976):

$$P = \frac{V}{a_o l}$$

in which V is the volume of the hydrocarbon part of the surfactant, l is the chain length of alkyl tail, and a_o is the mean cross-sectional head group surface area. A value of P smaller than 1/3 is indicative of the formation of micelles; P between 1/3 and 1/2 indicates the formation of wormlike micelles, whereas surfactants with P between 1/2 and 1 form vesicles. Inverted structures are formed when P is larger than 1 (Table 10.1).

Table 10.1 *The different types of surfactant aggregation with relation to their shapes (adopted from Israelachvili et al.,1976)*

Effective molecule	Shape of the surfactant	Packing parameter	Types of aggregation	Schematic structure
	Cone	<1/3	Spherical micelles	
	Truncated cone	1/3–1/2	Worm-like micelles	
	Cylinder	1/2–1	Bilayers vesicles	
	Inverted (truncated) cone	>1	Inverted micelles	

Recently, micelles have attracted the attention of researchers as drug delivery systems, because of their nanoscopic size, ability to solubilise hydrophobic drugs and site-specific delivery by passive and active targeting. Amphiphilic block copolymers with biodegradable and/or biocompatible chains have been used to incorporate hydrophobic drugs and target them to their site of action upon parenteral administration. Although much research has been carried out on micelles for parenteral delivery, their potential for oral drug administration remains largely untapped (Allen *et al.,* 1999; Yang, *et al.,* 2000; Rosler, *et al.,* 2001).

Block copolymers that have both hydrophilic and hydrophobic polymer chains in a molecule form micelles, in water, with hydrophilic chains outside and hydrophobic chains inside. The micelles are excellent drug carriers, because they can hold drugs firmly in their inner cores and control the drug release by changing the molecular structure of the inner cores. Protein antigens are mixed with detergent and the detergent slowly removed by dialysis (Moffitt, *et al.,* 1996; Munk, *et al.,* 1998; Tuzar *et al.,* 1993; Allen, *et al.,* 1999; Kataoka, *et al.,* 2001). The antigenic proteins orient with the hydrophilic residues facing outside and the hydrophobic residues inward. Since polyethyleneglycol (PEG) is used for the hydrophilic chains, the immune system does not recognise the micelles as foreign materials. The micelles also have an enhanced permeability and retention effect, useful for tumour targeting. Micelles are also used as non-viral carrier system for gene delivery. Polyethylene glycol-poly-aspartic acid as anion block copolymer mixed with polyethylene glycol-poly L-lysine (PEG-PLL) as cation block copolymer generates PIC with a diameter of dozens of nano-metres in a sharp diameter distribution. Micelles 80 nm in diameter were formed with plasmid DNA and PEG-PLL. Higher expression of luciferase in cultured cells was obtained with the micelles, compared with conventional (Cammas-Marion, T *et al.*, 1999; Kramarenko, *et al.*, 1999).

Although, pH-sensitive micelles may be advantageous for oral drug delivery as they can prevent burst drug release and precipitation upon dilution in the upper part of gastrointestinal tract, upon oral administration, these drug-loaded self-assemblies will remain in the aggregated form at low pH of stomach reducing the drug release. This may benefit the oral bioavailability of incorporated drug by enhancing its transport across the gut wall into the systemic circulation. Moreover, such micelles are advantageous over conventional nanoparticles because of the possibility of forming drug-loaded self-assemblies with an amphiphilic diblock copolymer as sole excipient. Thus, it is of interest to explore the potential of pH-sensitive micelles for improving oral bioavailability of poorly water-soluble drugs (Antonietti, *et al.*, 1997; Kataoka, *et al.*, 1993; Lynn *et al.*, 1999).

FORMATION OF MICELLES

At very low concentration (*e.g.* 10^{-4} M) many surfactants are soluble in water, forming solutions; if they are ionic, like fatty acid soaps or alkyl sulfate detergents, they will be dissociated as weak or strong electrolytes. As the concentration increases, the adsorption at the air in solution interface becomes stronger. Saturation is reached when the molecules are packed close together, with strong lateral interactions occurring between the hydrophobic chains, which tend to stick up out the water (see Figs. 10.1a to c). When the concentration of surfactant solute in the bulk of solution exceeds a limiting value, the formation of micelles is observed, globular or spherical structures, which are, organised aggregates of a large number of molecules. In the micelle, the hydrocarbon tails of the surfactant molecules point toward the centre of the sphere and the polar heads towards the water at its surface. The minimum concentration at which micelles begin to form in the solution is called the critical micellisation concentration (cmc). Micelle size is expressed as the micellar molecular weight or, more generally, as the aggregation number, i.e. the number of monomers making up the micelles. Generally this number is between 20 and 100 for single-chain anionic and cationic surfactants. Large aggregation numbers (> 1000) have been reported for non-ionic micelles, especially when the cloud point is approached. In these structures the hydrophobic portions of the surfactant molecule associate to form regions from which the solvent (water) is effectively excluded. The hydrophilic head groups remain on the outer surface to maximise their interaction with water and, in the case of ionic amphiphiles, with the oppositely charged ions (counterions). A significant fraction of the counterions remains strongly bound to the head groups, so that the lateral repulsive force between those groups is greatly reduced. The precise structure of the micelle depends upon not only the temperature and concentration but also on the molecular structure: the size of head group, the length and number of hydrocarbon chains, the presence of branches, double bonds or aromatic rings, etc are the factors that determine the shape of a micelle. Increasing the concentration of the surfactant leads to the formation of worm-like micelles and, subsequently, liquid crystals (Pramauro *et al.*, 1996).

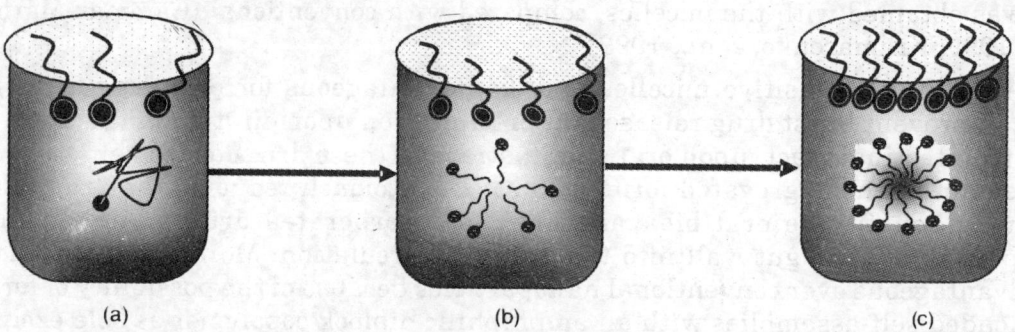

Fig. 10.1: *Formation of Micelles: (a) amphiphilic molecules at low concentration (b) amphiphile at higher concentration ≤ critical miceller concentration (CMC) (c) aggregated amphiphiles at above CMC*

THE CRITICAL MICELLAR CONCENTRATION (CMC)

The cmc is the concentration at which micelles first appear in the solution. Below this critical value, additional surfactant molecules added to the solution remain in monomeric form, and above this, essentially all additional surfactant form micelles. This transition

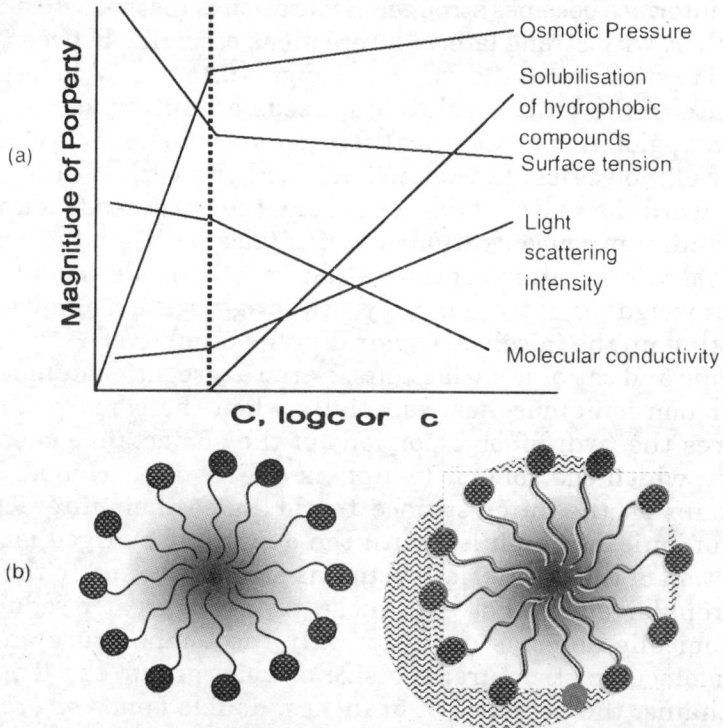

Fig. 10.2 *(a) Schematic illustration of how a range of experimentally accessible parameters changes with the surfactant concentration and how this can be used to detect the cmc. (b) Schematic illustration of spherical micelles*

from pre micellar to micellar solution at the cmc occurs over a narrow concentration range. Surfactant solutions exhibit a striking characteristic when quantitative data of their physical properties are plotted against concentration. Each curve shows a break, an inflection, occurring within a narrow concentration range. Among the properties that have been employed to determine the cmc are surface tension, optical turbidity, electric conductivity, osmotic coefficient, density, sound velocity, diffusion, viscosity, solubilisation, and NMR chemical shifts. Usually, the selected property is plotted against amphiphile concentration; the functions are selected so that the graph resembles as close as possible to a pair of straight lines whose intersection can be taken as the cmc (Lobanov, *et al.,* 1996).

The cmc can be used quantitatively as well as qualitatively to determine the average molecular weight and the net charge (if the amphipathic species are ionic) of the micelle. Factors that are affecting the cmc are the nature of the hydrophilic group and of the counterion, the presence of organic molecules, and the effect of temperature and pressure.

A low cmc indicates that it is thermodynamically favourable for the hydrophobic domain of the surfactant molecule to leave the aqueous solution, which will result in both an excess concentration at the interface and the formation of micelles. This ability to adsorb at an interface and reduce interfacial tension is of great importance for many processes of technological interest, such as emulsification, foaming, wetting, solubilisation, detergency, particle suspensions, and surface coatings (Preston, *et al.,* 1948).

Factors Affecting the Micelles Formation

Given the delicate balance between opposing forces, it is not surprising that surfactant self-assembly is affected by a range of factors, such as the size of the hydrophobic moiety, the nature of the polar head group, the nature of the counterion (charged surfactant), the salt concentration, pH, temperature, and presence of cosolutes. Probably the most universal of all these is the size of the hydrophobic domain(s) in the surfactant molecules. With increasing size of the hydrophobic domain, the hydrophobic interaction increases, thereby promoting micellisation. As a general rule, the cmc decreases a factor of 2 for ionic surfactants and with a factor of 3 for nonionic surfactants on addition of one methylene group to a surfactant alkyl chain. The extent of the decrease also depends on the nature of the hydrophobic domain in terms of both structures (e.g. single chain vs. double chain surfactants) and composition (e.g. fluorinated surfactant), but qualitatively, the same effect is observed for all surfactant.

PROTOCOL: 10.1

Mixed Micells for Drug Solubilisation

Sodium taurocholate
Sodium desoxycholate
Sodium cholate

Oleic acid

Glycerol

Monostearate

Stearic acid

Procedure

- Dissolve the bile salt, 40 mM in phosphate buffer in pH 7.4 with equimolar concentration of lipid in various composition ratios. Add the drug in excess to each system and sonicate at 37°C for 3 min at 10,000 MHz for every 30 sec with 30 sec resting time.

- Filter the solution through a 0.45µm filter and estimate the drug in micellar system.

PROTOCOL: 10.2

Solubilisation of Timolol Maleate in Reversed Micelles

Principle

Reversed micellar systems (RMS) consisting of 30% lecithin in isopropyl myristate (IPM) transform into liquid crystals on the addition of water.

Materials

The lecithin used is phospholipon 90®, which contains at least 90% phosphatidylcholine.

Isopropyl myristate (IPM)

Timolol maleate (TM)

Procedure

- To prepare a reversed micellar stock solution, dissolve 30% lecithin in 70% IPM at a temperature of 60°C while being stirred.

- As TM is insoluble in IPM, the drug needs to be dissolved 1:16 in water before being added to the RMS. By this way the drug is inserted in the resulting liquid crystal. Remove the water at a temperature of 60°C under continuous stirring for 36 h. After this time, a clear yellowish solution without visible particles is obtained (Scheme 10.1).

- The declared percentages of drug concentrations further in the text refer to the 30% stock solution. Characterise the particle size of reverse micelles containing the anti-glaucoma drug TM in varying concentrations by small angle X-ray scattering (SAXS) and photon correlation spectroscopy (PCS).

PCS

Take the PCS measurements with a Zeta Sizer 3 (Malvern, D-Herrenberg). Due to the large viscosity of the stock solution, dilute the systems 1:6 with IPM, resulting in RMS solutions which contain 5% lecithin. Collect the scattering light at an angle of 90°. For each sample the PCS measurements 3–5 times for at least 300 s each. PCS is based on the measurement of intensity changes in the scattering pattern, which are results of the diffusion of particles in the solution. Hence the gained values are the hydrodynamic diameters of the micelles.

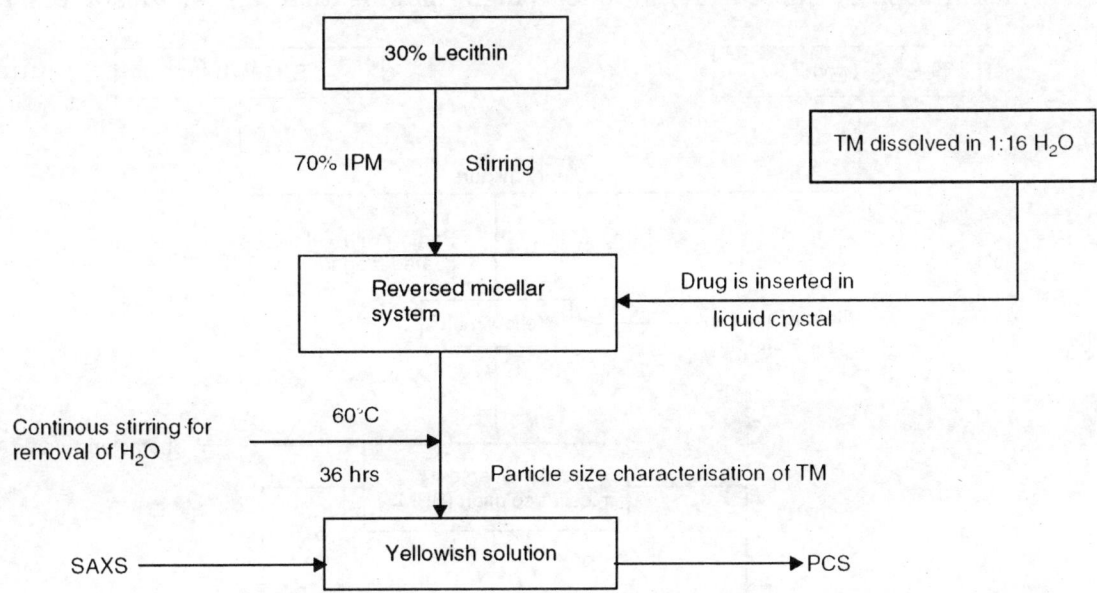

Scheme 10.1: *Solubilisation of timolol maleate in reversed micellar system*

Small Angle X-ray Scattering

There are two methods possible to obtain the micellar size, the Guinier approximation and the electron distance distribution, the latter provides information about the particle shape in addition. The Guinier approximation is based on the fact that the scattering curve shows Gaussian shape at small angles, of which the slope depends on the radius of gyration (Glatter and Kratky, 1982). Assuming a spherical symmetry, it is possible to calculate the micellar diameter.

The electron distance distribution $p(r)$ is obtained from the sample electron density by a Fourier transformation (Glatter, 1977). $p(r)$ describes the number of electron pairs with distance r, which means that the maximum extension of the micellar core is found at the first point of intersection with the abscissa. The primary scattering curve consists of the interference patterns from the scattering light of electron pairs. Therefore only those parts of the micelle can be recognised which differ from the solvent in electron density, in the samples of this study this is the hydrophilic micellar core. To avoid interparticular interferences, dilute the primary 30% samples 1:15 to gain 2% RMS, where no concentration effects are discernible (Muller and Glatter, 1982).

PROTOCOL: 10.3

Solidified Reverse Micellar Solutions

Principle

Liquid RMS enable controlled release of solubilized drugs after their transformation into a lamellar mesophase Moreover, they offer a high solubilisation rate for substances. Drug

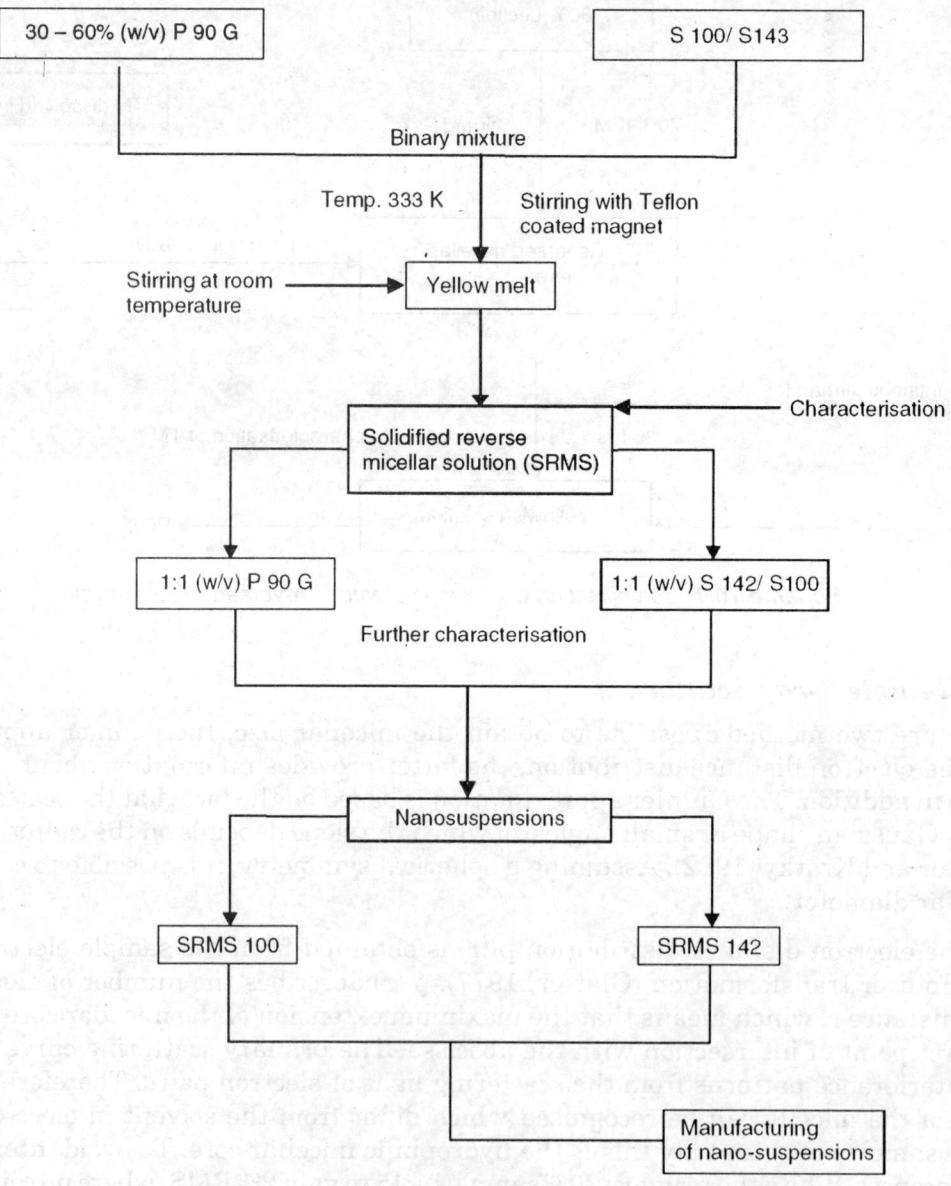

Scheme 10.2: Solidified reverse micellar solution

solubility is also high in the melt of SRMS, hence, SRMS represent a potent carrier for different types of drugs

Solidified reverse micellar solutions, i.e. binary mixtures of 30–60% (w/w) lecithin and two different hard fats were investigated regarding their physicochemical properties and the influence of lecithin on solid lipids.

For production of SRMS-based nanosuspensions, a PS80/SRMS ratio of 1:5 is sufficient for particle size reduction.

Materials

Softisan® 100 (S100) and Softisan® 142 (S142),

Solid triglyceride mixtures with a m.p. of 309 and 316 K,

Phospholipon® 90 G (P90G), a purified soybean lecithin with at least 90% (w/w) Phosphatidylcholine

Phospholipid GmbH

Polysorbate 80 (PS80) and sorbitol

Thimerosal

Pilocarpine base (PB) and hydrochloride (PHCl)

17β-oestradiol-hemihydrate (EST)

Water bidistilled quality.

Procedure

- Stir binary mixture of 30–60% (w/w) P90G and S100 or S142, respectively, with a Teflon coated magnet at a temperature of 333 K until a transparent yellow melt is obtained. Then stir the homogeneous mixture at room temperature until solidification. Solid 1:1 (w/w) mixtures are abbreviated to SRMS100 and SRMS142, respectively, depending on the type of solid lipid (Scheme 10.2).

Manufacturing of Nanosuspensions

Grind the SRMS100 or SRMS142 in melting nitrogen for 15–20 min (seven grinding processes). Disperse the frozen SRMS powder in an aqueous solution of PS80 under stirring for 20 min with a Teflon coated magnet (during screening of emulsifier concentration) or for 90 s at 13,000 rpm with an Ultra-Turrax T25 basic (Ika, Staufen, Germany) to yield a content of 5 or 15% (w/w) of SRMS in the dispersion. After screening of the emulsifier concentration preserve the suspensions with an emulsifier/SRMS ratio of 1:5 (w/w) and preserve the systems with 0.005% (w/w) thimerosal except for those, which were cooled in an ice bath. Pass the coarse suspension through the apparatus first without pressure for two cycles in order to disrupt greater agglomerates and then homogenise discontinuously at a pressure of 1000 or 1500 bar, respectively, for up to 30 cycles. Use the following conditions for temperature equilibration of the homogenisation procedure: 1. No temperature equilibration (room temperature, RT). 2. Immerse just a cooling coil behind the outlet tubing into ice water (CC). 3. Place the whole homogeniser including the cooling coil (see condition 2) an ice bath (ICE). For screening of emulsifier concentration condition 3. After manufacturing, the suspensions should be at a temperature of 278–281 K overnight. Systems produced for thermal and X-ray analysis isotonised with 4.75% (w/w) sorbitol related to the aqueous phase and homogenise continuously for 20 cycles at 1000 (SRMS100 systems) or 1500 bar (SRMS142 systems).

SUGGESTED READINGS

- Allen C., Maysinger D., Eisenberg A., (1999) Nano-engineering block copolymer aggregates for drug delivery, Colloids Surf. 16, 3–27.

- Antonietti M., Goltner C., (1997) Superstructures of functional colloids: chemistry on the nanometer scale, Angew. Chem. Int. Ed. Engl. 36, 910–928.

- Bader H., Ringsdorf H., Schmidt B., (1984) Water soluble polymers in medicine, Angew. Makromol. Chem. 123/124 457–485.

- Cammas-Marion S., Okano T., Kataoka K., (1999) Functional and site-specific macromolecular micelles as high potential drug carriers, Colloids Surf. B 16, 207–215.

- Friedrich, C.C. Mula-Goymann, 2003.

- Glatter and Kratky, 1982.

- Glatter, 1977.

- Israelachvili J. N., Mitchel D. J., and Ninham B. W., J. Chem. Soc., (1976) Faraday Trans. II. 72, 1525, p-p.

- Kataoka K., Harada A., Nagasaki Y., (2001) Block copolymer micelles for drug delivery: design, characterization and biological significance, Adv. Drug Deliv. Rev. 47, 113–131.

- Kataoka K., Kwon G.S., Yokoyama M., Okano T., Sakurai Y., (1993) Block copolymer micelles as vehicles for drug delivery, J. Controlled Release 24, 119–132.

- Kramarenko E Y., Potemkin I.I., Khokhlov A.R., Winkler R.G., Reineker P., (1999). Surface micellar nanopattern formation of adsorbed diblock copolymer system, Macromolecules 32, 3495–3501.

- Kratky and Kratky, 1984

- Kunitake T., (1992) Angew. Chem. 104, 692, p-p.

- Lobanov P. C. T. V. S., Katritzky A. R., Shah D. O., and Karelson M., (1996) Langmuir, 12, 1462, p-p.

- Lynn J. L. and Bory B. H., (1999) In: Concise Encyclopaedia of Chemical Technology, R. Kirk, Ed., Wiley, New York, p. 1949.

- Mackeben S., Miiler-Goymann C. C., (2000). Solubilization of timolol maleate in reversed micellar systems. Measurement of particle size using SAXS and PCS, International Journal of Pharmaceutics 196, 207–210.

- Moffitt M., Khougaz K., Eisenberg A., (1996). Micellization of ionic block copolymers, Acc. Chem. Res. 29, 95–102.

- Muller and Glatter, 1982.

- Munk P., Prochazka K., Tuzar Z., Webber S.E., (1998). Exploiting polymer micelle technology, Chemtech 28, 20–28.

- Nostrum C.F.V. (2004) Advanced Drug Delivery Reviews 56, 9–16.
- Papantoriou, 1995.
- Pramauro E. and Pelizzetti E., (1996) Surfactants in Analytical Chemistry: Applications of Organized Amphiphilic Media, Elsevier, Amsterdam.
- Preston W. C., (1948) J. Phys. Colloid Chem. 52, 84.
- Rigsdorf, 1984.
- Rosler, G.W.M. Vandermeulen, H. A. Klok, (2001). Advanced drug delivery devices via self-assembly of amphiphilic block copolymers, Adv. Drug Deliv. Rev. 53, 95–108.
- Tuzar Z., Kratochvil P., (1993). Micelles of block and graft co polymers in solutions, Surf. Colloid Sci. 15, 1–83.
- Yang L., Alexandridis P., (2000). Physicochemical aspects of drug delivery and release from polymer-based colloids, Curr. Opin. Colloid Interface Sci. 5, 132–143.

Liposomes are concentric bilayered vesicles in which an aqueous core is entirely enclosed by a membranous lipid bilayer mainly composed of natural and synthetic phospholipids. The lipid molecules are usually phospholipids-amphipathic moieties with a hydrophilic head group and two hydrophilic lipidic tails. On the addition of excess water, such lipidic moieties spontaneously originate to give the most thermodynamically stable conformation, in which polar head groups face outwards into the aqueous medium, and the lipidic chains turns inwards to avoid the water phase, giving rise to double layer or bilayer lamellar structures. Both water and lipid soluble drugs can be entrapped into the liposomes. Hydrophilic drugs can be entrapped in the aqueous environment and lipophilic drugs remain within the bilayer region. Liposomes may also contain the glycerol, glycolipids, organic acids, membrane proteins, hydrophilic polymers and other agents depending upon the type of vesicle required.

COMPOSITION OF LIPOSOMES

Phospholipids

Phospholipids are amphipathic (having affinity for both aqueous and polar moieties) molecules as they have a hydrophobic tail and a hydrophilic or polar head. The hydrophobic tail is composed of two fatty acid chains containing 10–24 carbon atoms and 0–6 double bonds in each chain. The polar end of the molecule is mainly phosphoric acid bound to a water-soluble molecule. The hydrophilic and hydrophobic domains/segments within the molecular geometry of amphiphilic lipids orient and self organise in ordered supramolecular structure when confronted with solvents (Lasic, 1988) (Table 11.1).

Cholesterol

Cholesterol is known to have important modulatory effect on the bilayer membrane (Papahadjopoulos *et al.*, 1973; Kirby and Gregoriadis, 1980; New, 1989). Cholesterol acts as "fluidity buffer", since below the phase transition it tends to make the membrane less ordered while above the transition it tends to make the membrane more ordered, thus suppressing the tilts and shift in membrane structure specifically at the phase transition. Though cholesterol it self does not form bilayers, but it can be incorporated into phospholipid membrane in very high concentrations up to 1:1 or even 2:1 molar ratio of cholesterol to PC.

Table 11.1. Compositional lipids of liposomes

Name of lipid	Carbon: unsaturation	Transition temperature	Net charge
DLPC	12:0	−1	0
DMPC	14:0	23	0
DPPC	16:0	41	0
DSPC	18:0	55	0
DOPC	18:1	−20	0
DMPE	14:0	50	0
DPPE	16:0	63	0
DOPE	18:0	−16	0
DMPA.Na	14:0	50	−1.3
DPPA.Na	16:0	67	−1.3
DOPA.Na	18:1	−8	−1.3
DMPG.Na	14:0	23	−1
DPPG.Na	16:0	41	−1
DOPG.Na	18:1	−18	−1
DMPS.Na	14:0	35	−1
DPPS.Na	16:0	54	−1
DOPS.Na	18:1	−11	−1
DPPE-mPEG-2000.Na	16:0	N/A	−1
DPPE-mPEG-5000.Na	16:0	N/A	−1
DPPE-Carboxy PEG-2000.Na	16:0	N/A	−2
DOTAP	18:1	−0	+1

CLASSIFICATION OF LIPOSOMES

Liposomes may be produced by a wide variety of methods. Their nomenclature also depends upon the method of preparation, structural parameters or special functions assigned to them (Table 11.2).

Table 11.2: Classifications of liposomes

1. Based on the size and number of lamellae

Type of vesicles	Unit of Size (nm)
Multilamellar Vesicles (MLVs)	500
Oligolamellar Vesicles (OLVs)	100 to 1000
Unilamellar Vesicles (ULVs)	20 to >1000
Multi Vesicular System (MVs)	>1000
Double liposomes	>1000
Depofoam	>1000

2. Based on the method of liposome preparation

REV	Single/oligomer vesicles made by reverse phase evaporation method
SPLV	Stable plurilamelar vesicles
FATMLV	Frozen and thawed MLV
VET	Vesicle prepared by extrusion technique
DRV	Dehydration-rehydration vesicles

3. Based on composition and application

Conventional liposomes	Natural or negatively charged phospholipid and cholesterol
Fusogenic liposomes	Reconstituted sendai virus envelop
PH sensitive liposomes	Phospholipid such as PE or DOPE with CHEMS or OA
Stealth liposomes	PEGylated long circulatory liposomes
Immuno liposomes	Monoclonal antibody anchored liposomes

Liposomes are manufactured in majority using various procedures in which the water soluble (hydrophilic) materials are entrapped by using aqueous solution of these materials as hydrating fluid or by the addition of drug/drug solution at some stage during the manufacturing of the liposomes (Ostro, 1987; New, 1989; Talsma and Crommelin, 1992). The lipid soluble (lipophilic) materials are solubilised in the organic solution of the constitutive lipid(s) and then evaporated to a dry drug containing lipid film followed by its hydration. These methods involve the loading of the entrapped agents before or during the manufacturing procedure (passive loading) (New, 1989). However, certain types of compounds with ionisable groups, and those, which display both lipid and water solubility, can be introduced into the liposomes after the formation of intact vesicles (remote loading) (Lasic *et al.*, 1995).

Passive Loading Techniques

Passive loading techniques include three different groups of methods working on different principles namely, mechanical dispersion, solvent dispersion and detergent solubilisation.

Mechanical Dispersion Methods of Passive Loading

All methods covered under this category begin with a lipid solution in organic solvent and end up with lipid dispersion in water. The various components are typically combined by co-dissolving the lipids in an organic solvent and the organic solvent is then removed by film deposition under vacuum. When all the solvent is removed, the solid lipid mixture is hydrated using aqueous buffer. The lipids spontaneously swell and hydrate to form liposomes. At this point methods incorporate some diverge processing parameters in various ways to modify their ultimate properties. These post-hydration treatments include vortexing, sonication, freeze thawing and high-pressure extrusion.

Thin Film Hydration Using Hand Shaking (MLVs) and Non-shaking Methods (ULVs)

In these methods, the lipids are casted as stacks of film from their organic solution using rotary flash evaporator under reduced pressure (or by hand shaking) and then the casted film is dispersed in an aqueous medium. Upon hydration the lipids swell and peel off from the wall of the round bottom flask and vesiculate forming multilamellar vesicles (MLVs) (Fig. 11.1). The mechanical energy required for the swelling of lipids and dispersion of casted lipid film is imparted by manual agitation (hand shaking technique) or by exposing the film to a stream of water-saturated nitrogen for 15 min followed by swelling in aqueous medium without shaking (non-shaken vesicles). It is interesting to note that as compared to hand-shaking method (that produces MLVs) the vesicles produced by non-shaken methods are large uni-lamellar vesicles (LUVs). The per cent encapsulation efficiency as high as 30% (at 100 mg lipid ml^{-1}) is achieved.

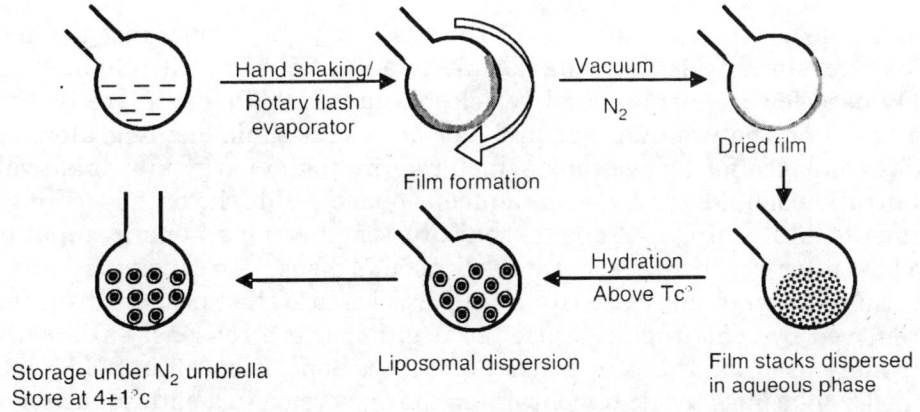

Fig.11.1 Preparation of MLVs by hand shaking technique using rotary flash evaporation

However, large amounts of water-soluble compounds are wasted during swelling as only 10–15% of the total volume gets entrapped. On the other hand, lipid soluble compounds can be encapsulated at 100% efficiency, provided they are present in adequate quantities, and does not disturb structural composition of the membrane.

PROLIPOSOMES

In order to increase the surface area of dried lipid film and to facilitate instantaneous hydration, the lipid is dried over a finely divided particulate support, such as powdered sodium chloride, or sorbitol or other polysaccharides. These dried lipid coated particulates are called proliposomes. Proliposomes form dispersion of MLVs on adding water into them, where support is rapidly dissolved and lipid film hydrates to form MLVs. The size of the carrier influences the size and heterogeneity of the liposomes. This method also overcomes the stability problems of liposomes encountered during their storage as dispersion, dry or frozen form. It is ideally suited for preparations where the material to be entrapped incorporates into lipid membrane. The method is applicable in cases where 100% entrapment of components is not a requirement rather the stability is preferred.

Mechanical Treatment of MLVs

Multilamellar vesicles formed on hydration of dried lipids could be further engineered or modified for their size and other characteristics. A large number of methods are devised to reduce their size and to convert liposomes of the large size range into smaller homogenous vesicles. These include techniques such as microemulsification, extrusion, ultrasonication and use of French pressure cell. A second set of methods is designed to increase the entrapment volume of hydrated lipids, and/or reduce the lamellarity of the vesicles formed. These include procedures such as freeze-drying, freeze thawing, or induction of vesiculation by ions or pH change.

Sonicated Unilamellar Vesicles (SUVs)

At high energy level, the average size of the vesicles is further reduced. This was first achieved on exposure of MLVs to ultrasonic irradiation and still remains the method most widely used for producing small vesicles (Huang, 1969). There are two methods of sonication based on the use of either probe or bath ultrasonic disintegrators (Fig. 11.2). The probe is employed for dispersions, which require high energy in a small volume (e.g. high concentration of lipids, or a viscous aqueous phase) while the bath is more suitable for large volumes of diluted lipids. Probe tip sonicators supply a high-energy input to the lipid dispersion but suffer from overheating of the liposomal dispersion causing lipid degradation. Sonication tips also tend to release titanium particles into the liposome dispersion, which must be removed by centrifugation prior to use. For these reasons, bath sonicators are the most widely used for the preparation of SUVs. Sonication of an MLV dispersion is accomplished by placing a test tube containing the dispersion in a bath sonicator (or placing the tip of the sonicator in the test tube in a probe sonicator) and sonicating for 5–10 min (1,00,000 g) above the Tc° of the constituent lipid. The lipid dispersion should begin to clarify to yield a slightly hazy transparent solution. The haze is due to light scattering induced by residual large particles remaining in the dispersion. These particles can be removed using centrifugation to yield a clear SUV dispersion.

Liposome dispersion after sonication is placed in a clear plastic walled ultracentrifuge tube. The dispersion is generally centrifuged at 100,000g (30 min, 20°C) to sediment titanium particles and large MLVs followed by higher speed centrifugation (1,59,000g for 3–4 h). After spinning the tube is carefully removed from the rotor and with the help of a Pasteur pipette, the liquid with top clear layer is decanted leaving the central opalescent layer (containing small multilamellar vesicles) and a pellet behind. The top layer constitutes pure dispersion of SUVs with varying diameters (in nanometric range) as the size and distribution is influenced by composition and concentration, temperature, sonication time and power, volume and sonication tuning.

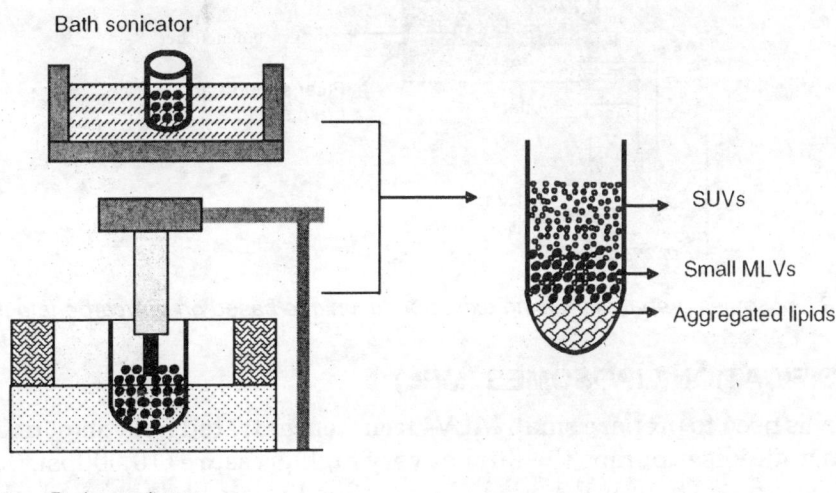

Fig. 11.2. *Preparation of small unilamellar vesicles (SUVs) by bath/probe sonication processes from MLVs*

FRENCH PRESSURE CELL LIPOSOMES

The ultrasonic radiation not only degrades the lipids but also macromolecules and other sensitive compounds, which are to be entrapped in liposomes. One of the first and still very useful methods developed is extrusion of preformed large liposomes in a French press under very high pressure (Barenholtz *et al.,* 1979; Hamilton *et al.,* 1980). This technique yields rather uni- or oligo- lamellar liposomes of intermediate size (30–80nm in diameter depending on the applied pressure). These liposomes are more stable as compared to sonicated liposomes. The method however, suffers some drawbacks, which include high initial cost of the press that consists of an electric hydraulic press and pressure cell (Fig. 11.3).

The sizes of resulting French press extruded liposomes (FPL) are variable, depending on the lipid composition, the temperature and most important, on the pressure. The liposomes prepared by this technique are less likely to suffer from the structural defects and instabilities as observed in sonicated vesicles. Leakage of contents from liposomes prepared using French press is slower and lower than sonicated liposomes. French press has also been used to reduce the heterogeneity of populations of proteoliposomes obtained by detergent dialysis technique.

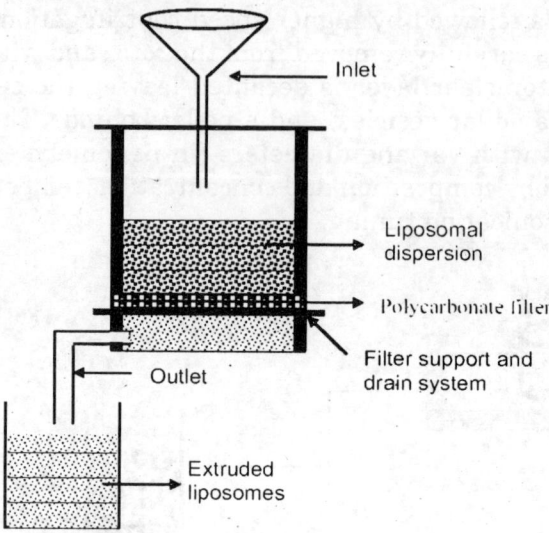

Fig. 11.3 Liposomes preparation using extrusion technique based on polycarbonate filters

MICROEMULSIFICATION LIPOSOMES (MEL)

"Micro fluidiser" is used to prepare small MLVs from concentrated lipid dispersion (Mayhew *et al.,* 1984). Microfluidiser pumps the fluid at very high pressure (10,000psi, 600–700 bar) through a 5–μm orifice. Then, it is forced along defined micro channels, which direct two streams of fluid to collide together at right angles at a very high velocity, thereby affecting an efficient transfer of energy. The lipids can be introduced into the fluidiser, either as a dispersion of large MLVs, or as slurry of unhydrated lipid in an organic medium. The fluid collected can be recycled through the pump and interaction chamber until vesicles of the spherical dimension are obtained.

After a single pass, the size of vesicles is reduced to a size 0.1 and 0.2 μm in diameter. The exact size distribution however depends on the nature of the components of the membrane and hydration medium. The presence of negative lipids tends to decrease their size, while increasing cholesterol concentration gives larger liposomes. In addition to the high rate of production, this method has the advantage of being able to process samples with a very high proportion of lipids (20% or more by weight). This process is efficient for encapsulation of water-soluble materials. Percentage capture values up to 70% have been reported, starting with lipid concentration of approximately 200mg/ml.

Vesicles Prepared by Extrusion Techniques (VETs)

In membrane extrusion method, the size of liposomes is reduced by gently passing them through membrane filter of defined pore size (Hope *et al.,* 1985). This can be achieved at much lower pressure (<100psi.) than required in case of French pressure cell.

The membrane extrusion technique can be used to process LUVs as well as MLVs. In this process, the vesicle contents are exchanged with the dispersion medium during breaking and resealing of phospholipid bilayers as they pass through the polycarbonate membrane. In order to achieve high entrapment, the water-soluble compounds should be present in suspending medium during the extrusion process. The material, which is not entrapped, can be removed subsequently. The liposomes produced by this technique have been termed LUVETs. The 30% capture volume can be obtained using high lipid concentration (300 mM PC). The trapped volume in this process is 1–2 litre/mol of lipids.

Extrusion technique is the most widely used method for SUV and LUV production for *in vitro* and *in vivo* studies. It is due to their ease of production, readily selectable vesicle diameter (dictated by the nominal pore size of the track-etch membranes used for extrusion, typically between 50–120 nm for *in vivo* experiments), batch-to-batch reproducibility, and freedom from solvent and/or surfactant contamination.

Dried-reconstituted Vesicles (DRVs)

This method starts with freeze drying of a dispersion of empty SUVs and then rehydrating it with the aqueous fluid containing the material to be entrapped (Kirby and Gregoriadis, 1984). This leads to a dispersion of solid lipids in finely subdivided form. However, the step of freeze-drying is used to freeze and lyophilize a preformed SUVs dispersion rather than to dry the lipids from an organic solution (as in the case of other methods). This leads to an organized membrane structure as compared to random matrix structure, which on addition of water (one tenth the volume of the original SUVs) can rehydrate, fuse and reseal to form vesicles with a high capture efficiency (Fig. 11.4). The water-soluble materials to be entrapped are added to the dispersion of empty SUVs and they are dried together, so the material for inclusion is present in the dried precursor lipid before the final step of addition of aqueous medium.

Liposomes obtained by this method are usually uni- or oligo- lamellar of the order of 1.0 μm or less in diameter. Entrapment yield can vary, but 40% is fairly standard compared with 2–10% for MLVs prepared by hand-shaking method.

Various advantages proposed for the DRV technique are high entrapment of water soluble component and the use of mild conditions for the preparation and loading of bioactives (Gregoriadis *et al.*, 1990). However, this method is suitable only for unilamellar vesicles, i.e. the liposomes to be freeze-dried should be in the form of vesicles as the incorporation rates with multilamellar vesicles are quite low.

Freeze Thaw Sonication (FTS) Method

The FTS method is an extension of classical DRV method (Mayer *et al.*, 1985, Ohsawa *et al.*, 1985). The method is based upon freezing of a unilamellar (mainly SUV) dispersion and then thawing by standing at room temperature for 15 min (cf. DRV method where the freeze-dried lipids are rehydrated with aqueous buffer) and finally subjecting to a brief sonication cycle. Thus the process ruptures and re-fuses SUVs during which the solute equilibrates between inside and outside, and the liposomes themselves fuse and increase markedly in size.

The entrapment volume can be up to 30% of the total volume of the dispersion (10 μl/mg phospholipids). Similar to DRV, the starting preparation of empty liposomes is made by sonication and after thawing, the liposomes are subjected to brief sonication again (Fig. 11.4). The second step sonication considerably reduces the permeability of the liposome membrane, perhaps by accelerating the rate at which packing defects are eliminated. In order to prepare giant vesicles of diameter between 10 and 50 μm, the freeze thaw technique has been modified to incorporate a dialysis step against hypo-osmolar buffer in place of second step sonication (Oku and MacDonald, 1983). In this case, SUVs (prior to freeze-thawing step) are first mixed with salt solution followed by freeze thawing several times. During subsequent dialysis, the large vesicles formed by freeze thawing swell and rupture as a result of osmotic lyses whereupon they fuse with each other to yield a large number of giant vesicles.

The inclusion of some negatively charged lipids gives yet higher trapped volume (20 μl/mg as compared to 10 μl/mg for neutral phospholipids). The FTS method has several disadvantages compared to DRVs in regard to encapsulation efficiency. Since the presence of charge is required for the formation of ice crystals to aid in the rupture/fusion process, neutral liposomes cannot be subjected to freezing and thawing method. For similar reasons sucrose (a cryo-protectant), divalent metal ions (which can neutralise the surface charge) and high ionic strength salt solutions cannot be entrapped efficiently. Nevertheless, the method is simple, rapid and mild for entrapped solutes, and results in a high proportion of large unilamellar vesicles formation, which are useful for study of membrane transport phenomenon.

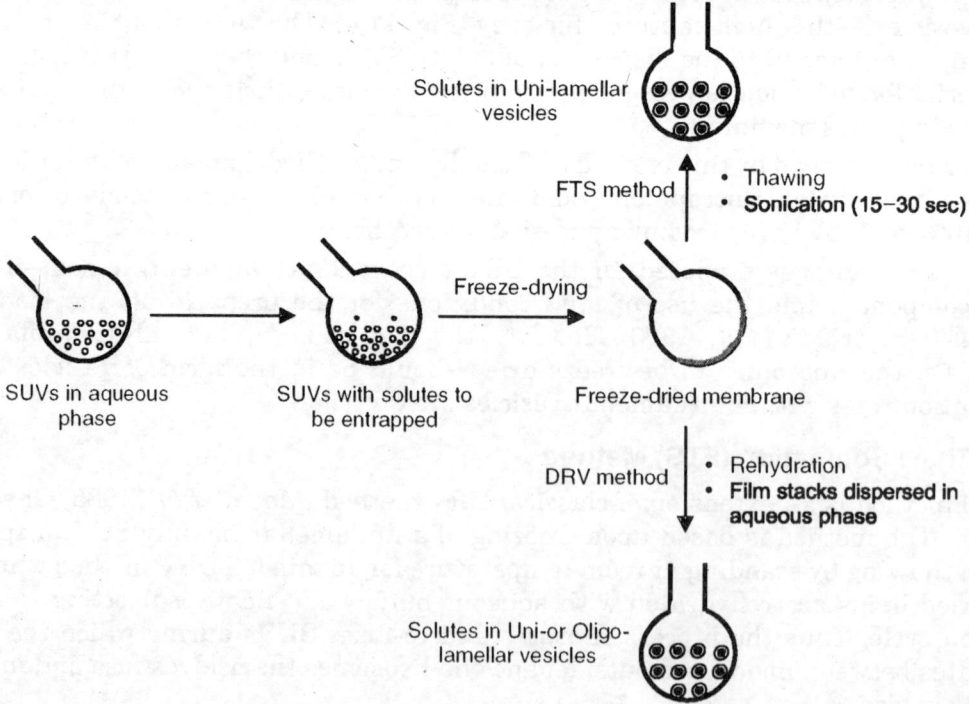

Fig.11. 4 *Preparation of dried-reconstituted vesicles (DRVS). membrane restructures enclosing a proportion of solute, which was originally present in extra-liposomal medium*

Liposomes from Preformed Vesicles

Several methods of liposome preparation use preformed vesicles and are intended mostly to increase the encapsulation efficiency of the preformed vesicles by using fusion of SUV's by fusogenic agents or by change in the microenvironment of the system.

pH Induced Vesiculation

This method is used to transform MLVs to LUVs using a change in the pH of the dispersion thus avoiding the use of sonication or high-pressure application. The process is an electrostatic event and termed "pH induced vesiculation". The transient change in pH brings about an increase in the surface charge density of the lipid bilayer, which induces spontaneous vesiculation (Hauser and Gains, 1982).

The preformed MLVs (prepared using hand shaking followed by freeze-thawing and having a pH of 2.5 – 3.0) are exposed to high pH (1M NaOH) to bring the pH 11.0. The period of exposure of liposomes to high pH should be less than 2 min. The exposure time should not be long enough to cause any detectable degradation of the phospholipid. Then the pH is reduced by addition of 0.1M HCl until a value of pH 7.5 is achieved.

Phospholipid dispersion with similar properties is obtained if concentrated NaOH solution is added directly to the dry lipid film to give dispersion without freeze thawing. The resultant dispersion is consisted of a relatively homogenous population of SUVs with an average outer diameter of 20 – 60 nm.

Calcium Induced Fusion

Calcium induced fusion method is principally based upon the concept of aggregation and fusion of acid phospholipid vesicles in the presence of calcium (Papahadjopoulos *et al.*, 1975).

In this method, SUVs are formed using sonication buffer (NaCl 0.385g, histidine 31.0 mg, Tris-base 24.2 mg, EDTA 3.72 mg, water 100 mL, pH 7.4) as the hydrating fluid. The large liposomes and lipid particles are removed by centrifugation at 100,000g. Equimolar proportion of calcium solution ($CaCl_2$) is added to phospholipids in the supernatant resulting in the formation of a white flocculent precipitate. It is incubated for 60 min at 37°C and the precipitate (pellet) is separated by spinning the contents at 3000g for 20 min at room temperature where the supernatant is discarded. The pellet is resuspended in a buffered saline containing the material to be entrapped, and incubated at 37°C for 10 min. The addition of EDTA to the pellet suspension with mixing, results in the formation of a cloudy dispersion, which clears rapidly and incubated for 15 min at 37 °C and further 15 min at room temperature. Finally, the Ca-EDTA complex is removed by dialysing the dispersion overnight against a litre of phosphate saline buffer.

The method has the advantage that it does not expose lipids or entrapped materials to deleterious chemical or physical conditions. Its principal drawback is the requirement of acidic phospholipids and the presence of calcium inside the liposomes, even after dialysis.

Cochleate Method

Cochleates are formed when small unilamellar vesicles made from negatively charged lipids mainly phosphatidylserine (PS) fuse into cylindrical rolls, termed as cochleate cylinders, upon addition of Ca^{++} ions. Subsequent removal of Ca^{++} by EDTA or by ion exchange or precipitation, results in the formation of large unilamellar vesicles. Concentration of Ca^{++} required to reproduce such effects vary for the nature of lipids used, for PS, it should be slightly above the half of the lipid concentration, while cardiolipin (CL) and especially PG require higher averages.

Solvent Dispersion Methods for Passive Loading

In solvent dispersion method, lipids are first dissolved in an organic solution, which is then brought into contact with an aqueous phase containing materials to be entrapped within the liposomes. The lipids align themselves at the interface of organic and aqueous phase forming monolayer of phospholipids, which forms the half of the bilayer of the liposome. Methods employing solvent dispersion can be categorised on the basis of the miscibility of the organic solvent and aqueous solution. These include the conditions where the organic solvent is miscible with the aqueous phase; the organic solvent is immiscible with the aqueous phase, the latter being in excess; and the cases where the organic solvent is in excess, and immiscible with the aqueous phase.

Ethanol Injection

This method has been reported as one of the alternatives used for the preparation of SUVs without sonication (Batzri and Korn, 1973). An ethanol solution of lipids is injected rapidly through a fine needle into an excess of saline or other aqueous medium. The rate of the injection is usually sufficient to achieve complete mixing, so that the ethanol is diluted almost instantaneously in water, and phospholipid molecules are dispersed evenly throughout the medium (Fig. 11.5). This procedure yields a high proportion of SUVs (~25 nm), although lipid aggregates and larger vesicles may form if the mixing is not thorough enough. This method is extremely simple and has low risk of degradation of sensitive lipids. The vesicles of 100 nm size may be obtained by little modification in this method, i.e. by varying the concentration of lipid in ethanol or by changing the rate of injection of ethanol solution in preheated aqueous solution.

The major shortcoming of the method is the limitation of the solubility of lipids in ethanol and volume of ethanol that can be introduced into medium (7.5% v/v maximum), which in turn limits quantity of lipid dispersed, so that resulting liposomal dispersion gets diluted. Another drawback is difficulty to remove residual ethanol from phospholipid membrane.

Ether Injection

Ether injection method is similar to the ethanol injection method however; it contrasts markedly with ethanol injection in many respects. It involves injecting the immiscible organic solution very slowly into an aqueous phase through a narrow needle at the temperature of vapourising the organic solvent (Fig. 11.5). This method may also treat sensitive lipids very gently. It has little risk of causing oxidative degradation provided ether is free from peroxides. The disadvantages of the technique are the long time taken to produce a batch of liposomes and a careful control needed for introduction of the lipid solution, requiring a mechanically operated pump. If substances are degraded at elevated temperature (60 °C), then the fluorinated hydrocarbons (Freons) may be used instead of ether. The efficiency of encapsulation is relatively low, although the captured volume per mole of lipid remains high, 8–17 l/mol.

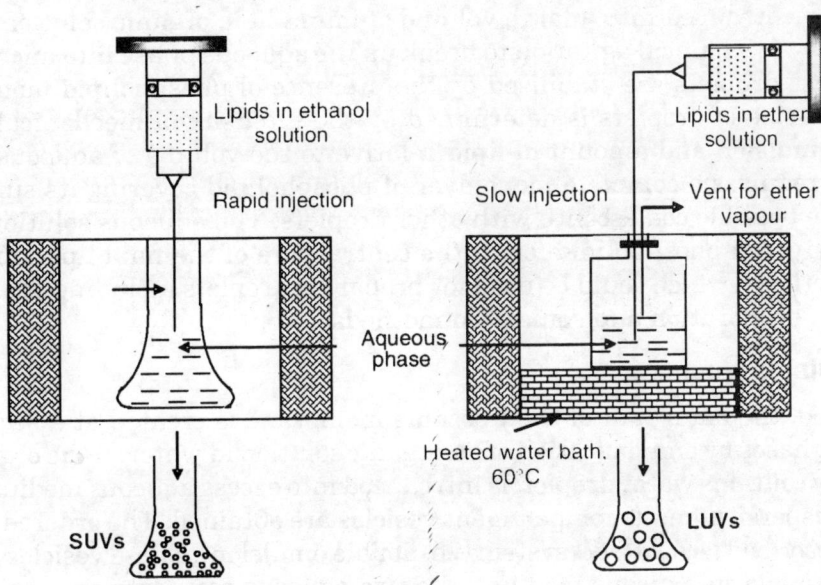

Fig.11.5 *Principle of vesicle formation by solvent dispersion methods in which two phases (aqueous and organic) are miscible with each other and form different types of vesicles*

Rapid Solvent Exchange Vesicles (RSEVs)

Rapid solvent exchange method has been a recent addition to the field of methodology of liposome preparation (Buboltz and Feigenson, 1999). In this method principally, the lipid mixture is quickly transferred between an essentially pure solvent environment and a pure aqueous environment. This method is specifically designed to form compositionally homogenous dispersion by sudden precipitation of a lipid mixture in an aqueous buffer. Phospholipid/cholesterol dispersion turns to be free of artifactual crystals when prepared by rapid solvent exchange method.

The method involves passing the organic solution of the lipids through the orifice of blue-tipped syringe (injection needle) under the vacuum into a tube containing aqueous buffer. The tube is mounted on the vortexer. Bulk solvent vapourises and is removed within seconds before coming in contact with aqueous environment, while the lipid mixture rapidly precipitates in aqueous buffer. Since the method is devised specifically for the fast and efficient removal of organic solvent, it does not require a highly volatile solvent. RSEV liposomes require not more than a minute for preparation and manifest high entrapment volumes with a high fraction of external surface area with no evidence of artifactual demixing as observed with conventional solvent dispersion methods.

De-emulsification Methods

This method requires two steps for the preparation of liposomes, first the inner leaflet of the bilayer, then the outer half. The common feature of this method is the formation of "water in oil" emulsion by introduction of a small quantity of aqueous medium containing material to be entrapped into a large volume of immiscible organic solution of lipid. This was followed by mechanical agitation to break up the aqueous phase into microscopic water droplets. These droplets are stabilised by the presence of phospholipid monolayer at the interface. The size of droplets is determined by the intensity of mechanical energy used to form the emulsion and amount of lipid relative to the volume of aqueous phase, since each droplet requires a complete monolayer of phospholipid covering its surface in order to prevent the possible coalescence with other droplets. The aqueous solution surrounded by the monolayer of phospholipid forms the central core of the final liposome. There are number of methods, which could be used for preparing droplets including double emulsion, reverse phase evaporation and sonication methods.

Double Emulsion Vesicles

In this method, the outer half of the liposome membrane is created at a second interface between two phases by emulsification of an organic solution in water. If the organic solution, which already contains water droplet, is introduced into excess aqueous medium followed by mechanical dispersion, multi compartment vesicles are obtained. The ordered dispersion so obtained is described as a W/O/W system (i.e. double emulsion). These vesicles with aqueous core are suspended in aqueous medium, the two aqueous compartments being separated from each other by a pair of phospholipid monolayers whose hydrophobic surfaces face each other across a thin film of organic solvent. Removal of this solvent clearly results in an intermediate sized unilamellar vesicle. The theoretical entrapment may reach up to 90%.

The double emulsion is prepared by rapidly injecting the dispersion of micro-droplets into hot aqueous solution of Tris-buffer with the help of 22-gauge hypodermic needle under vigorous stirring. The organic solvent is evaporated using strong jet of nitrogen thus forming double emulsion. The last traces of organic solvent are removed by evaporation and finally the volume is adjusted by adding extra-distilled water and then the product is centrifuged at 20 °C for 30 min at 37,000g to remove lipid aggregates.

Reverse Phase Evaporation Vesicles

The essential feature of this method, established by Szoka and Papahadjopoulos (1978), is the removal of solvent from an emulsion by evaporation. The droplets are formed by bath sonication of mixture of the two phases, then the emulsion is dried down to a semisolid gel in a rotary evaporator under reduced pressure. At this stage, the monolayers of phospholipids surrounding each water compartment are closely opposed by each other and in some cases probably already form part of a bilayer membrane separating adjacent compartments. The next step is to bring about the collapse of a certain proportion of the water droplets by vigorous mechanical shaking using a vortex mixer. In these circumstances, the lipid monolayer, which enclosed the collapsed vesicle, is contributed to adjacent intact vesicle to form the outer leaflet of the bilayer of a large unilamellar liposome. The aqueous content of the collapsed droplet provides the medium required for dispersion of these newly formed liposomes. After conversion of the gel into a homogenous free flowing fluid, the dispersion is dialysed to remove the last traces of solvent. The vesicles formed are unilamellar and have an average diameter of 0.5 μm. The encapsulation per centage is found to be nearly 50%.

Stable Plurilamellar Vesicles (SPLVs)

The method of plurilamellar vesicle formation involves preparation of water-in-organic phase dispersion with an excess of lipid followed by drying under continued bath sonication with an intermittent stream of nitrogen. The redistribution and equilibration of aqueous solvent and solute occurs in between the various bilayers in each plurilamellar vesicle. The internal structure of SPLVs is different from that of MLV-REVs, in that they lack a large aqueous core, the majority of the entrapped aqueous medium being located in the compartment in between adjacent lamellae. The per cent entrapment normally ranges around 30% (compared with > 60% for MLV-REVs).

Detergent Depletion (Removal) Methods of Passive Loading

In these methods, the phospholipids are brought into intimate contact with the aqueous phase via detergents, which associate with phospholipid molecules and serve to screen the hydrophobic portions of the molecule from water. The structures formed as a result of this association are known as micelles, and can be composed of several hundreds of component molecules. Their shape and size depend on chemical nature of the detergent, the concentration and other lipids involved. The concentration of detergent in water at which micelles just start to form is known as the 'critical micelle concentration' (CMC). Below the CMC, the detergent molecules exist entirely in free solution. As detergent is dissolved in water in concentration higher than the CMC, micelles form in more and more numbers, while the concentration of detergent in the free form remains essentially the same as it is at the CMC. Micelles containing other participating components in addition to the detergent (or composed of two or more detergents) in their formation are known as "mixed micelles".

As a general rule, membrane-solubilising detergents have a higher affinity for phospholipid membranes than for the pure detergent micelles. Thus, as detergent is added in increasing amounts to the membrane preparation, more and more detergent gets incorporated into the bilayer, until a point is reached where a transition from the lamellar to the spherical micellar phase configuration takes place. As the detergent concentration increases further, the micelles are reduced in size until they become saturated with detergent, whereupon the concentration of free molecules equals the CMC and simple detergent micelles are formed. It is usually found that a high concentration is advantageous for solubilising membrane phospholipids although one might expect the converse, since a high affinity for lipid membranes should be reflected by a low CMC. A three-stage model of the interaction for detergents with the lipid bilayers with increasing detergent/lipid ratio was proposed.

- At low (sublytic) concentrations detergent equilibrates between vesicular lipid and water phase (stage-I). At this stage, mean vesicle size increases and functional properties of the bilayer change.

- After reaching a critical detergent concentration ('saturation' of the bilayers), membrane structure tends to be unstable and transforms gradually into micelles (stage-II). In this stage detergent saturated bilayers coexist with lipid-saturated micelles.
- At stage-III, all lipid exists in mixed micelle form.

Invariably in all methods, which employ detergent in the preparation of liposomes, the basic feature is to remove the detergent from preformed mixed micelles containing phospholipid, whereupon unilamellar vesicles form spontaneously. The detergent methods are not very efficient in terms of percentage entrapment values. On the other hand, they are certainly the best methods for preparing liposomes with lipophilic proteins inserted into the membranes. Another special feature is the ability to vary size of the liposomes by precise control of the conditions of detergent removal. Three methods are applied for the removal of detergent and transition of mixed micelles to concentric bilayered form. These include, dialysis, column chromatography and the use of biobeads.

Dialysis

In contrast to phospholipids, detergents are highly soluble in both aqueous and organic media and there is equilibrium between the detergent molecules in the water phase, and in the lipid environment of the micelle. The critical micelle concentration can give an indication to the position of this equilibrium. Upon lowering the concentration of detergent in the bulk aqueous phase, the molecules of detergent can be removed from mixed micelle by dialysis. A higher CMC indicates that the equilibrium is strongly shifted towards the bulk solution, so that removal from the mixed membrane by dialysis becomes relatively easy.

Detergents commonly used for this purpose exhibit reasonably high CMC (~10–20 mM) so that their removal is facilitated. They include the bile salts sodium cholate and sodium deoxycholate and synthetic detergents such as octylglucoside. The treatment of egg PC with a 2:1 molar ratio of sodium cholate followed by dialysis results in the formation of vesicles (~100 nm). A commercial version of the dialysis system is available under the trade name LIPOREP^{TM}.

Column Chromatography

Phospholipids in the form of either sonicated vesicles or as a dry film, at a molar ratio of 2:1 with deoxy-cholate form unilamellar vesicles of 100 nm on removal of deoxycholate by column chromatography (Enoch and Strittmatter, 1976). This could be achieved by passing the dispersion over a Sephadex G-25 column pre-saturated with constitutive lipids and pre- equilibrated with hydrating buffer.

Detergent Adsorption using Bio-beads

Detergent (non-ionic)/phospholipid mixtures can form large unilamellar vesicles upon removal of non-ionic detergent (Triton X-100) using appropriate adsorbents for the detergent (Levy *et al.*, 1990). The ability of Bio-beads SM-2, to adsorb Triton X-100 selectively and rapidly, makes them a suitable candidate for LUV preparation by detergent solubilisation method. On hydrating the casted lipid film with 0.5–1.0 % Triton X-100, washed Bio-beads are added to the dispersion (0.3 g wet Bio-beads per ml of dispersion) and rocked for about 2 h at 4±1°C.

REMOTE (ACTIVE) LOADING

A general scheme describing various types of liposomes is presented with their formation methodology. The utilisation of liposomes as drug delivery systems is stimulated with the advancement of efficient encapsulation procedures. The membrane from lipid bilayer is in general impermeable to ions and larger hydrophilic molecules. Ions transport can be regulated by the ionophores while permeation of neutral and weakly hydrophobic molecules can be controlled by concentration gradients. Some weak acids or bases however, can be transported through the membrane due to various transmembrane gradients, such as electrical, ionic (pH) or specific salt (chemical potential) gradients. Several methods exist for improved loading of the drugs, including remote (active) loading methods, which load drug molecules into preformed liposomes using pH gradients and potential difference across liposomal membranes. A concentration difference in proton concentration across the membrane of liposomes can drive the loading of amphipathic molecules. Active loading methods have the following advantages over passive encapsulation techniques:

- High encapsulation efficiency and capacity
- Reduced leakage of the encapsulated compounds
- "Bed side' loading of drugs thus limiting loss of retention of drugs by diffusion, or chemical degradation during storage
- Flexibility for the use of constitutive lipids, as drug is loaded after the formation of carrier units
- Avoidance of biologically active compounds during preparation steps in the dispersion thus reducing safety hazards
- The transmembrane pH gradient can be developed using various methods depending upon the nature of the drug to be encapsulated
- For amphipathic weak bases by remote loading procedures such as using a proton gradient or an ammonium sulphate gradient
- For amphipathic weak acids by remote loading procedures using a calcium acetate gradient.

Weak amphipathic bases accumulate in the aqueous phase of lipid vesicles in response to a difference in pH between the inside and outside of the liposomes (pH_{in} and pH_{out}). The pH gradient is created by preparing liposomes with a low pH inside, followed by the addition of the base to the extraliposomal medium. Usually, a two-step process generates this pH imbalance and remote loading: first, the vesicles are prepared in a low pH solution, thus generating a low-pH within the liposomal interiors, followed by the addition of the base to the extraliposomal medium. Basic compounds, carrying amino groups are relatively lipophilic at high pH and hydrophilic at low pH. In a two-chambered aqueous system separated by membrane liposomes, accumulation occurs at the low pH side, under dynamic equilibrium conditions. Thus the unprotonated form of basic drug can diffuse through the bilayer. At the low-pH side the molecules are predominantly protonated, which lowers the concentration of the drug in the unprotonated form, and thus promote the diffusion of more drug molecules at the low-pH side of the bilayer. The second step involves the exchange of external medium by gel-exclusion chromatography with a neutral solution. Weak bases like doxorubicin, adriamycin and vincristine which co-exist in aqueous solutions in neutral and charged forms have been successfully loaded into preformed liposomes via the pH gradient method. Similarly, short modified peptides and insulin (FITC-insulin) were also loaded successfully in large unilamellar vesicles through pH gradients (inside acidic). Recently, the approach has been further modified using transmembrane differences in salt concentrations, such as ammonium sulphate gradient method or calcium acetate gradient method. This technique takes advantage of the large differences in the permeability coefficients across lipid bilayer of the sulphate anion (P<10–12 cm/s) and of the ammonia molecule (P=0.13 cm/s), generated by the dissociation of the ammonium cation. This results into an increase in liposomal internal pH. In addition, the sulphate salt of this molecule has a very low solubility and aggregates inside the liposomes, resulting in even larger encapsulation efficiencies and the stabilisation of the loading.

Table 11.3: *Properties of various vesicular systems*

Properties	Large unilamellar vesicles (LUVs)	Small unilamellar vesicles (SUVs)	Multilamellar vesicles (MLVs)
Entrapped volume	Higher	Lower	Medium (<LUVs)
Thermodynamic Stability	Less stable	Unstable	Stable
Energy requirement	Less	Higher	Less
RES Uptake	Rapid clearance	Long circulating higher T1/2	Rapid clearance (less T1/2)
Preparation Methods	Reverse phase evaporation method ether injection double emulsion detergent dialysis	Solvent injection french pressure cell method probe sonication	Thin film hydration method

CHARACTERISATION OF LIPOSOMES

Liposomal formulations after their formulation and processing for a specified purpose are characterised to ensure their predictable *in vitro* and *in vivo* performances (Ostro, 1987, New 1989, Weiner *et al.,* 1989). The liposomes produced by different techniques may have different physicochemical characteristics. These differences do have an impact on their behaviour *in vivo* (disposition) and *in vitro* (e.g. sterilisation and shelf life) (Table 11.3). The characterisation parameters for the purpose of evaluation could be classified into three broad categories, which include physical, chemical and biological parameters. Physical characterisation evaluates various parameters, including size, shape, surface features, lamellarity, phase behaviour and drug release profile. Chemical characterisation includes those studies, which establish the purity and potency of various liposomal constituents. Biological characterisation parameters are helpful in establishing the safety and suitability of the formulations for the *in vivo* use or for therapeutic applications.

Some of the parameters characterized in liposome product development are size and size

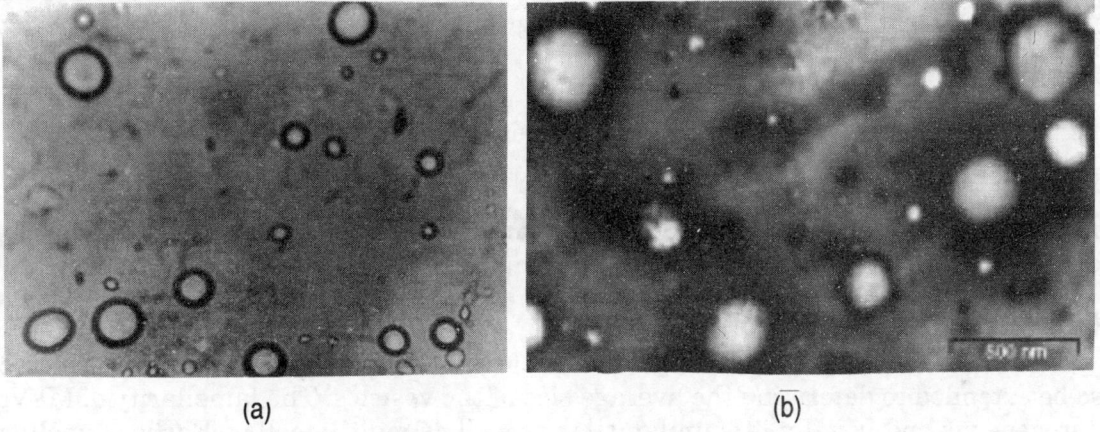

(a)   (b)

Fig 11.6: Optical photomicrographs (a) and TEM (b) images of liposomes

distribution, surface topology, encapsulation efficiency, capture volume, lamellarity and *in vitro* drug release profile (Talsma and Crommelin, 1992; Barenholz and Cromellin, 1994).

Size

Various techniques are used to determine the size and size distribution of liposomes.

Light scattering technique: It is based on a dynamic laser light scattering. It is generally used for monodisperse phase. The method relies on algorithms to determine particle size.

Optical Microscopy

This method is used for the determination of gross size distribution of large vesicles preparation such as MLVs. Various methods included are bright field microscopy phase contrast and fluorescent microscopy.

Electron Microscopy

Electron microscopy is used to determine size of vesicles, but this method is especially useful for observing the morphological structure of liposomes. Various types of electron microscopy used are (Fig. 11.6):

Freeze Fracture Electron Microscopy

Freeze etched and fracture electron microscopy is suitable for the measurement of a small vesicle-diameters as the effects of random cleavage that can occur through and around the vesicle, can be compensated for each step. For large size vesicles, freeze fracture techniques can be useful for examining the morphological changes that occur in the bilayer surface as the PL pass through the gel liquid crystalline transition.

Negative Stain Electron Microscopy

Negative stain electron microscopy is also a useful method, which is simple to perform and require only limited equipment. It can provide important information whether the liposomes produced are multi or unilamellar. This technique visualises relatively transparent liposomes as bright areas against a dark background (Lopez *et al.*, 1983).

Transmission Electron Microscopy

This method is mostly used for visualising uniformity and shape of vesicles.

Scanning Electron Microscopy

This method is less frequently used due to sample distortion during preparation, as it requires dehydration of sample prior to examination.

Vesicle Shape and Lamellarity

Vesicle shape can be assessed using various electron microscopic techniques, which can also be extended to determine the average size of the vesicles. The lamellarity of MLVs is heterogeneous and usually it is unilamellar as well as multilamellar. Earlier lamellarity calculations were based on techniques that detected proportion of lipids exposed to the external medium (New, 1989). This led to approximately half of the total lipid in LUVs and an even smaller fraction in MLVs. Labelling or binding studies are now employed to determine the proportion of outer monolayer lipid. However, lamellarity of the vesicles, i.e. the number of bilayers present in the liposomes is determined using Freeze-fracture electron microscopy (Ostro, 1987) and ^{31}P nuclear magnetic resonance analysis (Hope *et al.*, 1985).

Freeze-fracture and freeze-etch Electron Microscopy

Freeze-fracture electron microscopy can be used not only to assess the shape and lamellarity but also the surface morphology (topology) of the liposomes (Mandal and Downing, 1993). In this technique the fracture plane passes through the vesicles, which are randomly positioned in the frozen state. Thus, the fracture plane may not necessarily pass through the mid-plane and thus non-mid plane fracture may result in erroneous readings. The observed distribution profile thus depends on the distance of vesicle centre from the plane of fracture. Furthermore, heterogenous populations require a careful monitoring before analysing the final results. However, quick-freeze and deep etching techniques give much better lamellarity evaluation (Nakata *et al.*, 1990). It is reported that ethching of freeze-fractured specimen can provide information about fractures of vesicles that are unilamellar in a given population. After 5 min of etching, cross-fractured vesicles are clearly seen and the number of lamellae can readily be determined.

^{31}P Nuclear Magnetic Resonance Analysis

^{31}P nuclear magnetic resonance analysis has been one of the most accurate and straightforward techniques that determine the lamellarity of liposomes (Arica *et al.,* 1995). The technique exploits ^{31}P nuclear magnetic resonance (NMR) to monitor the phospholipid phosphorus signal intensity. In particular, adding an impermeable paramagnetic shift or nonpermeable broadening agent (such as Mn^{++}) to the external medium will decrease the intensity of the initial ^{31}P NMR signal by an amount proportional to the fraction of lipid exposed to the external medium. Manganese ions interact with the outer leaflet of the outermost bilayer. Thus, a 50% reduction in NMR signal intensity indicates a unilamellar whereas subsequent reductions indicate a multilamellar vesicular preparation.

Vesicle Size and Size Distribution

The average vesicle size and size distribution are important parameters as far as *in vitro* characterisation of the liposomal product is concerned. This is because they influence the physicochemical properties and biological fate of the liposomes and/or entrapped materials after *in vivo* administration. Various techniques are described in the literature for the determination of size and size distribution. These include light microscopy, fluorescent microscopy (if a fluorescent probe is included in either lipid or aqueous domain), electron microscopy (specially transmission electron microscopy and freeze-fracture microscopy), laser light scattering, photon correlation spectroscopy, field flow fractionation, gel permeation and gel exclusion and zetasizer. Most of the methods used in the size, shape and distribution analysis can be grouped into various categories, namely microscopic, diffraction and scattering and hydrodynamic techniques.

MICROSCOPIC TECHNIQUES
Optical Microscopy

The microscopic methods include the use of Bright-field, phase contrast microscope and fluorescent microscope (if liposomes are loaded with fluorescent probes) and are useful in evaluating the vesicle size of large vesicles (>1µm) particularly the upper end of the size distribution for multilamellar vesicles. Vesicular dispersion appropriately diluted are wet mounted on a haemocytometer and photographed with a phase contrast microscope. The negatives then can be projected on a piece of calibrated paper using a photographic enlarger at x1250 (Vyas and Katare, 1991). Diameters of approximately 500 vesicles are measured and thus this method is tedious and coupled with the limitation of resolution, hence electron microscopic methods with greater resolutions are preferred.

Negative Stain Transmission Electron Microscopy (TEM)

Electron microscopic techniques used to assess liposome shape and size are mainly negative-stain transmission electron microscopy (New, 1989) and scanning electron microscopy

(Barenholz and Cromellin, 1994). However, the latter technique requires dehydration of the sample prior to examination and is less preferred. Negative stain electron microscopy visualises relatively electron transparent liposomes as bright areas against a dark background (hence termed as negative stain). Liposomes are embedded in this method in a thin film of electron-dense heavy metal (salt) stain.

The negative stains used in the TEM analysis are ammonium molybdate ($(NH_4)_6$ Mo_7O_{24}, AM, 0.5–2%) or phosphotungstic acid (H_3PO_4. $12WO_3$. $24H_2O$, PTA, 0.5–2.0%) or uranyl acetate ($UO_2(CH_3COO)_2$. $2H_2O$, 0.2–0.5%). Both PTA and AM are anionic in nature and thus do not bind to liposomes composed of either neutral (PC) or negatively charged phospholipids (e.g. PA, PG or PS) however, they may precipitate or aggregate liposomes composed of positively charged lipids. In the latter case, cationic uranyl acetate should be used. However, it should be noted that uranium salts are precipitated by phosphate ions, and therefore, liposomes prepared in phosphate buffer should be washed before being stained with uranyl acetate (New, 1989).

The use of negative stain electron microscopy facilitates estimation of the liposome size range at the lower end of the frequency distribution. For SUVs, sizing by negative staining compares favourably with measurements determined by coulter counter or by freeze-fracture techniques. However, for larger sizes, or for heterogeneous populations of liposomes, negative staining electron microscopy offers real advantage over freeze-fracture technique. In the latter technique, the fracture plane passes through liposomes, oriented randomly in the frozen specimen, hence non-midplane sectioning is a possibility which will result in an observed diameter of vesicles different from real diameter of liposome (Ostro, 1987).

Negative staining electron microscopy alleviates this drawback in that complete structure is observed, although the liposome morphology may be deformed from spherical. Irregular or ellipsoid shapes can be treated mathematically to correct for perimeter irregularities thus estimations of original spherical diameters can be calculated.

Cryo-Transmission Electron Microscopy Technique (Cryo-TEM)

Cryo-TEM has been used to elucidate the surface morphology and size of the vesicles. This method is also used to characterise liposomal formulations where the drug is loaded by remote loading in order to ensure their stability. The method involves freeze fracturing of samples followed by their visualisation using transmission electron microscopy. Thin sample films are prepared under controlled temperature (25 °C) and humidity conditions within a custom-built environment chamber. The films are thereafter vitrified by quick freezing in liquid ethane and transferred to TEM analysis. To prevent sample preparation and formation of ice crystals; specimens are kept below 108K during both transfer and reviewing procedures.

Schmidtgen *et al.*, 1998 used cryo-TEM to examine the morphology of vesicles formed from lipids of the human stratum corneum (hSC). Gustafsson *et al.*, 1995 studied the association structures formed by cationic liposomes and DNA-plasmids based gene carriers by cryo-TEM (cryo-transmission electron microscopy).

Freeze-fracture Electron Microscopy

Freeze-fracture electron microscopy though is used mainly to assess the surface features and lamellarity, it can also be used to calculate the true vesicle diameter. If the angle of disposition of the shadowing material is 45° to the fracture plane, then vesicle faces that are 50% shadowed are cleaved equatorially and thus may reflect the true vesicle diameter.

Scanning Electron Microscopy (SEM)

Scanning electron microscopy is less frequently used, although SEM has been reported in the literature. The distortion during sample preparation can be cited as the reason of non-acceptability of SEM as one of the evaluation method. Scanning tunneling microscopy (or atomic force microscopy) on the other hand offers excellent improvisation in resolution. Monolayers under water can be resolved at the level of individual lipid molecules using these techniques.

Diffraction and Scattering Techniques

Laser Light Scattering

Light scattering techniques, particularly laser-based, quasi-elastic light scattering techniques are useful in analysing the homogeneous colloidal particulate populations (Kolchens *et al.,* 1993; Barenholz and Cromellin, 1994). The technique is based on the time-dependent coherence of light scattered by a vesicle, sensitive to vesicle diffusion, which in turn is dependent upon the viscosity of the aqueous medium and vesicle size. This technique can be applied to unimodel systems (homogeneous or monodisperse) with mean diameters less than 1µm. Moreover, its application in case of heterogeneous systems exhibiting bimodal or more complex size distributions should be crosschecked using other methods. This is because light scattering methods rely on algorithms to determine the vesicle size distributions and the results obtained thus are not well correlated with hetero-dispersed systems. Furthermore, such techniques cannot distinguish between a large particle and a flocculated mass of smaller particles. Most importantly, it is imperative in these methods to remove micron-sized (or beyond µm) particles that are present in the dispersion prior to analysis. Recently, multi-angle quasi-elastic light scattering based (QELS) methods are used to avoid errors due to the angular dependence of the scattering function of the particles. The experimentally determined auto-correlation function was analysed by multiple mathematical procedures, i.e. single exponential, CUMULANT, exponential sampling, non-negatively constrained least square and CONTIN, in order to select suitable models for vesicle characterisation (Barenholz and Cromellin, 1994).

Photon correlation spectroscopy is the major technique based upon laser scattering analysis that exploits the time dependence of intensity fluctuations in scattered laser light due to the different Brownian motions of the particles in liposomal dispersion. This differential diffusion profile of the particles of small and larger dimensions accordingly influences the rate of fluctuations of scattered light intensity, which is a function of the mean hydrodynamic radius of the particles (vesicles) determined using Stokes-Einstein equation.

Hydrodynamic Techniques

Field-Flow-Fractionation (FFF) Techniques

The applicability of hydrodynamic method like FFF for characterisation of liposomes is recently introduced (Moon and Giddings, 1993). Because of fundamental differences in their driving forces, sedimentation FFF and flow FFF measure different vesicle properties. Sedimentation FFF, although used to measure vesicle sizes and size distributions, is fundamentally a technique that measures the effective mass and mass distribution of particles. It is sensitive to small changes in the effective mass of either the biomembrane or its encapsulated load. It is useful in characterising properties such as drug loading, biomembrane volumes and areas, and distributions of these properties. Size characterisation by sedimentation FFF can only be done by deducing size from effective mass. Flow FFF, in contrast, provides a direct measurement of vesicle size and size distribution. The effect of ionic strength and pH of carrier solutions on the separation of liposomes by flow field-flow fractionation (flow FFF) has been studied for the determination of accurate vesicle size distribution of liposomes.

Gel Permeation

Gel permeation or gel-exclusion chromatography is preferably used techniques for the size distribution determination of liposomes. The ability to separate various components of heterodispersed preparations could be exploited to estimate various sized particles present in the dispersion. However, it is also used for the separation of unentrapped drug or separation of various heterodispersed liposomal preparations (Lesieur *et al.,* 1991; Andrieux *et al.,* 1998). While practically any gel medium can separate liposomes from non-encapsulated molecules gel media with larger porosities, such as Sepharose 4B or 2B, and Sephacryl S500 and S1000, allows fractionation of liposomes in the working volume of the column.

The largest inclusion volume is found in Sephacryl 1000, which separates particles with diameters between 0.4 µm in the void volume and ~10 nm in the total volume. A proper calibration of the gel column offers valuable data for size distribution of liposomes, as well as interactions such as fusion, lipid mixing and size growth.

Ultracentrifuge

Ultracentrifuge can yield valuable data on size-distribution of liposomes. It is however, used for the analytical purposes. The density of egg PC bilyer is 1.0135 g/ml (with 50 mol% of cholesterol it increases to 1.0142 g/ml), and since physiologic saline is having a density of 1.0048, liposomes can be pelleted. Because of the small differences in density, SUV's have very small sedimentation coefficient. Therefore, to pellet SUV's, centrifugation at 2,00,000 g for 10–12 h is required.

Surface Charge

Liposomes are usually prepared using charge imparting constituting lipids and hence it is imperative to study the charge on the vesicle surface. In general two methods are used to assess the charge, namely free-flow electrophoresis and zeta potential measurement. From the mobility of the liposomal dispersion in a suitable buffer (determined using Helmholtz-Smoluchowski equation), the surface charge on the vesicles can be calculated (Adamson, 1967).

Encapsulation Efficiency and Trapped Volume

Encapsulation efficiency and trapped volume determine the amount and rate of entrapment of water-soluble agents in the aqueous compartment of liposomes (Fry *et al.,* 1978; Gunter *et al.,* 1982; Weiner *et al.,* 1989; New, 1989; Barenholz and Cromellin, 1994).

Encapsulation Efficiency

The encapsulation efficiency describes the per cent of the aqueous phase and hence the percent of water-soluble drug that becomes ultimately entrapped during preparation of liposomes and is usually expressed as % entrapment/mg lipid. Encapsulation efficiency is assessed using two techniques including minicolumn centrifugation method and protamine aggregation method (Fig. 11.7).

Minicolumn centrifugation is generally used both as a means of purification and separation of liposomes on a small scale and analysis of a liposomal dispersion to determine encapsulation efficiency (Fry *et al.,* 1978). A Sephadex or Sepharose column pre-saturated with the dispersion medium in 1.0 ml disposable syringe is run while applying liposomal dispersion (200 µl) first and saline (250 µl) thereafter and centrifuging the column at 2000 rpm for 3 min and assaying the elutes. Depending upon the different molecular weights of solutes entrapped, various medium and their cut off point should be chosen. The concentration of free or entrapped material in elutes can be assessed by disrupting liposomes using ethanol (2 ml ethanol for 10 µl of liposomes) or Triton X-100 (10 µl of 10% Triton X-100 for 10 µl of liposomes) and estimating the liberated contents using standard methods. The lipid concentration can be assessed using Barlett assay.

Protamine aggregation method may be used for neutral and negatively charged liposomes (Gunter *et al.,* 1982). Liposomal dispersion (~100 µl) can be precipitated with a protamine solution (100 µl, 10 mg ml^{-1}) and subsequent centrifugation at 2000 rpm. By analysing the material in the supernatant and in the liposome pellet (after disrupting liposomal pellet with 0.6 ml of 10% Triton X-100), the encapsulation efficiency of the entrapped material can be estimated.

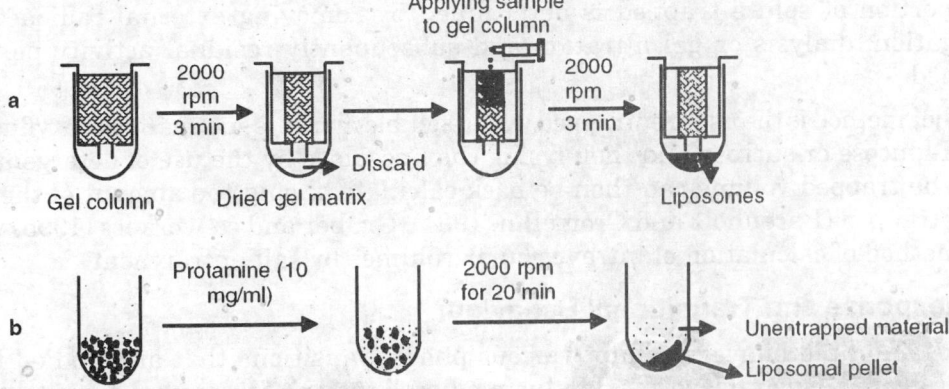

Fig. 11.7. *Determination of entrapment efficiency of liposome entrapped material using (a) minicolumn centrifugation technique and (b) protamine aggregation methods.*

Trapped Volume

Trapped volume is an important parameter that governs the encapsulation efficiency and morphology of the vesicles (Ostro 1987, Perkins *et al.,* 1988; Weiner *et al.,* 1989). Measurement of captured volumes by solute entrapment is pivotal for most types of vesicles. While estimating the encapsulation, it is assumed that no solute has leaked out of the liposomes after separation of unentrapped material. However, such assumptions sometime may prove invalid. For example in two phase methods of preparations, the aqueous phase (water) can be lost from the internal compartment during the drying down process that removes organic solvent or otherwise water can be expelled from the internal compartment as a result of unanticipated osmotic gradients. The measurement of the quantity of aqueous buffer is the best way to calculate trapped volume.

The internal or trapped volume is the aqueous entrapped volume per unit quantity of lipid and expressed as µl/µmol or µl/mg of total lipid. This can vary from 0.5 µl/µmol for some MLVs and SUVs to as much as 30µl/µmol for certain LUVs. Various materials including spectroscopically inert fluid, radioactive markers and fluorescent markers are used to determine the internal volume (entrapped volume) (Ostro, 1987).

The best way to measure internal volume is to measure the quantity of water directly, and this may be done by replacing the external medium (water, H_2O) with a spectroscopically inert fluid (deuterium oxide, D_2O), and then measuring the water signal, for example, using NMR. The permeability of the liposomal membrane to water is such that H_2O and D_2O equilibrate very rapidly throughout the whole volume of the medium. The NMR scan of this medium can be used to assess the peak height, which can be related to concentration by comparison with standards containing known amount of H_2O in D_2O.

The validity of atomic absorption spectrophotometry for measuring markers of trapped volume is also investigated and its superiority against determinations of markers with established optical spectrophotometry methods has been established (Yoss *et al.,* 1985).

Trapped volumes are also determined experimentally by dispersing lipid in an aqueous medium containing non-permeable radioactive solute such as [22Na] and [14C] inulin. The proportion of solute trapped is determined by removing external radioactivity by centrifugation, dialysis or gel filtration and subsequently residual activity per lipid is determined.

Another method is the use of entrapped water-soluble markers such as 6-carboxyfluorescein, [14C] or [3H]-glucose or sucrose and then lysing the liposomes by the use of detergent (Triton X-100). The trapped volume can then be back calculated using the amount of the marker that is entrapped (Barenholz and Cromellin, 1994). Gruber and co-workers (1995) reported a novel method of calculation of intravesicular volumes by salt entrapment.

Phase Response and Transitional Behaviour

Liposomes and lipid bilayers exhibit various phase transitions that are studied for their roles in triggered drug release or stimulus-mediated fusion of liposomal constituents with the target cells. Lipid bilayers can exist in a low-temperature solid-ordered phase and, above a certain temperature, in a fluid-disordered phase, the temperature of this phase transition can be tailored by selecting the proper lipids (Chapman, 1975). Various phase transition situations are studied in liposomal behaviour. An understanding of phase transitions and fluidity of phospholipid membranes is important both in the manufacture and exploitation of liposomes, since the phase behaviour of a liposomal membrane determines such properties as permeability, fusion, aggregation, and protein binding. Moreover, these phase behaviours are important to characterise while formulating the liposomes with lipids having different phase transition temperatures and for polymer (PEG) grafted liposomes where polymer grafting as such provides a stealthing effect deterring them from macrophagic uptake (and hence long circulation) (Lasic, 1998).

Thermodynamic Methods

These phase transitions have been evaluated using freeze-fracture electron microscopy; They are more comprehensively verified by differential scanning calorimetry (DSC) analysis (New, 1989). In differential scanning microcalorimeter, the heat required by liposomes to maintain a steady upward rise in temperature is plotted as a function of temperature. In basic terms, two small aluminium paths are compared, one empty, and one containing a concentrated liposomal dispersion. Transmitter monitors the temperature of each pan, as the pans are heated up separately.

The heat input of the sample pan is adjusted so that its temperature matches those of the reference pan. At the phase transition point, extra heat is required to maintain the rise in temperature of the sample pan equal to that of the reference, and this is recorded directly. The area under the peak is recorded as the enthalpy of the phase transition.

Vesicle Fusion Measurements

Liposomal fusion with cells and with intracellular contents has been a major area of research especially in the case of fusogenic liposomes, like pH sensitive liposomes, pH sensitive immunoliposomes, virosomes and cationic liposomes (Jones and Cossins, 1989). Fusion has been monitored using a fluorescence resonance energy transfer (RET) between two lipid analogues originally placed in separate vesicle population or in the same vesicle population (termed as fluorescence probe dilution assay) that measures intermixing of membrane lipids (Uster and Deamer, 1981; Morgan *et al.*, 1983). This technique depends upon an overlap in the emission spectrum of one fluorophore (the donor) and the excitation spectrum of a second fluorophore (the acceptor). Excitation of acceptor molecules can then occur by direct energy transfer of energy from the excited donor molecule, which is manifested as a reduction in the emission intensity of the donor fluorescence and a corresponding increase in emission intensity of the acceptor fluorescence. Thus, by incorporating donor and acceptor molecules into different liposome populations, the fusion could be detected by the onset of RET. The relative change of RET on fusion is linearly related to the extent of fusion. The fluorescent lipid analogues most frequently used in the fusion assay are:

- N-(-7-nitro-2,1,3-benzoxadiazol-4-yl) phosphatidylethanolamine (N-NBD-PE), which acts as a donor
- N-(Lissamine rhodamine B sulphonyl) phos-phatidylethanolamine (N-Rh-PE), which acts as an acceptor.

A variation in the RET method (also termed as probe dilution assay) is to premix the donor and acceptor lipid analogues in the same liposomes (0.5 mol %) and to induce fusion in the presence of an excess of unlabelled liposomes.

The dilutions of the fluorophores as they disperse through the unlabelled membranes (increased distance between the NBD-PE and Rh-PE) then leads to a decrease in RET. Because RET decreases as the sixth power of distance between donor and acceptor molecules, it occurs only when the two molecules come into close contact, as in the case when both occupy the same bilayer. The maximum fluorescent intensity (F_{max}) in each sample can be calculated following the solubilisation of vesicles with Triton X-100 to reach an infinite dilution of the probe. The per cent of fusion can be calculated using the following equation:

$$\% \text{ Fusion} = \frac{F_t - F_o}{F_{max} - F_o}$$

Where, F_t is the fluorescence intensity at each time point and F_0 is the initial fluorescence intensity.

Chemical Characterisation of Liposomes

Various chemical analysis methods used for quantitative and qualitative tests of liposomal components prior to and after the preparation are critical characteristics of liposomes (Barenholz and Cromellin, 1994). These methods become more essential to characterise liposomes, which require lipid stability cropping up from oxidation, lipid peroxidation, hydrolysis and degradation in various environments used in their manufacturing.

Phospholipid concentration is determined in terms of lipid phosphorus content using Barlett assay/Stewart assay (Barlett, 1959; Stewart, 1959) and thin layer chromatography (Terao *et al.*, 1985); cholesterol concentration is determined using Cholesterol oxidase assay/Ferric perchlorate method (Wybenga *et al.*, 1970) and GLC (Brooks *et al.*, 1984); and drug concentration can be determined using appropriate methods given in the monograph. Lysolecithin, which is one of the major product of hydrolysis of lecithin (egg PC) is estimated using densitometry (New, 1989). However, phospholipid peroxidation is quantitatively determined using UV absorbance, TBA reagent (for endoperoxidase), iodometry (for hydroperoxidase) and GLC techniques (New, 1989). Phospholipid hydrolysis is determined using HPLC and TLC and cholesterol auto oxidation can be assessed using HPLC and TLC (New, 1989).

PROTOCOL: 11.1

Preparation of Liposomes by Hand Shaking Method

Procedure

- Take egg lecithin, cholesterol and drug* to be entrapped in a 50 ml round bottom quick-fit flask and dissolve in 10 ml of chloroform: methanol (1:1). Flush the flask with nitrogen and maintain controlled vacuum.

Note: if the drug to be entrapped is lipophilic in nature it should be added in the first step of the procedure only.

- Rotate the flask to evaporate the solvent leaving a thin layer on the wall of round bottom of flask.
- Keep the flask for 6 hour to ensure complete removal of solvent system.
- Add 10ml of phosphate buffer saline in which drug[†] is previously dissolved.

[†]*Note:* if the drug to be entrapped is water soluble in nature dissolve it in the hydrating aqueous buffer.

- Seal the flask and hydrate the lipid film with manual shaking or using a manual shaker for 72 hours.
- Centrifuge the liposomal suspension, discard the supernatant.
- Redisperse in phosphate buffer saline and again centrifuge.
- Repeat the step 3–4 times to ensure removal of un-entrapped drug and lipids (Scheme 11.1).

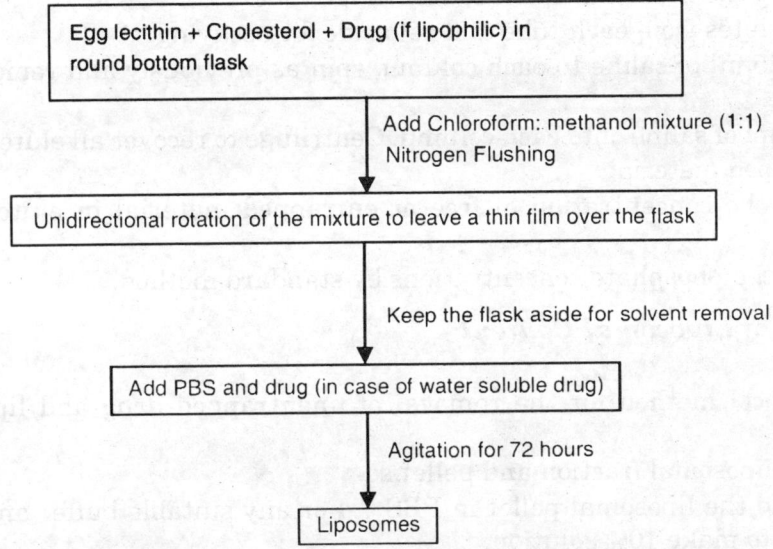

Scheme 11.1: *Liposome preparation by hand shaking method*

PROTOCOL: 11.2

Removal of Unentrapped Drug from Liposomes by Size Exclusion Chromatography

Procedure

Preparation of Column

- Allow 10 g of Sephadex G-50 to swell in 120 ml of 0.9% NaCl in a glass screw capped bottle for at least 5 h at room temperature. Store at 4°C until required for use.

- Remove the plunger from 1 ml of disposable plastic syringes and plug each barrel with a Whatman GF/B filter pad.
- Rest each barrel in a 13X10 mm centrifuge tube.
- Fill the barrels to the top with hydrated gel, using a Pasteur pipette with the tip removed.
- Place the tubes containing the column in a bench centrifuge, and spin at 2000 rpm for 3 min to remove excess saline solution. After spinning, the gel column should be dry and have come away from the sides of the barrel. The height of the bed should be level with the 0.9 mark.
- Empty the eluted saline from each collection tube.

Processing the Sample

- Apply exact 0.2 ml of liposome suspension dropwise to the top of the gel bed. Take care not to let the sample trickle down the sides of the column bed.
- Spin the column at 2000 rpm for 3 min in a bench centrifuge to expel the void volume containing the liposomes into the centrifuge tube.
- Remove elutes from each tube and set aside for assaying.
- Apply 0.25 ml of saline to each column, spin as previously and remove elates from each tube.
- Load 0.1 ml of saline onto each column. Centrifuge to recover all elute containing the unentrapped material.
- Measure the concentration of free or entrapped material in elutes by standard methods.
- Measure the phosphate concentrations by standard method.

Measurement of Liposomal Content
Direct Method

- Use protocol method for the removal of unentrapped drug and lipids from liposomes.
- Take the liposomal fraction and pelletise.
- Resuspend the liposomal pellet in PBS 7.4 or any suitable buffer and add triton X 100 so as to make 10% solution.
- Again centrifuge and take the supernatant.
- Measure the concentration of entrapped material in by standard methods.

PROTOCOL: 11.3

Liposome Preparation by REV's

Materials

Cholesterol
HEPES buffer
Deionised water

Chloroform
Sodium bisulfite
Diethyl ether

Procedure

- Weigh cholesterol into a 50 ml round bottom flask with a 24/40-ground joint.
- Add phospholipids previously dissolved in chloroform to the flask and allow the cholesterol to dissolve in the chloroform by gentle swirling.
- Attach the flask to rotary evaporator and purge nitrogen through the flask to maintain an inert atmosphere.
- Apply a vacuum of about 700 mm Hg to evaporate the chloroform and to form a thin film of lipid/cholesterol mixture on the walls of the flask.
- Add HEPES buffer (25 ml) containing 0.1 g sodium bisulfite to a separatory funnel. Then add diethyl ether (3 ml per 66 µmol lipid) to the funnel.
- Mix the HEPES and the ether together by gentle swirling and then allow to separate. This step removes any free radicals present in the ether.
- Remove the aqueous fraction and add the ether to the lipid film in the round bottom flask. Swirl the flask gently to dissolve the lipid completely in the ether.
- Then add the aqueous phase (1 ml per 66 µmol lipid) containing the material to be entrapped to the lipid solution.
- Cover the flask with a rubber septum with an 18G and a 26G needle fitted through it. Attach polypropylene tube to the 26G needle such that the free end of the tube is immersed in the liquid. Bubble argon slowly into the liquid through the tubing to maintain an inert atmosphere inside the flask. The 18G needle acts as an exit for the gas.
- Sonicate the two-phase mixture in a bath sonicator while maintaining the temperature of the sonication process around 4°C. The sonication should be performed with gentle swirling of the flask to make sure that the contents of the flask are uniformly subjected to the sonication process. Continue sonication till a stable emulsion of the aqueous phase in the ether phase forms (~2–3 minutes).
- Attach the flask with the two-phase emulsion to the rotary evaporator and maintain nitrogen purge through the flask while stirring. To evaporate the ether slowly expose the content to a low vacuum (~200 mm Hg).
- Continue the process till a semisolid gel forms in the flask. Remove the flask and stir the contents to break the gel.
- Slightly increase vacuum pressure (~300–350 mm Hg) and maintain at that level for about 15 minutes. The gelled material gradually converts into a smooth suspension as the ether is removed. Remove the flask and mix the contents again.
- Further increase the vacuum in steps until it finally reaches 700 mm Hg, maintain it for about 30 minutes to evaporate all of the remaining ether. Extrude the liposomes after which separate the entrapped material by gel permeation chromatography and/or centrifugation (Scheme 11.2).

PROTOCOL: 11.4
Preparation of DRV's

Procedure

- Weigh cholesterol into a 50 ml round bottom flask with a 24/40-ground joint. Add phospholipids previously dissolved in chloroform to the flask and allow the cholesterol to dissolve in the chloroform by gentle swirling.

- Attach the flask to rotary evaporator and purge nitrogen through the flask to maintain an inert atmosphere. Apply a vacuum of about 700 mm Hg to evaporate the chloroform and to form a thin film of lipid/cholesterol mixture on the walls of the flask.

- Add distilled water (1 ml per 33 µmol lipid) to the thin film of lipid in the flask in order to hydrate it and form MLV's. Stir the mixture to speed up the hydration process. Purge nitrogen through the flask in order to maintain an inert atmosphere inside the flask. Continue the stirring for 2 hours.

- Extrude the MLV's thus formed through polycarbonate membranes in order to convert them to SUV's. Extrude the MLV's several times through membranes with pore sizes 0.4 µm, 0.2 µm and 0.1 µm in that order.

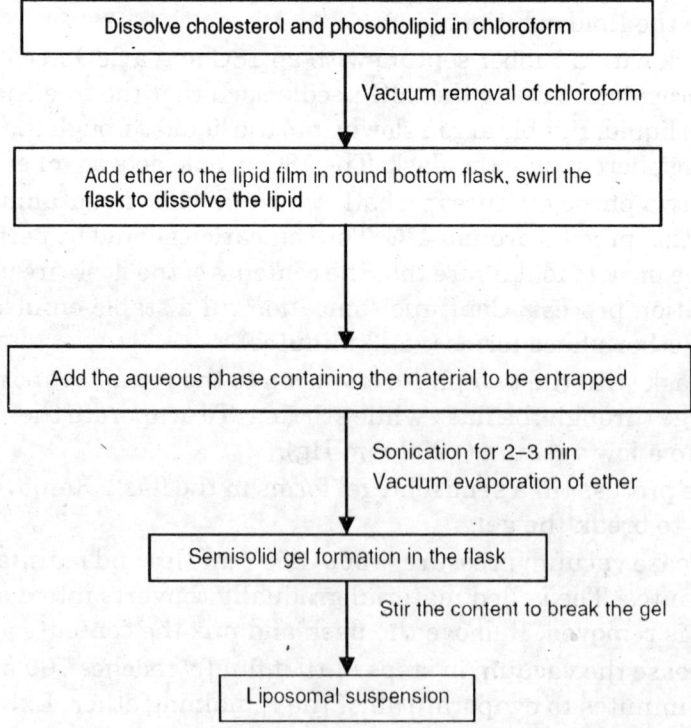

Scheme 11.2: *Preparation of liposomes by REV method*

- Then mix the SUV's with an equal volume of a solution of the material to be entrapped (in distilled water) in another 50 ml round bottom flask. Stir the mixture for about 15 minutes under a nitrogen purge to ensure proper mixing.

- Lyophilise the mixture of SUV's and the material to be entrapped in a freezing mixture of dry ice and isopropanol. Gently swirl the flask in the dry ice-isopropanol mixture so that the mixture in the flask is frozen on the walls of the flask in the form of a thin shell, which aids in the hydration of the mixture further in the preparation.

- Then lyophilise the mixture overnight in a bench top freeze dryer operating at −75°C and a vacuum of about 20 millitorrs.

- Following freeze-drying, rehydrate the preparation with distilled water. The amount of distilled water added in this step is very critical to the amount of solute entrapped in the MLV's. Distilled water is added in the amount of 1 ml per 4 ml of SUV's used.

- Gently vortex the mixture in order to speed up mixing of the contents and to aid hydration of the preparation. Allow to stand for 30 minutes after which dilute with HEPES buffer (higher osmolality) in 212 order to prevent leakage of entrapped material. Centrifuge the unentrapped material by centrifugation.

PROTOCOL 11.5:
Preparation of Liposomes by the Ethanol Injection Method
Procedure

- Dissolve 30 mg of PC in 1 ml of ethanol.

- Introduce 10 ml of nitrogen purged aqueous medium (water, saline, solute solution etc.) into a 25 ml conical flask, and stir rapidly with a magnetic stirrer.

- Fit a fine gauge needle to a 1 ml glass syringe and draw up 750 µl of the lipid solution.

- Position the tip of needle below the surface of the stirred aqueous solution and inject the organic solution as rapidly as possible into the medium. Liposomes will be formed immediately. The final concentration is approximately 2 mg of PC/ml, which is the maximum attainable without further processing.

PROTOCOL: 11.6
Preparation of Liposomes by the Ether Injection Method
Procedure

- Prepare a solution of lipid in diethyl ether by dissolving 13.5 mg of egg PC, 1.5 mg of PA and 5 mg of cholesterol in 10 ml of ether.

- Place 5 ml of aqueous solution containing the material to be entrapped inside a 10 ml glass vial closed with a silicone rubber injection cap.

- Prepare the needle for ether injection by taking a long 19 gauge disposable hypodermic needle, and crimping it tightly with a silicone rubber injection cap.

- Break the tip off by bending and file the crimped surface to give a narrow slit approximately 0.1 mm across.

- Introduce the needle into the vial, through the rubber cap until the tip of the needle i.e. the newly formed slit is well below the surface of the aqueous solution.

- Introduce a second needle (19 gauge or wider) through the cap, projecting 1 cm into the vial, to act as a gas release vent.

- Fill a 10 ml glass syringe with 2 ml of the ether solution, and fit the syringe into a Harvard infusion pump apparatus.

- Attach the injection needle to the syringe head, and orient the pump and needle so that the vial hangs vertically below the pump.

- In this orientation place the pump in a clamp so that the vial is suspended in a shaking water bath set at 55 °C. Ideally the water bath should be located in a fume hood, in order to remove ether vapour as soon as it is produced. Set the pump working so as to introduce ether solution into the vial at a rate no faster that 2.2 ml /min.

- After all the ether has been introduced, remove residual vapour by withdrawing the syringe tip from the aqueous phase and passing a stream of nitrogen though the gas space above the liquid in the vial.

- Remove aggregates by low speed centrifugation, unentrapped material, as well as the last traces of ether, may be removed either by dialysis or gel permeation chromatography.

PROTOCOL: 11.7

Preparation of LUVs From MLVs

In membrane extrusion method, the size of liposomes is reduced by gently passing them through a membrane filter of defined pore size. This can be achieved at much lower pressure (<100psi.) than required for French pressure cell.

The membrane extrusion technique can be used to process LUVs as well as MLVs. In this process, the vesicle contents are exchanged with the dispersion medium during breaking and resealing of phospholipid bilayers as they pass through polycarbonate membrane. In order to achieve high entrapment, the water-soluble compounds should be present in suspending medium during the extrusion process. The material, which is not entrapped, can be removed subsequently. The liposomes produced by this technique have been termed LUVETs. The 30% capture volume can be obtained using high lipid concentration (300 mM PC). The trapped volume in this process is 1–2 litre/mol of lipids.

Extrusion technique is the most widely used method for SUV and LUV production for *in vitro* and *in vivo* studies. It is due to their ease of production, readily selectable vesicle diameter (dictated by the nominal pore size of the track-etch membranes used for extrusion, typically between 50–120 nm for *in vivo* experiments), batch-to-batch reproducibility, and freedom from solvent and/or surfactant contamination.

PROTOCOL: 11.8
Preparations of Giant Unilamellar Vesicles (GUVs)

Materials

L-α-Phosphatidylcholine (Lecithins Type XVI-E from fresh egg yolk, lyophilised powder app. 99% pure packaged under argon)

L-α-Phosphatidylcholine (synthetic, lyophilised powder app. 99% pure)

β- Arachidonoyl L-α-Phosphatidylcholine

γ-palmitoyl L-α-Phosphatidylcholine.

Methods

- Dissolve the lipid in different molar ratio in chloroform (0.1M) and take 20µl of this solution in a 50ml round bottom flask containing 980µl of chloroform and 100–200µl of methanol.

- Evaporate the organic phase with the rotary evaporator under reduced pressure. For organic solvent evaporation, maintain the pressure, temperature and rotation 10mmHg (1.3 kPa) at 40°C and 40rpm respectively.

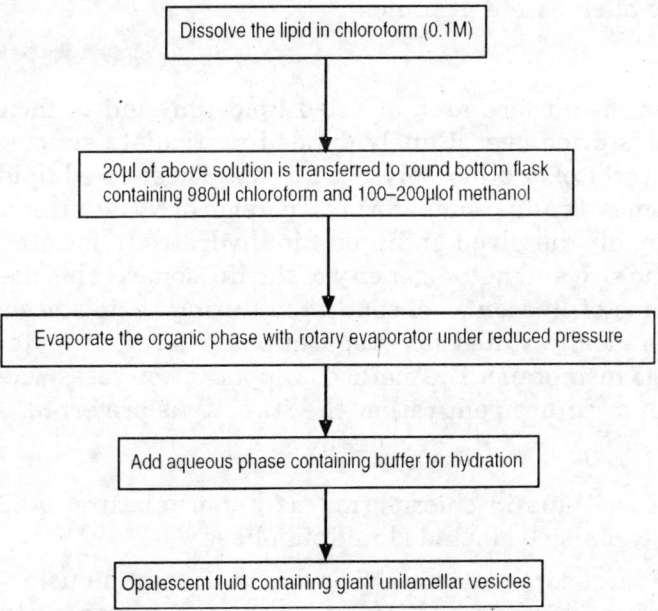

Scheme 11.3: *Preparation of giant unilamellar vesicles*

- Then carefully add aqueous phase consisting of 7 ml of water or buffer along the flask walls. Different buffers can also be used for hydration of organic film such as HEPES buffer (10mM, pH 7.4) sodium phosphate buffer (10mM, pH 7.4), sodium borate buffers (50mM, pH 9.2), etc. for the entrapment of proteins or enzymes use 10 mg/ml solution of it in buffer.

- After evaporation for 2 min an opalescent fluid with a volume of approximately 6.5 ml will be obtained. The resulting aqueous solution contained giant unilamellar vesicles (GUVs) in high concentration.

- Thus formed liposomes will be characterised for bright field, fluorescence and electron microscopy to measure size distribution, membrane seal and the detailed membrane structure (Scheme 11.3).

PROTOCOL 11.9

Proliposomes of Effervescent Granules

Materials

Soya lecithins

Cholesterol

Stearylamine

Chloroform: methanol mixture (70:30 ratio)

Sodium chloride effervescent granules

Principle

In order to increase the surface area of dried lipid film and to facilitate instantaneous hydration, the lipid is dried over a finely divided particulate support, such as powdered sodium chloride, or sorbitol or other polysaccharides. These dried lipid coated particulates are called pro-liposomes. Pro-liposomes form dispersion of MLVs on adding water into them, where support is rapidly dissolved and lipid film hydrates to form MLVs. The size of the carrier influences the size and heterogeneity of the liposomes. This method also overcomes the stability problems of liposomes encountered during their storage as dispersion, dry or frozen form. It is ideally suited for preparations where the material to be entrapped incorporates into lipid membrane. The method is applicable in cases where 100% entrapment of components is not a requirement rather the stability is preferred.

Procedure

- Dissolve soya lecithins in chloroform: methanol mixture (70:30). Cholesterol and stearylamine can also be included in lipid phase.

- Coat the solid inert core material using this lipid solution using fluidised bed drying to provide uniform drying condition under an inert nitrogen atmosphere.

- Spray the lipid solution over the core materials (Sodium chloride effervescent granules) in different aliquots.

- The factors that may affect the proliposomes preparation are operational formulation and drying parameters (liquid nitrogen inlets and pressure). The size of the core material is generally within the range of 75–590 μm.

- Store the prepared dry granular products in sealed containers under the inert atmosphere of nitrogen in a dark place at 20°C. These products were reconstituted in distilled water just one hour prior to use.

- *Cast film method:* Prepare liposomes using soya lecithin with or without cholesterol and stearyl amine in different compositions. Dissolve the lipids in chloroform: methanol mixture (70:30) and dry in a round bottom flask under a stream of nitrogen. Hydrate the dried lipid film with a hydrating medium (phosphate buffer saline pH 7.4) for 24 hours with intermittent shaking (Scheme 11.4).

Liposome Size Distribution

Liposomes obtained either from proliposomes or from cast film method, are studied for their homogeneity in size. Wet mount the liposomal suspension on a haemocytometer and count the vesicle population (number of vesicles/mm^3).

Cytoprotective Evaluation

Prepared products can be evaluated for their cytoprotective activity by measuring ulcerogenicity produced by anti-inflammatory drugs in rats.

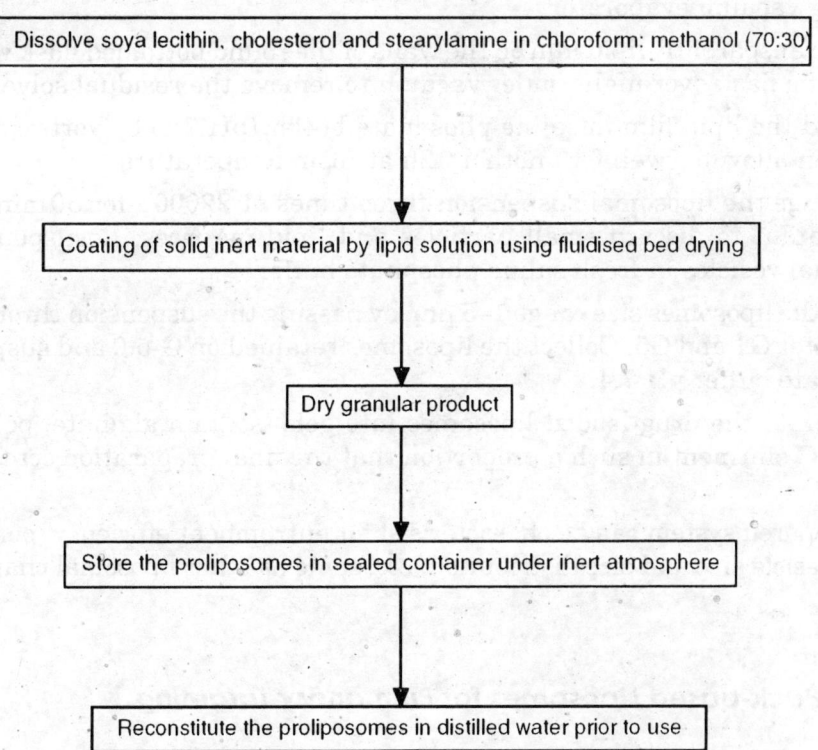

Scheme 11.4. *Preparation of proliposomes of effervescent granules*

PROTOCOL 11.10

Topical Liposome System Bearing Local Anaesthetic

Principle

Multi-lamellar liposomes are prepared by the film casting method

Materials

Drug (Lipophilic, i.e. Lidocaine)

Soya lecithins

Cholesterol

Stearylamine

Diacetylphosphate (DCP)

Sodium alginate

Polyacrylamide

Procedure

- Take lipophilic drug (lidocaine) and phospholipids in 1:1 ratio and dissolve in organic solvent containing chloroform and methanol (7:3) and dry under nitrogen using a rotating vacuum evaporator.

- A thin transparently lipid film on the walls of the round bottomed flask will be formed. Leave the flask over night under vacuum to remove the residual solvent.

- Suspend the lipid film in saline phosphate buffer (pH 7.4) by vortexing for 10 min, and then allow to swell for another 12h at room temperature.

- Centrifuge the liposomal suspension three times at 22000 g for 30 min. Remove the supernatant to discard small particles and lipid matrices. Resuspend the settled liposomal vesicles in fresh saline phosphate buffer.

- Isolate the liposomes size range 1–5 µm, by passing the suspension through a sintered glass filter G1 and G5. Collect the liposomes retained on G-5.0 and suspend in saline phosphate buffer pH 7.4.

- Incorporate the drug-loaded liposomes into gels (sodium alginate, polyacrylamide) and PEG ointment in such a proportion that the final preparation contains 5% w/w drug.

- The prepared system can be characterised for entrapment efficiency, per cent drug release, vesicle size and size distribution, etc. same as other liposomal characterisation.

PROTOCOL: 11.11

Pressurised Pack-based Liposomes for Pulmonary Targeting

Materials

Soya lecithins

Egg lecithins (Type X)

Dicetylphosphate

Phosphatidyl ethanolamine

Cholesterol

Drug (lipophilic drug, i.e. isoprenaline)

Procedure

Step 1. Preparation of Liposomes by the Ether Injection Method

- Take the phospholipids egg lecithins, cholesterol and drug to be encapsulated in 3:1:0.5 molar ratio respectively and dissolve in diethyl ether.
- Then inject this ether solution into an aqueous solution at 55–60°C under reduced pressure to enhance the evaporation of ether.
- Adjust the rate of injection at 0.2 ml/min. Filter the preparations through a sintered glass filter with 1 µm pore size.
- Discard the filtrate while re-disperse the liposomes retained over the filter in PBS (phosphate saline buffer, pH 7.4).

Step 2. Preparation of Aerosolised Packed Liposomes

- Prepare solution phase pressure packs (30 ml volume) containing lipid/ isoprenaline or isoprenaline solubilised in a chlorofluorocarbon (CFC) blend using a previously reported method (Farr *et al*).
- Weigh accurately the quantity of each ingredient into a glass bottle and propellent (P_{11}) is filled in excess.
- Evaporate the P_{11} until the required weight attained; this procedure also evacuates air from within the bottle.
- Seal the unit hermetically using a metering valve, and add the required quantity of P_{12}, with the help of pressure burettes (Scheme 11.5).

Characterisation of Aerosol Device

- Liposomal size distribution
- Entrapment efficiency
- Leak test with the container immersed into a water bath at 55°C for 5 min.
- Internal pressure by pressure gauze
- Aerosol valve discharge rate and spray pattern
- Airways penetration efficiency
- Lung disposition study

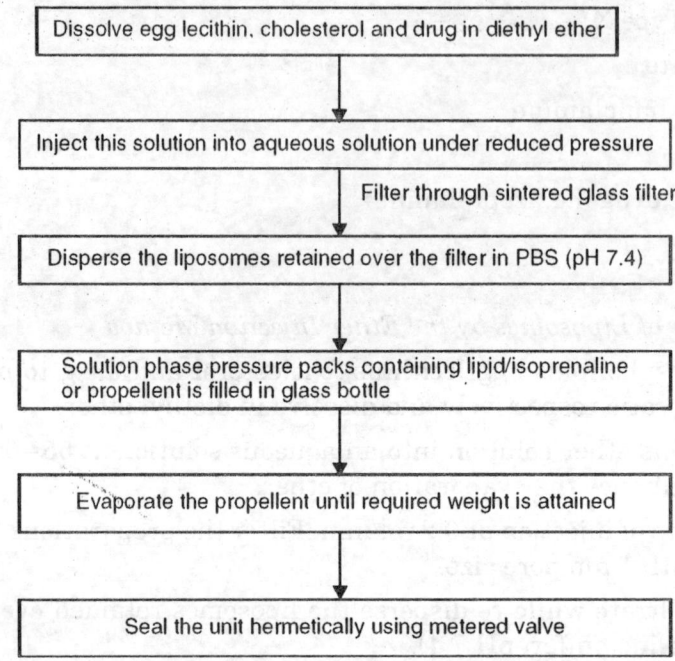

Scheme 11.5: Preparation of pressurised pack-based liposomes for pulmonary targeting

---

PROTOCOL: 11.12

Gelospheres for Oral Controlled Delivery

Materials

  Sebacoyl chloride

  1,6 hexamine

  Polyvinyl alcohol

  Polyacrylamide

  Span 60

Procedure

  Drug loaded gellospheres are prepared by the method used in the following step.

Step 1. Formation of Drug-polymer Composite Biphasic Systems

 • Prepare drug-polymer composite biphasic systems by conventional emulsion formation method. Add 2.0 ml of aqueous 0.4 M hexamethylenediamine solution in 0.45 M $NaHCO_3$–Na_2CO_3 buffer (pH 9.8) to an equal volume of 10% w/v drug containing polyvinyl alcohol (PVA) solution. In the case of polyacrylamide (PAA), replace the buffer with hydrochloride (pH 1.2). Then emulsify this aqueous solution with 20 ml of a cyclohexane-chloroform (4:1) organic phase using 1% w/v span 60 as emulsifier.

Step 2. Formation of Nylon Capsule Membrane

- Cool the emulsion formed in the step 1 to 10°C under continuous stirring. Slowly add 0.02M sebacoyl chloride (20ml) in the cylohexane: chloroform (4:1) to the emulsion under constant stirring. The interfacial nylon membrane will be obtained.

Step 3. Gelling of Encapsulated Polymers

- In the case of PVA subject the internal phase containing the polymer to a freeze thaw cycle for gelling. Cool the mixture at –4°C for 18 h and allow thawing at room temperature for 8 h. This constituted one freeze thaw-cycle (FTC) the mixture was exposed to twice to FTC's

Step 4. Removal of Organic Phase

- Remove the organic phase that is left after completion of step 3 by decantation to obtain wet slurry. Transfer this slurry to a flash evaporator and remaining organic phase is removed. Store the resultant free flowing drug containing spherical capsules in amber coloured bottles to protect the nylon from photodegradation.

PROTOCOL: 11.13

Liposome Preparation by Organic Solvent Removal Method

Materials

Ceramide (50%)

Cholesterol (28%)

Palmitic acid (17%)

Cholesteryl sulphate (5%)

Procedure

- Take 10 mg of lipid mixture containing lipid at the following concentrations (w/w) ceramide (50%), cholesterol (28%), palmitic acid (17%) and cholesteryl sulphate (5%) in close approximation of the composition of SC lipids in a flask. Add 1.0 mol% of α-tocopherol to this lipid mixture as an antioxidant.

- Dissolve the lipidic mixture in a mixture of diethyl ether: chloroform mixture (1:1 volume ratio) to a volume of 50 ml and sonicate for 20–30 min. For sonication, maintain temperature between 5–10 °C using a ice bath.

- Dissolve the lipid mixture completely, and add the aqueous phase (sodium acetate buffer pH 5.0) containing drugs to yield a ratio of drug lipid 1:3.

- Sonicate the resulting two-phase system for 20–30 min in a bath type sonicator and place on a rotor evaporator at 20–25 °C to remove the organic solvent under reduced pressure.

- Heat the preparation at 70°C (using thermo barrel attached to a circulating water-bath); this temperature is above to gel-liquid-crystal transition temperature of the hydrated SC lipids (Tc= 65 °C).

- Extrude the preparation containing 5mg lipid/ml using a stainless steel extrusion device at 70°C through polycarbonate filters to an initial pore size of 5µm and subsequently of 1µm (Scheme 11.6).

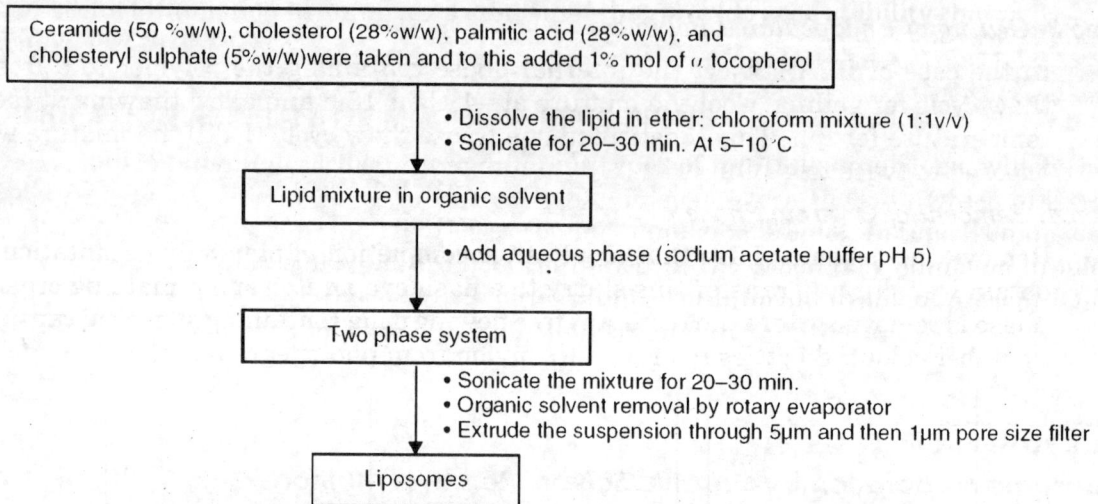

Scheme 11.6: *Liposome preparation by organic solvent removal method*

PROTOCOL: 11.14

Liposomes Preparation by Modified Freeze-thaw Method

Materials

Dipalmitoyl phosphatidylcholine (DPPC)

Cholesterol (CHOL)

Dimyristoyal phosphatidyl glycerol (DMPG)

Procedure

- Use lipids at a molar ratio of 3 DPPC: 1 CHOL: 0.25 DPMG. Form a thin lipid film onto round bottom flasks using a rotary evaporator.

- The volume of lipids used for dry film preparations are given as—1.95 ml of DPPC (16 mg/ml) in chloroform, and 2.2 ml of DPMG (1.1 mg/ml) in mixture of methanol and chloroform (1:3).

- Incubate the flask at 43°C in vacuum oven (230 mmHg) overnight to remove the residual solvent.

- Rehydrate the lipids with 2.0 ml of PBS containing 300 µg of drug/peptides. Incubate flasks at 53°C in a water bath and vortex until lipids dissolves from the sides of the flasks and the solution appears homogeneous.

- Perform five cycles of the following: freeze flask in dry ice/acetone, thaw for 40 minutes at room temperature, incubate at 41°C in a water bath 5 min, vortex for 30s.

- Collect the liposomes by ultracentrifugation, at 50,000 g for 20 minutes and wash twice with PBS. Collect supernatant after each centrifugation for analysis of peptide content. Resuspend liposomes pellet in a replacement volume of PBS (Scheme 11.7).

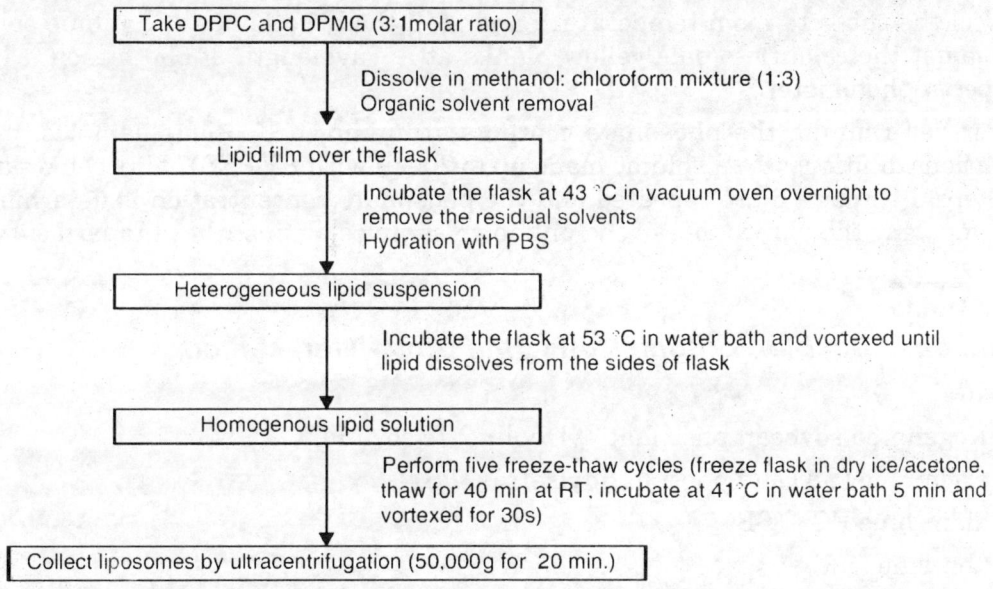

Scheme 11 7: *Preparation of liposomes by modified freeze-thaw method*

PROTOCOL: 11.15

Phosphate Assay

Procedure

- Prepare a 10% ascorbic acid solution in deionised water (0.88g in 50 ml). Store the solution in a dark coloured bottle and preferably covered with aluminum foil to prevent exposure to light. The solution can be used until it develops a pale yellow colour. Prepare 0.08 M solution of ammonium molybdate in deionised water (0.5g in 50 ml) and separately 20% solution of perchloric acid in deionised water.

- Use a phosphorus standard solution (Sigma) as the reference for measuring phosphate concentrations. Pipette out various amounts of the phosphorus standard solution containing 25 to 125 nmol of phosphorus into test tubes.

- Dilute the various amounts of the phosphorus solution to 200 µl using HEPES buffer followed by addition of 300 µl of 20% perchloric acid. Also, tubes containing just 200 µl of HEPES and 300 µl of perchloric acid serve as blanks. Digest these mixtures on a hot plate at 180–210°C for 30 minutes.

- Allow the test tubes to cool and add 3 ml of deionised water, 200 µl of ammonium molybdate and 100 µl of ascorbic acid orderly to each of the tubes including the blanks.

- Vortex the tubes to mix the contents and then place in a boiling water bath for 15 minutes during which a blue colour develops depending on the amount of phosphorus present.

- Cool the tubes to room temperature and read the absorbance of the blue solutions against the colourless/pale yellow blanks at a wavelength of 830 nm on a UV/Vis spectrophotometer.

- For determining the phosphate contents of unknown liposome samples, prepare various dilutions (total volume made up to 200 µl with HEPES) of liposome samples. Steps 3 through 6 are repeated and the phosphate concentration is determined by comparing the absorbance of the unknown samples against the standard curve.

PROTOCOL: 11.16

Preparation of Double Liposomes Using the Glass-filter Method

Materials

Hydrogenated soybean phosphatidylcholine (H-soya PC)

Stearylamine (SA) and phosphatidylserine (PS)

Brilliant blue FCF (BB)

Erythrosine (ER)

Procedure

- Dissolve twenty-six micromole H-soya PC alone or with 2.6 mM SA or 2.6 mM PS as lipids with electrical charges in chloroform. Pour BB or ER in ethanol (1 mM) into the lipid solution.

- Filter the mixture into a G4 glass filter (pore size: 10 to16 mm) and evaporate chloroform with a gentle stream of nitrogen gas at room temperature. The lipid layer forms on the glassfilter after hydration with 1 ml of phosphate buffered saline (pH 7.4) for 10 min.

- Soak the glass filter in a water bath and sonicate for 30 min at 60°C. Then pass 3 ml of buffer solution through the filter repeatedly by alternately pressing syringes connected to both sides of the filter to form the liposomes. Double liposomes will be obtained by filtering a suspension of liposomes prepared using a G4 filter into a G3 filter (pore size: 40–100 mm) coated with a similar lipid layer.

Characterization

Size and Shape

Confirm the liposomal preparation by light microscopy. For the detailed morphological structure of the double liposomes freeze-fracture microscopy is performed.

The diameter of liposomes prepared using the G4 filter was 0.8–2 mm and that of liposomes prepared using the G3 filter or double liposomes was 5–10 mm.

Drug Loading

Add 4 ml of PBS to 1ml of suspension of liposomes containing BB or ER, centrifuge the suspension (1800 rpm, 10 min) and remove the supernatant. Repeat the process twice. To destroy the liposomes, add 1 ml of 10% Triton X-100 to the pellet. Analyse the solution spectrophotometrically at 630 or 524 nm for BB or ER, respectively.

Encapsulation efficiency (%) can be calculated by the following formula:

Encapsulation efficiency (%)=Elemental drug in pellet/Elemental drug added × 100

PROTOCOL: 11.17

Polysaccharide Coated Liposomes for Oral Delivery

Materials

Egg phosphatidylcholine (PC)

Cholesterol

Phosphatidylethanolamine (PE)

Model protein (BSA)

Pullulan (polysaccharide)

Palmitoyl chloride

Procedure

Step 1. Synthesis and Characterisation of O-palmitoylpullulan (OPP)

- Take 1.0 g pullulan and dissolve in 11.0 ml dry dimethylformamide at 60°C.
- Add 1.0 ml dry pyridine and 0.1 g palmitoyl chloride in this mixture, and dissolve in 0.24 ml dry dimethyl formamide.
- Stir the mixture for 2 h at 60°C followed by 1 h at room temperature. Pour slowly drop wise this mixture into 70 ml absolute ethanol under stirring.
- Collect the precipitate and wash with 80 ml absolute ethanol and 60ml dry diethyl ether. Collect the white solid material and then dry in vacuum at 50°C for 2 h.
- Characterise the synthesised polymer by FTIR and pNMR. Take 1% OPP and incorporate it into a compressed KBr Pellet and determine the IR spectra of OPP.
- Obtain the pNMR spectra of OPP in deuterated dimethylsulfoxide solution (DMSO-d6) using tetramethylsiane (TMS) as internal standard.

Step 2. Preparation of Liposomes by Reverse Phase Evaporation Method

- Take phosphatidylcholine, cholesterol and phosphatidylethanolamine in 7:2:1 molar ratio and dissolve in 5 ml diethyl ether. Add aqueous phase, i.e. phosphate buffer saline (pH7.4) containing 1.0 mg/ml BSA.

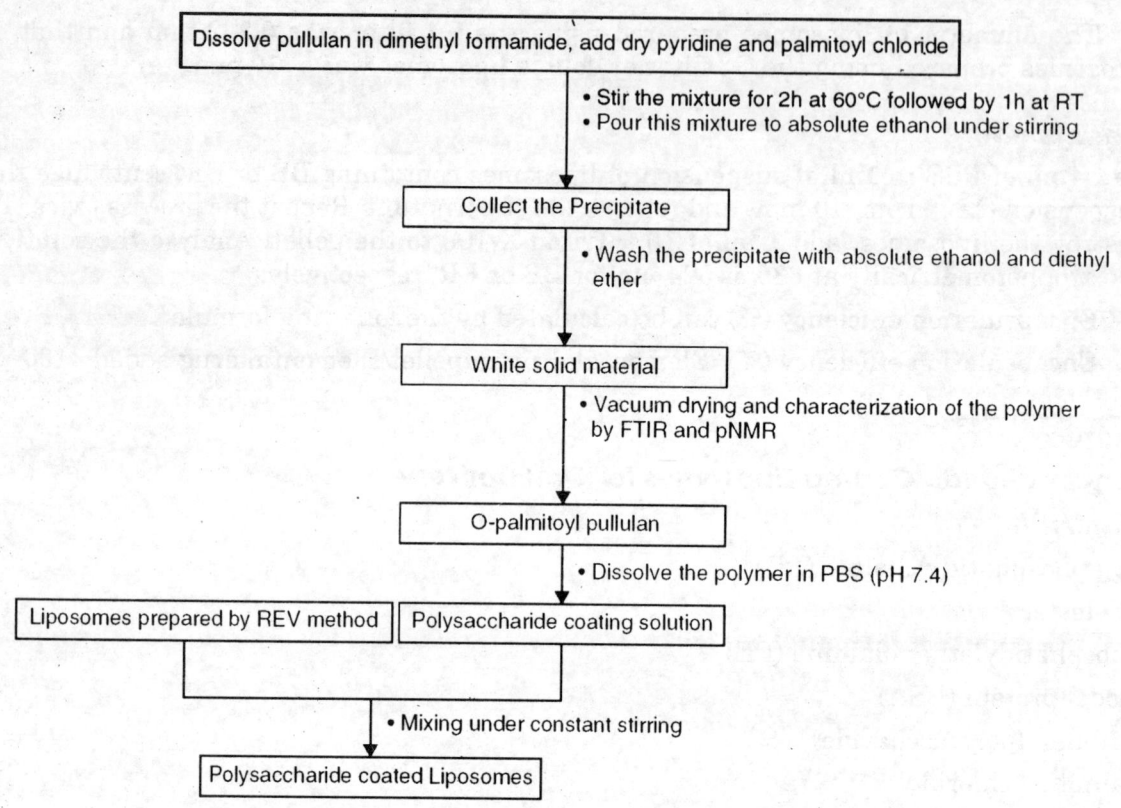

Scheme 11.8: *Preparation of polysaccharide-coated liposomes*

- Sonicate the mixture for 10 min (with an interval of 2 min after 5 min). A thick white emulsion forms. Keep the emulsion over a vortex mixer in order to remove any residual ether.

- Add 3.0 ml of warm phosphate buffer saline (pH7.4) to this emulsion to hydrate the vesicles.

Step 3. Coating of Liposomes with OPP

- Dissolve the OPP in PBS (pH 7.4) to obtain 100µg/ml solution. Add this 2.0 ml OPP solution into the 4ml of liposome dispersion under constant stirring.

- Continue this constant stirring for 1 h in order to ensure complete coating on the liposomal surface (Scheme 11.8).

Encapsulation Efficiency

Take the prepared liposomes and separate the free (unentrapped) antigen/drug by a sephadex G-25 minicolumn using centrifugation. Repeat the method thrice with a fresh syringe packed with Sephadex G-25 gel each time. Finally collect the fractions and estimate the amount of free antigen or drug.

Encapsulation efficiency can also be determined by isolating the liposomes by the centrifugation at 60,000 rpm for 4 h. Treat the pellets with 2 ml of 0.2 % Triton X-100 in distilled water solution to disrupt the vesicles. Estimate the liberated antigen by the Bradford method or drug by respective spectrophotometric or HPLC method.

PROTOCOL 11.18
Preparation of Proliposomes
Materials

Phosphatidyl choline from egg yolk,

Phosphatidyl ethanolamine

Cholesterol

Indomethacin (model drug)

Phosphate buffer saline (PBS)

Procedure

- Take the lipids PC: CH: PE in molar ratio of 1: 0.5: 0.16 and mix the lipid mixture thoroughly in dry form and dissolve in warm ethanol. Add the drug solution in PBS (pH 7.4, 2 mg/ml) to yield a lipid ethanol water mixture.

- Heat this mixture to 60°C for few minutes and then cool the mixture at the room temperature to facilitate the formation of a proliposome in the mixture.

- Add drop wise the buffer with the continuous stirring to this proliposome mixture that finally converts into a liposome suspension.

- Sonicate the prepared MLVs with a probe sonicator for 3 mins and extruded six times through a 0.22μm pore size polycarbonate membrane filter.

- Dialyse the liposome suspension to remove the unencapsulated drug against PBS (pH 7.4) and observe under transmission electron microscope.

- To determine the encapsulation efficiency, dissolve the measured volume of liposome in methanol and determine the drug concentration HPLC determination.

PROTOCOL: 11.19
Preparation of Multivesicular Liposomes (DEPOFOAM)
Materials

Recombinant human insulin

Phospholipids, 1,2-dioleoyl-*sn*-glycero-3-phosphocholine (DOPC or DC18:1 PC),

1,2-dierucoyl-*sn*-glycero-3-phosphocholine (DEPC or DC22:1 PC)

2-dinervonoyl-*sn*-glycero-3-phospho-choline (DNPC or DC24:1 PC)

1,2-dipalmitoyl-*sn*- glycerol-3-phosphoglycerol (DPPG)

Triolein

Tricaprylin

Cholesterol

L-Lysine

Normal saline (0.9% sodium chloride)

50% glucose

1 M hydrochloric acid

Acidified isopropyl alcohol (IPA)

Procedure

The multivesicular DepoFoam particles containing protein or peptide drugs can be prepared by a two-step water-in-oil-in-water double emulsification process.

Step 1. The First Step is to Prepare 'Water-in-oil' Emulsion

- Emulsify A lipid combination solution made of 13.20 mM DCn:1PC (n518, 22, or 24), 19.88 mM cholesterol, 2.79 Mm DPPG, and 2.44 mM triolein or tricaprylin in chloroform with an equal volume of an aqueous solution (the first aqueous solution) containing drugs (insulin, metenkephalin, octreotide, or leuprolide,) in 50 mM HCl (for insulin), or 25 mM citric acid (for enkephalin and octreotide), or 100 mM phosphoric acid (for leuprolide), and varying amounts of sucrose (ranging from 2.5–7.5%), to produce a 'water-in-oil' emulsion (the first emulsion).

Step 2. A Subsequent Emulsification with a Second Aqueous Solution, such as 1.5% Glycine containing 40 mM Lysine, resulted in a 'water-in-oil -in water' Double Emulsion (the Second Emulsion)

- Transfer the second emulsion and add into another aliquot of the second aqueous solution. Remove the chloroform by flushing nitrogen over the surface of the mixture at 37°C.
- Wash the resulting multivesicular liposomes to remove unencapsulated drug and harvest by centrifugation for 10 min at 600 × g and then re-suspend in buffered saline solution.
- After harvesting the DepoFoam particles, determine the amount of free drug in the supernatant, which reflects the amount of drug released subsequent to the wash steps, and is an indication of the stability of the DepoFoam matrix.

Characterisation of DepoFoam Formulations

Determination of Per cent Encapsulation (or per cent Yield)

Per cent encapsulation (or per cent yield) of drug is defined as the per cent ratio of the amount of drug in the final liposome suspension to the total amount of drug used in the first aqueous solution.

Lipocrit

Lipocrit is defined, in analogy to hematocrit, as the per cent ratio of the pellet volume to the suspension volume (see conditions below for obtaining the pellet volume). Lipocrit is calculated by the hematocrit method. In this method, approximately 50 ml of the multi-vesicular liposome suspension into a capillary tube is taken. Seal the one end of the tube while ensuring that there are no air bubbles. Upon centrifugation at 600g for 10 min, separate the suspension into a pellet layer and a supernatant layer. The per cent ratio of the length occupied by the pellet to that by the supernatant plus pellet gives the lipocrit.

Drug Loading and Per cent Free Drug

Per cent free drug is defined as the per cent ratio of the amount of drug in the supernatant to the amount of drug in the final suspension times (1-lipocrit). Drug loading is defined as the amount of drug encapsulated in each unit of the encapsulated volume, and can be estimated as the ratio of the drug concentration of the final DepoFoam suspension to the lipocrit. To determine the free drug concentration in the formulation product, collect the supernatant by centrifugation for 10 min at $600 \times g$ and then extract with acidified isopropyl alcohol (IPA) solution, typically 2–4-fold, followed by rigorous mixing to obtain a clear solution. For determination of the total concentration, extract the DepoFoam suspension with the same extraction solution as for the supernatant except that a higher extraction dilution, typically 10-fold with the acidified IPA can be used. Estimate the concentration of insulin at 280 nm with a UV spectrophotometer. Determine the drug concentrations in the supernatant and suspension using a standard curve previously prepared by known concentrations of appropriate drug.

Particle Size Distribution

Particle size distribution and the median diameter can be determined by the method of laser light diffraction using a particle size analyser.

In vitro Release

To determine the *in vitro* release experiments, dilute the DepoFoam suspensions 5-fold into human plasma containing 0.01% NaN_3. Take a 0.5-ml sample of the diluted suspension in 3 screw-cap Eppendorf tube for each time point; incubate the samples under gentle rotating conditions (12 cycles /min) at 37° C. Withdraw the samples in duplicate for analyses according to the planned schedule and add 0.9 ml of normal saline. Collect the particle pellets by centrifugation in a micro-centrifuge at $16,000 \times g$ for 4 min and stored at –20 °C. Extract the particle pellets with acidified isopropyl alcohol (IPA) as described above, and the extracts analysed by RP-HPLC.

SUGGESTED READINGS

- Andrieux, K., Lesieur, S., Ollivon, M., Grabielle-Madelmont, C. (1998) J. Chromatogr. Biomed. Sci. Appl., 706,141.
- Barenholtz, Y., Amselem, S. and Lichtenberg, D. (1979) FEBS Lett., 99, 210.

- Barenholz, Y. and Cromellin, D.J.A. (1994) Encyclopedia of Pharmaceutical Technology (Swarbrick, J., Ed.), Marcel Dekker, pp 1.
- Barlett, G.R. (1959) J. Biol. Chem., 234, 466.
- Batzri, S. and Korn, E.D. (1973) Biochim. Biophys. Acta, 298, 1015.
- Brooks, C.J.W., MacLachlan, J., Cole, W.J. and Lawrie, T.D.V. (1984) Proceedings of symposium on Analysis of Steroids, Szeged, Hungary, pp. 349.
- Buboltz, J.T. and Feigenson, G.W. (1999) Biochim. Biophys. Acta, 1417, 232.
- Chapman, D. (1975) Quart. Rev. Biophys. 8, 185.
- Enoch, H.G., Stritamatter, P. (1976) Proc. Natl. Acad. Sci. USA, 76, 145.
- Fry, D.W., White, C. and Goldman, D.J. (1978) Anal. Biochem., 90, 809.
- Gregoriadis, G., de Silva, H. and Florence, A.T. (1990) Int. J. Pharm., 65, 235.
- Gruber, H.J., Wilmsen, H.U., Schurga, A., Pilger, A. and Schindler, H. (1995) Biochim. Biophys. Acta 1240, 266.
- Gunter, K.K., Gunter, T.E., Jarkowski, A. and Rosier, R.N. (1982) Anal. Biochem., 120, 113.
- Hamilton, R.L., Goerke, J., Guo, L.S.S., Williams, M.C. and Havel, R.J. (1980) J. Lipid Res., 21, 981.
- Hauser, H. and Gains, N. (1982) Proc. Natl. Acad. Sci. USA, 79, 1683.
- Hope, M.J., Bally, M.B., Webb, G. and Culis, P.R. (1985) Biochim. Biophys. Acta, 812, 55.
- Hope, M.J., Bally, M.B., Webb, G. and Culis, P.R. (1985) Biochim. Biophys. Acta, 812, 55.
- Huang, C. (1969) Biochemistry, 8, 344.
- Jones, G.R. and Cossins, A.R. (1989) Physical methods of study, Liposomes: A practical approach (New, RRC, Ed.), OIRL Press, Oxford, pp. 184–191.
- Katayama K., Kato Y., Onishi, H., Nagai T., Machida, Y., Int. J. Pharm.248 (2002) 93.
- Kirby, C. and Gregoriadis, G. (1984) Biotechnology, 2, 979.
- Kolchens, S., Ramaswami, V., Birgenheier, J., Nett, L. and O'Brien, D.F. (1993) Chem. Phys. Lipids, 65,1.
- Lasic, D.D. (1998) Trends in Biotechnology, 16, 307.
- Lasic, D.D., Ceh, D.D., Stuart, M.C.A., Guo, L., Frederik, P.M. and Barenholz, Y. (1995) Biochim. Biophys. Acta, 1239, 145.
- Lesieur, S., Grabielle-Madelmont, C., Paternostre, M.T. and Ollivon, M. (1991) Anal. Biochem. 192, 334.
- Levy, D. *et al.,* (1990) Biochim. Biopyhs. Acta, 179, 1025.
- Lopez-Berestein, G., Mehta, R., Hopffer, R., Mills, K., Kasi, L., Mehta, K., Fainstein, V., Luna, M., Harsh, E.N. and Juliano, R. (1983) J. Infect. Dis., 147, 939.
- Mandal, T.K. and Downing, D.T. (1993) Acta Derm. Venereol., 73, 12.
- Mayer, L.D., Hope, M.J., Cullis, R.P. and Janoff, A.S. (1985) Biochim. Biophys. Acta, 817, 193.
- Mayhew, E., lazo, R., Vali, W.J., King, J. and Green, A.M. (1984) Biochim. Biophys. Acta, 775, 169.
- Moon, M.H. and Giddings, J.C. (1993) J. Pharm. Biomed. Anal. 11, :911.
- Morgan, C.G., Thomas, E.W. and Yianni, Y.P. (1983) Biochim. Biophys. Acta, 728, 356.
- Nakata, T., Sobue, K. and Hirokawa, N. (1990) J Cell Biol. 110, 13–25.
- New, R.R.C. (1989) Liposomes: A practical approach, OIRL Press, Oxford, London, pp. 1.

- Ohsawa, T., Miura, H. and Harada, K. (1985) Pharm. Bull., 33, 2916.
- Oku, N. and MacDonald, R.C. (1983) Biochemistry, 22, 855.
- Ostro, M.J. (1987) Liposomes: From biophysics to therapeutics, Marcel Dekker, New York.
- Papahadjopoulos, D., Vali, W.J., Jacobson, K. and Poste, G. (1975) Biochim. Biophys. Acta, 394, 483.
- Perkins, W.R., Minchey, S.R., Ostro, M.J., Taraschi, T.F. and Janoff, A.S. (1988) Biochim. Biophys. Acta 943, 103.
- Schmidtgen, M.C., Drechsler, M., Lasch, J. and Schubert, R. (1998) J. Microsc. 191,177.
- Stewart, J.C.M. (1959) Anal. Biochem., 104, 10
- Szoka, F. and Papahadjopoulos, D. (1978) Proc. Natl. Acad. Sci. USA, 75, 4194.
- Talsma, H. and Crommelin D.J.A. (1992) Liposomes as Drug Delivery Systems, Part I: Preparation, Pharmaceutical Technology, 16, 96.
- Terao, J., Asano, I. and Matsushito, S. (1985) Lipids, 20, 312.
- Uster, P.S. and Deamer, D.W. (1981) Arch. Biochem. Biophys., 209, 385.
- Vyas, S.P., Katare, Y.K., Mishra, V. and Sihorkar, V. (2000) Int. J. Pharm., 210, 1.
- Weiner, N., Martin, F. and Riaz, M. (1989) Drug Dev. Ind. Phar., 15, 1523.
- Wybenga, D.R., Pileggi, V.J., Dirstine, P.H. and Di Giorgio, J. (1970) J. Clin. Chem., 16, 980.

Microspheres, Microparticles and Microcapsules

12

The term microcapsule is defined as a spherical particle with size varying from 50 nm to 2 mm, containing a core substance. Microspheres are, in technical sense, spherical empty particles. However, the terms microcapsules and microspheres are often used synonymously. In addition, some related terms are used as well viz; "microbeads" and "beads". Spheres and spherical particles are also used for microspheres of large size and rigid morphology. The microspheres are characteristically free flowing powders consisting of proteins or synthetic polymers, which may or may not be biodegradable in nature, and ideally having a particle size less than 200 μm. Solid biodegradable microspheres incorporating a drug dispersed or dissolved throughout particle matrix have the potential for the controlled release of drug. These carriers received much attention not only for prolonged release but also for the targeting of the anticancer drugs to the tumour (Widder et al., 1979).

MATERIAL(S) USED

A number of different substances both biodegradable as well as non-biodegradable have been investigated for the preparation of microspheres. These materials include the polymers of natural and synthetic origin and also modified natural substances. Synthetic polymers employed as carrier materials are methyl methacrylate (Kreuter, 1983), acrolein (Margel and Wiesel, 1984), lactide, glycolide and their copolymers, ethylene vinyl acetate copolymer, polyanhydrides, etc. The natural polymers used for the purpose include albumin (Lee et al, 1981), gelatin, starch, collagen and carrageenan, etc. Some of the commonly used polymers in the preparation of the microspheres are classified and listed in Table 12.1.

METHODS OF PREPARATION

Single Emulsion Technique

The microparticulate carriers of natural polymers, i.e. those of proteins and carbohydrates are prepared by single emulsion technique. The natural polymers are dissolved or dispersed in aqueous medium followed by dispersion in the non-aqueous medium, e.g. oil. In the second step of preparation, crosslinking of the dispersed globule is carried out. The crosslinking can be achieved either by means of heat or by using a chemical crosslinker. The chemical crosslinking agents used include glutaraldehyde, formaldehyde, terephthaloyl chloride, diacid chloride, etc. Crosslinking by heat is affected by adding the dispersion to previously heated oil. Heat denaturation is however, not suitable for the thermolabile drugs while the chemical crosslinking suffers disadvantage of excessive exposure of active ingredient to chemicals if added at the time of preparation their removal is a cumbersome process.

Table 12.1: Classification of polymers

---

1. **Synthetic polymers**

   Non-biodegradable

   - PMMA
   - Acrolein
   - Epoxypolymers

   Biodegradable

   - Lactides, glycolides and their polymers
   - Polyanhydrides
   - Polycyanoacrylates

2. **Natural**

   Proteins

   - Albumin
   - Gelatin
   - Collagen

   Carbohydrates

   - Starch
   - Agarose
   - Chitosan

   Chemically modified carbohydrates

   - DEAE cellulose
   - Poly (acryl) dextran

Double Emulsion Technique

Briefly, double emulsion method of microspheres preparation primarily involves the formation of the multiple emulsions or the double emulsion of type W/O/W and is the best-suited method to the water-soluble drugs, peptides, proteins and the vaccines. This method can be used with both the natural as well as the synthetic polymers. The aqueous protein solution is dispersed in a lipophilic organic continuous phase. This protein solution may contain the active constituents. The continuous phase is generally consisted of the polymer solution that eventually encapsulates the protein contained in dispersed aqueous phase. The primary emulsion is then subjected to homogenisation or sonication before it is added to the aqueous solution of the poly vinyl alcohol (PVA). This results in the formation of a double emulsion. The emulsion is then subjected to solvent removal either by solvent evaporation or by solvent extraction process. The solvent evaporation is carried out by maintaining emulsion at reduced pressure or by continuous stirring of the emulsion so that the organic phase evaporates out. In the latter case, the emulsion is added to the large quantity of water (with or without surfactant) into which organic phase partially or fully diffuses. The solid microspheres are subsequently separated by filtration and washing.

Polymerisation Technique

The polymerisation techniques conventionally used for the preparation of the microspheres are mainly classified as:

    I.   Conventional polymerisation

   II.   Interfacial polymerisation

Conventional Polymerisation

The two processes are carried out essentially in a liquid phase. The conventional polymerisation is carried out using different techniques such as bulk polymerisation, suspension precipitation, emulsion and miceller polymerisation processes.

In bulk polymerisation, a monomer or a mixture of monomers along with an initiator is usually heated to initiate the polymerisation and to carry out the process. The catalyst or the initiator is added to the reaction mixture to facilitate or accelerate the rate of the reaction. The polymer so obtained may be molded or comminuted mechanically to obtain microspheres. For loading of drug, adsorptive drug loading or adding drug during the process of polymerisation may be opted.

The suspension polymerisation, which is also referred to as the bead or pearl polymerization is carried out by heating the monomer or mixture of monomers with active principles (drugs) as droplets dispersion in a continuous aqueous phase. The droplets may also contain an initiator and other additives.

The emulsion polymerisation, however, differs from the suspension polymerisation in respect to presence of an initiator in the aqueous phase, which in process diffuses to and through the surface of the micelles or into the emulsion globules. The bulk polymerisation has an advantage of formation of the pure polymer, but it also suffers a disadvantage, as it can efficiently dissipate the heat of reaction, which can adversely affect the thermolabile active ingredients. On the other hand the suspension and emulsion polymerisation can be carried out at lower temperature, since continuous external phase is normally water, which allows heat to dissipate fast. The two processes also lead to the formation of the higher molecular weight polymer due to relatively faster rate of polymerisation. The major disadvantage of suspension and emulsion polymerisation is the association of polymer with the unreacted monomer and other additives, which are difficult to remove completely.

Interfacial Polymerisation

Interfacial polymerization essentially proceeds involving reaction of various monomers at the interface constituted of the two immiscible liquid phases to form a film of polymer that essentially envelops the dispersed phase. In this technique two reacting monomers are employed; one of which is dissolved in the continuous phase while the other being dispersed in the continuous phase. The continuous phase is generally aqueous in nature throughout, in which the second monomer is dispersed or emulsified. The monomers present in either of phases diffuse rapidly and polymerise rapidly at the interface. Two conditions arise depending upon the solubility of formed polymer in the emulsion droplet. If the polymer is soluble in the droplet it will lead to the formation of the monolithic type of the carrier on the other hand if the polymer is insoluble in the monomer or the dispersion media droplet, the formed carrier is of capsular (reservoir) type.

The degree of polymerisation can be controlled by controlling the reactivity of the monomers, their concentration, the composition of the vehicle of either phases and by the temperature of the system. The particle size can be controlled by controlling the droplets or globules size of the disperse phase. The polymerisation is generally controlled by maintaining the concentration of the monomers, which can be varied by addition of an excess of the continuous phase. The interfacial polymerisation is not widely used in the preparation of the microparticles because of certain drawbacks, which are associated with the process such as:

- Toxicity associated with the unreacted monomer
- High permeability of the film
- High degradation of the drug during the polymerisation
- Fragility of microcapsules
- Non-biodegradability of the microparticles

Phase Separation Coacervation Technique(s)

Phase separation method is specially designed for preparing the reservoir type of the system, i.e. to encapsulate water soluble drugs, e.g. peptides, proteins, however, some of the preparations are of matrix type particularly, when the drug is hydrophobic in nature, e.g. steroids. In matrix type device, the drug or the protein is dissolved in the polymer phase. The process is based on the principle of decreasing the solubility of the polymer in the organic phase by using physicochemical variants to affect the formation of the polymer rich phase referred to as the coacervate phase. The coacervation can be brought about by addition of the third component to the system which results in the formation of the two distinct phases, one rich in the polymer, while the other one, i.e. supernatant, depleted of the polymer. There are various means and methods, which are effectively employed for coacervate phase separation. The choice of method is largely dependent on the polymer being used and set of conditions. The methods could alternatively be based on salt addition, non-solvent addition, addition of the incompatible polymer or change in pH.

In this technique, the polymer is first dissolved in a suitable solvent and then drug is dispersed by making its aqueous solution, if it is hydrophilic or it may be dissolved in the polymer solution itself, in case it is hydrophobic; phase separation is then accomplished by changing the solution conditions by using any of the method mentioned above. The process is carried out under continuous stirring to control the size of the microparticles. The process variables are critical, since the rate of achieving the coacervate determines the distribution of the polymer film, the particle size and agglomeration of the formed particles. The agglomeration must be avoided by stirring the suspension using a suitable speed stirrer since as the process of microspheres formation proceeds; the formed polymerised globules tend to agglomerate. Therefore, the process variable should critically be monitored, as they seem to control the kinetic of particles formation.

Spray Drying and Spray Congealing

Spray drying and spray congealing methods are based on the drying of the mist of the polymer and drug in the air. Depending upon the removal of the solvent or the cooling of the solution, the two processes are named spray drying and the spray congealing respectively. The polymer is first dissolved in a suitable volatile organic solvent such as dichloromethane, acetone, etc. The drug in the solid form is then dispersed in the polymer solution under high-speed homogenisation. This dispersion is then atomised in a stream of hot air. The atomisation leads to the formation of the small droplets or the fine mist from which the solvent evaporates instantaneously leading to the formation of the microspheres in a size range 1–100 µm. Microparticles are separated from the hot air by means of the cyclone separator while the traces of solvent are removed by vacuum drying. One of the major advantages of the process is feasibility of operation under aseptic conditions. The two processes are rapid, requiring single stage operation, suitable for both batches and bulk manufacturing. The rate of solvent removal by evaporation strongly influences the characteristics of the formed microspheres and it depends on the temperature, pressure, and the solubility parameter of the polymer, the solvent and the dispersion media. Very rapid solvent evaporation, however leads to the formation of porous microparticles.

Solvent Extraction

Solvent extraction method used for the preparation of microparticles, is based on removal of the organic phase by extraction of the organic solvent. The method involves water miscible organic solvents such as isopropanol. Organic phase is removed by extraction with water. This process decreases the hardening time for the microspheres. One variation of the process involves direct addition of the drug or protein to polymer organic solution. The rate of solvent removal by extraction method depends on the temperature of water, ratio of emulsion volume to the water and the solubility profile of the polymer.

CHARACTERISATION

Particle Size and Shape

The most widely used procedures to characterise microparticles are conventional light microscopy (LM) and scanning electron microscopy (SEM) (Fig. 12.1). Both techniques can be used to determine the shape and outer structure (morphology) of the microparticles. Confocal laser scanning microscopy (CLSM) is applied as a nondestructive visualisation technique for microparticles, especially within biological system(s).

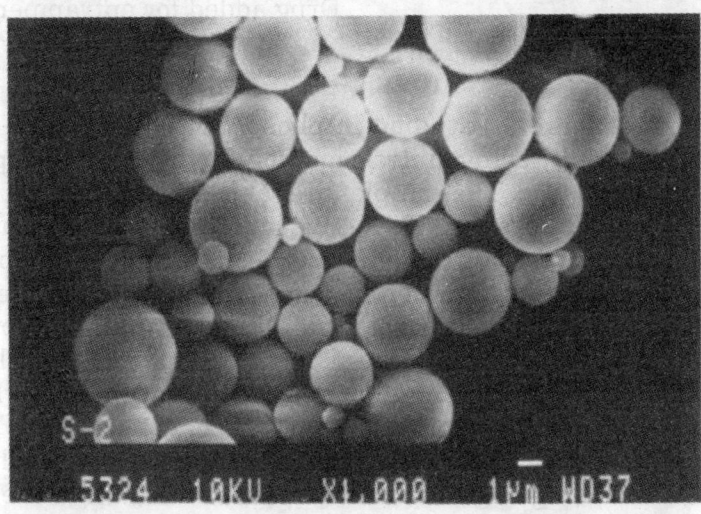

Fig 12.1: *SEM photographs of PLGA microspheres*

Degradation Behaviour

The surface chemistry of the microspheres can be determined using the electron spectroscopy for chemical analysis (ESCA). ESCA provides a means to the determination of the atomic composition of the surface. The spectrum obtained using ESCA determines the surfacial degradation of the biodegradable microspheres. Similarly, FTIR is successfully used to determine the degradation of the polymeric matrix of the carrier system.

Density Determination

Measured by using a multivolume pychnometer

Isoelectric Point

The microelectrophoresis is a method that measures the electrophoretic mobility of microspheres from which the isoelectric point can be determined and used for separation and qualitative surface electric property approximation.

Surface Functional Residue

The carboxylic acid functional group free (residue) is largely measured by using radioactive glycine whereas surface associated amino acid residue is determined by the radioactive [14]C - acetic acid conjugate based radioactive tracers techniques.

Capture Efficiency

The capture efficiency of the microspheres or the per cent entrapment can be determined by allowing washed microspheres lysis. The lysate is then subjected to the determination of active constituents as per monograph drug content requirement. The per cent encapsulation efficiency is calculated using following equation

$$\text{Encapsulation efficiency (\%)} = \frac{\text{Amount of drug entrapped}}{\text{Drug added for entrapment}}$$

Release Studies

Drug release from microspheres is studied in phosphate buffer saline of pH 7.4, using rotating paddle apparatus or by using dialysis method. In the case of the paddle apparatus the sample is agitated at 100 rpm. The samples are taken at specific time intervals and are replaced by the same amount of saline. The active ingredient in the sample withdrawn is analysed as per the monograph requirement and release profile is computed and plotted as amount of drug released as a function of time. The release profile of the drugs or proteins generally depends on the method of formulation, formulation conditions (process variable), and more importantly on the nature of the polymer used in their preparation. Degradation profile of the polymer is another important parameter, which determines, whether the release is sustained, prolonged or burst type. Alternatively, dialysis method can be used to study the release of the drugs/proteins from the microspheres. The microspheres are kept in a dialysing bag or tube with membrane, while the dialysing media is continuously stirred and samples of dialysate are periodically taken. The withdrawn samples are estimated for drug content. Each time the volume is replaced with equal fresh buffer solution.

Hydrophobicity

Angle of contact is measured to determine the nature of microspheres in terms of hydrophilicity or hydrophobicity.

PROTOCOL: 12.1

PLGA Microspheres

Materials

Poly-lactic-co-glycolic acid (PLGA) 80,000 MW

Polyvinyl alcohol (PVA) 78,000 MW

Isopropyl alcohol

Methylene chloride

Rhodamine G6 chloride (fluorescent lipophilic marker)

Procedure

Preparation of Microsphere Matrix

- Dissolve the polymer and the drug and dye mixture separately in methylene chloride in equal volumes.
- Sonicate it for 20 seconds to solubilise the polymer.

- Mix polymer solution to drug dye solution.

Preparation of Continuous Phase

- Dissolve 500 mg of PVA in 30 ml of distilled water and warm to 65°C.
- Add the solution to 70 ml of glycerol and mix.
- Add 4 ml of the polymer drug dye solution in methylene chloride to a 100ml of the continuous phase, chill at 4° and 10°C, and administer with a syringe attached to a 10-inch long needle. Agitate the mixture using a mechanical shaker at 5000 rpm.
- After 5 minutes, replace the ice bath with a water bath previously warmed to 45°C for 5 minutes to expedite the evaporation of organic solvent under continued stirring at 5000 to 6000 rpm.
- Subsequently, transfer the contents to a 5% isopropyl alcohol solution and stir vigorously for 30 minutes using a magnetic stirrer.
- Centrifuge the microspheres suspension at 12,000 rpm to remove residual isopropyl alcohol.
- Place the centrifuge vials overnight in a vacuum oven under a vacuum pressure of 27 mm Hg without heating.
- The microspheres can be obtained and collected on drying (Scheme 12.1).

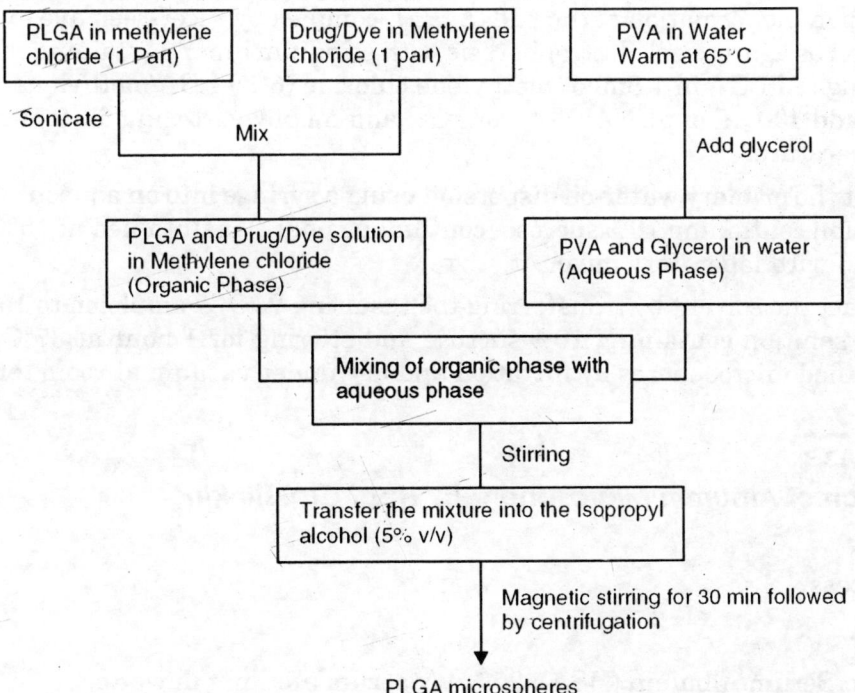

Scheme: 12.1 *Preparation of PLGA microspheres*

PROTOCOL: 12.2

Preparation of Plasmid DNA Loaded Microspheres

Microspheres of PLGA are biodegradable and biocompatible, and they offer many distinct advantages over conventional delivery systems. Encapsulation of therapeutic agents such as DNA in microspheres protects the agent from enzymatic degradation, enhances tissue specificity due to localised delivery, eliminates the need for multiple administration, and allows for controlled and sustained delivery. Microspheres preparation is based on water-oil-water (W/O/W) emulsion solvent evaporation/extraction method.

Material

pDNA (supercoiled, ~5 kilobase [kb]) encoding luciferase gene

PLL (poly-l-lysine)

Methylene chloride

Tris-EDTA (TE; 10mM/L Tris-HCl buffer containing 1mM/L EDTA, pH 7.4)

Procedure

* Prepare a pDNA: PLL complex (1:0.6,w/w) at room temperature by gently mixing 200 µL of pDNA (2.25–6.75 mg/ml) in Tris-EDTA buffer with an equal volume of PLL (1.35–3.75 mg/ml) in TE buffer.

* Confirm the formation of the pDNA: PLL complex by PicoGreen dye exclusion assay as well as agarose gel electrophoresis with ethidium bromide staining . Then, dissolve 150 mg of PLGA in 1.8ml of methylene chloride (6% PLGA/methylene chloride, w/v) and add 400 µL of pDNA: PLL complex and mix by vortexing for 2 minutes at room temperature.

* Inject the primary water-oil dispersion using a syringe into an aqueous 4% (w/v) PVA solution containing 10% sucrose (continuous phase) maintained at 15°C while being mixed with laboratory mixer or stirrer.

* Extract the solvent by transferring the resulting W/O/W emulsion to 150 ml of 0.35% PVA solution containing 10% sucrose and stirring for 1 hour at 37°C. Recover the solidified microspheres by filtration and dry under vacuum at room temperature.

PROTOCOL: 12.3

Preparation of Albumin Microsphere by Heat Crosslinking

Principle:

Batch process

Materials:

Human Serum Albumin (HSA): 25% w/v serum albumin in water
Cottonseed oil : 1 litre
Propeller type magnetic stirrer

Procedure

- Dissolve human serum albumin in water to achieve a final solution of 25% w/v.

- Inject 4ml of this solution into 1 litre of cottonseed oil, which has been preheated to 30–50°C with a 25-gauge hypodermic needle, and stirred at 500 rpm using a propeller type stirrer.

- Prepare water in oil type emulsion and raise the temperature of the oil bath to 110°C with continuous stirring until the microspheres are essentially dehydrated.

- After drying by dehydration at an appropriately selected temperature, i.e. above 100°C filter the microspheres from the oil bath on filter paper and wash with diethyl ether. The obtained microspheres are generally 10–20μm in diameter and are discrete may be a free flowing powder on drying (Scheme 12.2).

- Several factors that affect the microspheres preparation include stirring rate, higher temperature of oil bath, etc.

- A well classical study thus may be designed to study the effect of these parameters on resultant size of microsphere(s), drug loading efficiency and drug release profile.

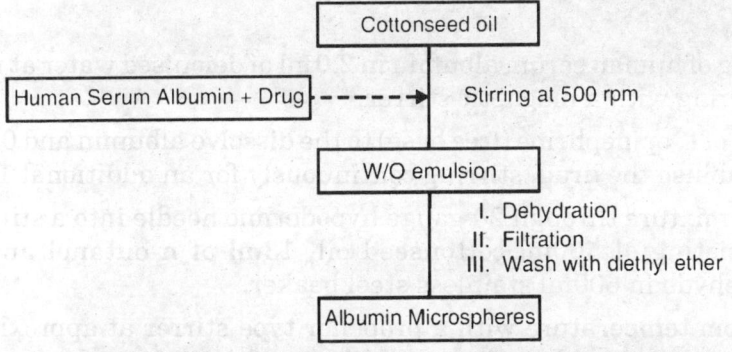

Scheme 12.2: *Preparation of albumin microspheres*

PROTOCOL: 12.4

Preparation of Drug Loaded Albumin Microspheres by Heat Induced Crosslinking

Procedure

- Dissolve 1g of human serum albumin in 2.0ml of deionised water by stirring with magnetic stirrer.

- Add 0.1g of 5-flurouracil (5-FU) or any other drug selected for entrapment/loading to the albumin aqueous solution (25% w/v) and stir continuously for an additional 15 min.

- Since 5-FU at this concentration does not completely dissolve in the albumin solution. place the aqueous mixture in a standard tissue grinder of 10ml capacity and further, disperse to ensure homogenous distribution of the remaining undissolved 5-FU particle through out the albumin solution.

- Then immediately inject with a tuberculin syringe equipped with a 20-gauge hypodermic needle into 500 ml of cottonseed oil contained in a 600ml stainless steel beaker at room temperature and stir with a propeller stirrer at approximately 2000rpm. The oil bath and its contents are then cooled at room temperature. Separate the resulting microspheres from the oil on Whatman No. 5 filter paper using vacuum filtration.

- Remove final traces of oil from the drug-loaded microspheres by washing them several times with 30 ml haptane.

PROTOCOL: 12.5

Preparation of Microsphere by Chemical Crosslinking at Room Temperature

The method is essentially used to load the drugs in albumin microspheres, which are characteristically thermolabile.

Procedure

- Dissolve 1g of human serum albumin in 2.0 ml of deionised water at room temperature under stirring with a magnetic stirrer.

- Add 0.15g of L-epinephrine (free base) to the dissolve albumin and 0.725 L (+) ascorbic acid to stabilise the drug, stirring continuously for an additional 15min.

- Inject the mixture through 20-gauge hypodermic needle into a stirred homogeneous bath consisting of 500ml cottonseed oil, 13ml of n-butanol and 2ml of 25 %v/v glutaraldehyde in 600ml stainless steel beaker.

- Stir at room temperature with a propeller type stirrer at approximately 1200rpm. Stir continuously for 4 h during which the resulting microspheres are dehydrated by n-butanol and crosslinked by the glutaraldehyde.

- The hardened microspheres so formed are separated from the bath medium on Whatman No. 5 filter paper using vacuum filtration. Final traces of oil are removed from the drug-loaded microspheres by washing them several times with 100-ml aliquots of heptane.

Note: additional chemical cross linking at room temperature

In addition to formaldehyde and glutaraldehyde other crosslinking agent may be utilized in preparing albumin microspheres (Abdella *et al.,* 1979). These crosslinkers include di, tri, and tetravalent metallic cations. More specifically cationic Fe^{3+} and Al^{3+} are found to be suitable for the purpose and they are readily dissolved in n-butanol and sec-butanol, 2-ethylhexanol, and other lipophilic drying alcohols. The latter are freely miscible with cottonseed or other vegetable oils. The resulting solution serves as a one step crosslinking bath especially for albumin microspheres.

PROTOCOL: 12.6

Chemical Crosslinking at Low Temperatures
Procedure

- Dissolve bovine serum albumin (600 mg) in 2.4 ml of a solution containing 0.1% sodium dodecyl sulphate (SDS) in 1mM sodium phosphate buffer (pH 7.5).
- Cool the solution to 4°C and disperse the drug in a fine dispersion form.
- Immediately add 5% (v/v) aqueous solution of glutaraldehyde.
- The resulting dispersion is rapidly pipetted off into a 150 ml, volume of a well stirred 1:4 mixture of corn oil and petroleum ether contained in a 250 ml beaker.
- Stirring continuously for 15min, at the end of which the solid microspheres are settled to the bottom of the beaker.
- Decant the spheronised bath mixture and wash three times with petroleum ether followed by drying the microspheres in vacuum desiccator.
- Incubate the dried microspheres twice for 15min time period in 25ml of a solution containing 0.1% (w/v) serum albumin dissolved in 0.05mM Tris buffer at pH 8.6.
- Wash the microspheres with 500ml of 1mM HCl using sintered glass funnel; Wash off the acidic solution with distilled water, and dry microspheres in a vacuum desiccator. The resulting microspheres containing drug are generally dark brown in colour and 100–200 μm diameter.

PROTOCOL: 12.7

Preparation of Magnet Responsive Albumin Microspheres

Magnetically responsive microspheres are prepared from albumin and other proteins polysaccharides and polypeptides. In general method given in previous protocols for the preparation of albumin microspheres can be utilised to prepare magnetic microspheres by simply dispersion of sufficient amount of magnetically responsive materials (e.g. Fe_2O_3, barium ferrite, etc.) in the initial albumin solution (which may or may not contain a drug) that is used in the microspheres preparation.

PROTOCOL: 12.8

Preparation of Hydrophilic Human Serum Albumin Microspheres
Materials

    Human serum albumin
    Distilled water
    Poly-methyl methacrylate (PMMA)
    Chloroform
    Toluene
    Glutaraldehyde

Instruments

    Ultrasonicator

Procedure

- Dissolve human serum albumin (150mg) in 0.5ml-distilled water in a test tube.

- Add the solution drop wise to a 25%w/v solution of PMMA previously dissolved in a mixture of 1.5ml chloroform and 1.5ml toluene in a screw cap test tube.
- Disperse the mixture with 1.0ml glutaraldehyde a vortex type mixer for 2 min (cross linking agent) and combine 1.0ml toluene in a separate test tube.
- Disperse the phases by ultrasonication for 20 sec at 50W.
- Add the resulting saturated solution of glutaraldehyde in toluene to albumin dispersion and mix with a rotary mixer at room temperature for 8 h.
- Wash the crossedlinked HSA/MS so as to remove all PMMA by the addition of 10.0ml of acetone, briefly agitate, and then centrifuge (2000 rpm, 2 min) following each washing.
- Discard the supernatant and resuspend HSA/MS pellet in additional 10.0ml of acetone. Repeat this wash procedure eight times. After the last wash allow HSA/MS to air vacuum dry (Scheme 12.3).
- The product obtained will be a brown free flowing powder with an average diameter of 30 ± 5µm.

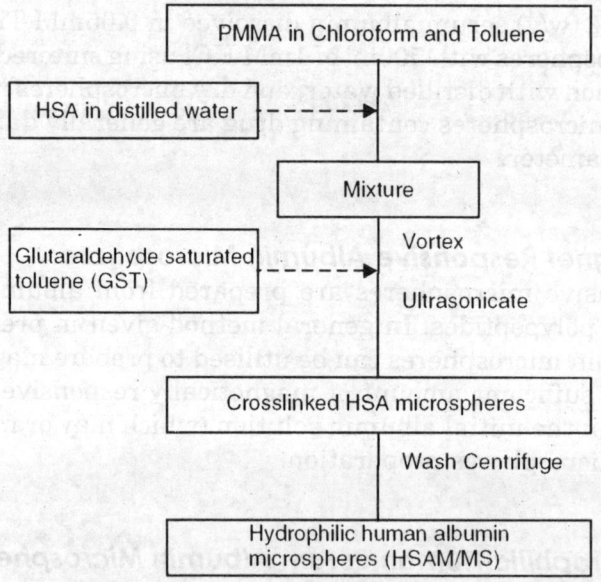

Scheme 12.3: *Preparation of hydrophilic human albumin microspheres*

PROTOCOL: 12.9

Incorporation of Water Soluble Drug in Albumin Microsphere

There appears to be two basic methods, which are available for the production of albumin microspheres. First, either a thermal denaturation of HSA at elevated temperatures (95-170°C) or chemical crosslinking in vegetable oil or isooctane, etc. emulsion. The latter method-which is claimed to produce hydrophilic microspheres (Longo *et al,* 1982; Przyborowsky *et al,* 1982; Miller *et al,* 1982) depends on the chemical crosslinking of HSA in a water in oil emulsion using concentrated polymer solutions as a dispersing phase.

Preparation

Human serum albumin microspheres may be prepared in the range of 0.2–100µm using the manufacturing process as outlined below:

- Add highly purified olive oil to a flat-bottomed glass beaker (diameter 60mm, height 110mm) equipped with four baffles (4mm depth) positioned against the wall of the beaker. Place a motor driven four bladed axial-flow impeller in the center of the beaker, two-third into the oil such that there is a distance of 3mm between the baffles and the impeller blade.
- After prestirring of the oil for 30 min at the desired speed, add an aqueous solution of HSA and drug in isotonic buffer (pH 7) drop wise through a hypodermic syringe in the olive oil.
- Generally this aqueous phase (including crosslinkers) constitutes a final volume of 0.5ml. Stir the resulting water in oil emulsion for an additional period of time depending upon the method of stabilisation.

PROTOCOL: 12.10

Polyacrolein Microspheres

Principle

Several types of hydrophilic polyacrylate microspheres containing a variety of functional groups on their surface such as carboxylate, hydroxyl, amide or pyridine groups, have been synthesised previously. The functional groups were used to bind proteins covalently to microspheres by means of a series of chemical reactions. The last step of microspheres derivatisation prior to protein binding, is a reaction with glutaraldehyde that introduces reactive aldehyde groups on the surface of microspheres. In order to simplify the derivatisation procedures, polyglutaraldehyde microspheres prepared formed. However, the polyglutaraldehyde microspheres possess several disadvantages, i.e.

- Low yield of microspheres (3% w/w)
- Instability of microspheres especially of those with diameter larger than 0.7µm
- Instability of microspheres with magnetic properties in PBS solution.

Recently polyacrolein (PA) microspheres were synthesised. These microspheres address above disadvantages and they can be considered as relatively more advanced polyaldehyde microspheres.

Procedure

Polyacrolein Synthesis

PA microspheres are prepared by aqueous polymerisation of acrolein in the presence of an appropriate surfactant. The polymerisation is carried out under alkaline condition.

Preparation of Surfactant Sodium Hydrogen Sulphite-Polyglutaraldehyde

- Allow the reaction of 5.0 gm polyglutaraldehyde with sodium bisulphate (12.5gm in 30ml of water) until all the polyglutaraldehyde dissolves.
- Dialyze the solution extensively against demineralised water and then lyophilise.

The obtained surfactant was specifically designed for stabilisation of alkaline microspheres, since it contains both electrostatic and appropriate steric stabilisation groups. Many other surfactants, e.g. poly(ethylene)oxide, poly(vinyl alcohol), Tween20, sodium dodecyl sulphates, however fail to stabilise these microspheres.

Preparation of Microspheres

- Add 0.2N NaOH drop-wise to an aqueous solution containing 0.8% (w/v) of acrolein and 0.5% (w/v) of surfactant sodium hydrogen sulfite-polyglutaraldehyde conjugates, until the pH reaches to 10.5.
- Keep it for 2 hr and then dialyse the mixture extensively against distilled water.
- Centrifuge through water four times at 2000g for 20 min. The PA microspheres of average diameter 0.1μm as reportedly determined by scanning electron microscopy (SEM) could be obtained which can be redispersed easily in PBS or in distilled water. Various factors such as the concentration of surfactant, or acrolein or pH of the polymerisation reaction may affect the size of the microspheres (Scheme 12.4).

The microspheres prepared by this alkaline mechanism are of extremely uniform diameter, ranging from 0.04 upto ~8μm. PA microspheres with fluorescent or magnetic properties were synthesised by carrying out the above described polymerisation procedures in the presence of appropriate ferrochromic or ferrofluidic compounds, respectively.

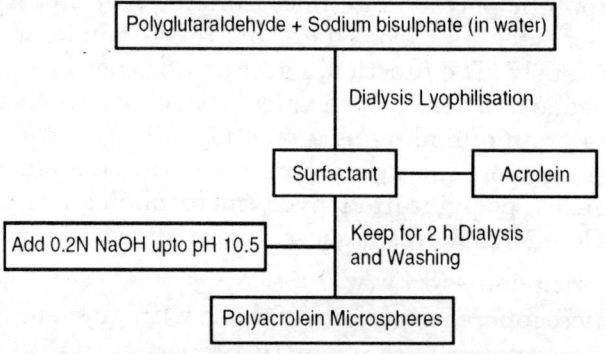

Scheme12.4: *Preparation of polyacrolein microspheres*

PROTOCOL: 12.11

Hybrido Microspheres

Principle

Hybrido microspheres can be prepared by grafting of preformed microspheres of approximately 0.1μm diameters, prepared by irradiation onto the surface of polyacrolein microspheres as obtained above under alkaline conditions (Protocol 12.10).

Procedure

- Mix 4.0ml of 4.5% v/v aqueous solution of acrolein, 0.5% of polyethylene oxide and 100mg of alkaline microspheres of 2.5μm diameters and de-aerate with argon.

- Irradiate the stirred solution with cobalt source (0.75Mrad). The PA grafted microspheres will form.
- Wash four times at 500 g for 10 min.

PROTOCOL: 12.12

Agarose-polyacrolein Microspheres Beads (APAMB)
Materials

- Agarose
- Polyacrolein microspheres [Prepare as per protocol 12.10]
- Peanut oil
- Divinyl sulfones

Agarose-Polyacrolein Microspheres Beads (APAMB) are prepared by encapsulating polyacrolein microspheres (Protocol 12.10) of approximately 0.15µm diameters within an agarose matrix.

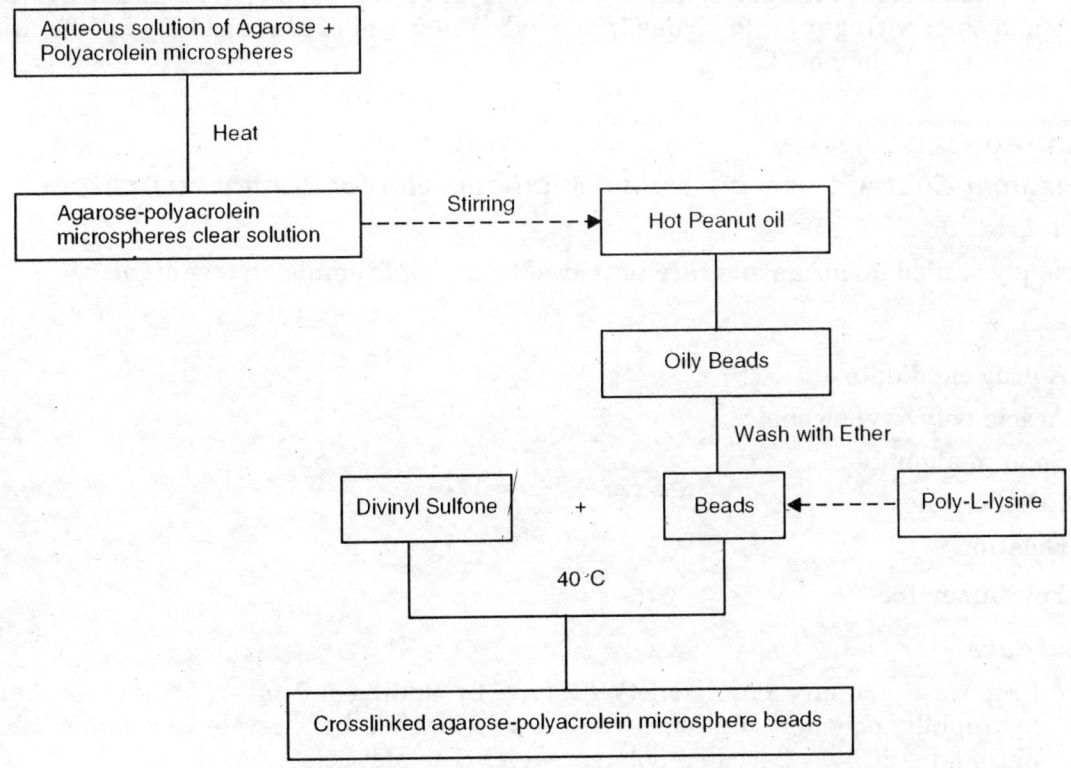

Scheme 12.5: *Preparation of agarose-polyacrolein microsphere beads*

Procedure

- Heat the aqueous solution containing 1g agarose and 25ml of polyacrolein microspheres (4% w/v) to 95°C until the agarose gel convert into a clear solution.

- Reduce the temperature of solution to 70°C and pour into a vessel containing peanut oil (previously heat upto 70°C) with stirring at 300 rpm.

- After ten minutes, cool the solution using ice.

- Wash the beads with ether thrice to remove the oil. Remove ether by evaporation.

- The diameter of beads, which are obtained, range from 50 to 250μm. Fractionations of beads can be done by passing them through appropriate sieves.

- Crosslinking of the APAMB is accomplished by interacting the beads with divinyl sulfone.

- Add 1ml of APAMB to an aqueous solution containing 2.0 ml of 0.5M sodium carbonate buffer at pH 11.0 and 20μl divinyl sulfone.

- Allow the reaction to proceed at 40°C. Wash the APAMB to remove divinyl sulfone by repeated decantation with water.

- The spacer arm of the polylysine-glutaraldehyde is bound to the APAMB by interacting the beads first with polylysine (1gm beads and 5 mg of polylysine in 2ml of water) and then with glutaraldehyde (1gm beads and 0.1ml of glutaraldehyde 50% in 2ml of water) (Scheme 12.5).

PROTOCOL: 12.13

Poloxamer Coated Three-ply-walled Microcapsules for Controlled Delivery

Principle

Three-ply-walled microcapsules are prepared by multiple emulsion technique.

Materials

A drug candidate

Acacia polyvinyl alcohol

Sodium alginate

Ethyl cellulose

Gelatin

Poloxamer 188

Procedure

- Prepare a primary emulsion (W/O type by adding 6.0 ml of 5% w/v solution of hydrophilic polymer solution to 18.0ml of 4% w/v ethyl acetate containing dibutyl phthalate (20% w/v based on polymer weight) as plasticiser.

- Stir the solution for 10 min.

- Add W/O primary emulsion to 36ml hydrophilic polymer solution under stirring in order to obtain a multiple emulsion; continue stirring for a period of 10 min.
- Then separate microcapsules by dialysing the multiple emulsions for a period of 2 days against PBS (pH 7.4) (Scheme 12.6).

Table 12.2 lists various formulation constituents of three-poly-walled microcapsule systems. The three plying system, based on acacia /ethyl cellulose/ acacia (AEA), acacia/ ethyl cellulose/acacia-gelatin and poly vinyl alcohol/ethyl cellulose/polyvinylachohol resulted in a stable three-walled system.

Table 12.2 *Formulation constituents of three-ply-walled microcapsules*

Acacia	Ethyl cellulose	Acacia-gelatin
Acacia	Ethyl cellulose	Acacia
Gelatin	Ethyl cellulose	Gelatin
Polyvinyl alcohol	Ethyl cellulose	Polyvinyl alcohol
Gelatin	Ethyl cellulose	Acacia
Sodium alginate	Ethyl cellulose	Acacia
Polyvinyl pyrrolidone	Ethyl cellulose	Acacia

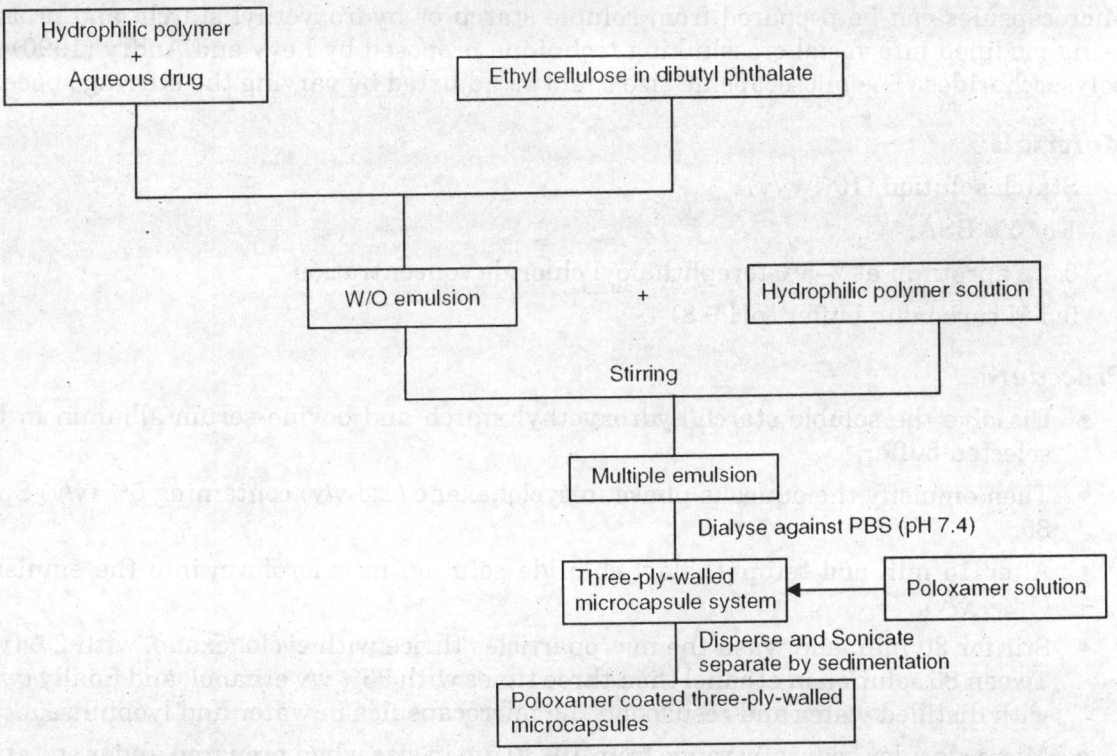

SCHEME 12.6: *Preparation of polyoxamer coated three-ply-walled microspheres*

Preparation of Drug Microcapsules

- To prepare 5% w/v drug solution, dissolve water-soluble drug in internal acacia solution.
- Disperse the internal phase into a 4% w/v solution of ethyl cellulose in ethyl acetate containing dibutylphthalate as a plasticiser.
- Subsequently the primary emulsion W/O type drop-wise to an aqueous acacia solution in order to obtain the secondary emulsion.
- The microcapsules can subsequently be collected as described earlier.

Coating of Poloxamer

- Disperse the drug-loaded microcapsules based on the acacia/ethyl cellulose/ acacia system into a 1% w/v poloxamer solution under constant stirring for 30 min.
- Sonicate for 30 sec. Separate the coated microcapsules by sedimentation and dry at room temperature.

PROTOCOL: 12.14

Preparation of Starch Microcapsules

Microcapsules can be prepared from soluble starch or hydroxyethyl starch, and protein using modified interfacial crosslinking technique proposed by Levy and Andry (1990) for polysaccharides. The microcapsule size could be adjusted by varying the stirring speed.

Materials

Starch solution (10% w/v)

1 or 5% BSA,

0.4% aprotinin at 2–5% terephthaloyl chloride concentration

0.5 M carbonate buffer (pH 9.8)

Procedure

- Dissolve the soluble starch/hydroxyethyl starch and bovine serum albumin in the selected buffer.
- Then emulsify the aqueous phase in cyclohexane (1:3 v/v) containing 5% (v/v) Span 80.
- After 15 min add terephthaloyl chloride solution in chloroform into the emulsion (1:2.4 v/v).
- Stir for 30 min. and wash the microparticles thrice with cyclohexane, with 2% (v/v) Tween 85 solution in ethanol then three times with 95% v/v ethanol, and finally twice with distilled water and resuspend the microcapsules in water and lyophilise.
- Microcapsules generally range from 10–30 μm in size when prepared under agitation at 1500 rpm and 50–100 μm when the stirring used is 500 rpm (Scheme 12.7).

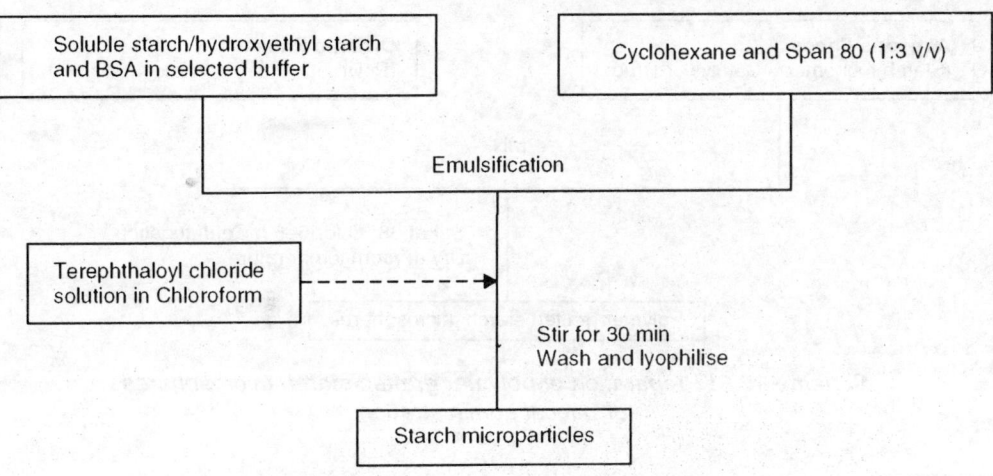

Scheme 12.7: *Preparation of starch microspheres*

PROTOCOL: 12.15

Polymer Grafted Starch Microspheres for Buccal Administration

Principle

Polymeric surfacial grafting of starch spherules is accomplished by surface polymerisation of acrylic acid and methyl methacrylic acid monomers.

Materials

Drug (isosorbide dinitrate)

Starch

Methyl methacrylic acid monomer

Acrylic acid

Sorbitan monooleate (Span 80)

Hexane and hydroxyquinone

Procedure

- Prepare organic phase, i.e. 10% polymethyl methacrylate and 1% Span 80 as a stabiliser.
- Prepare aqueous phase- starch monomer, a catalyst (0.01 M $FeSO_4$ and 0.2 M hydrogen peroxide) and drug (10% w/w of grafted starch weight).
- Disperse aqueous phase into an organic phase containing 5% w/v Span 80. Stir the mixture continuously while keeping temperature at $38 \pm 2\,°C$ for 5–6 h.
- Separate polymer-grafted starch microspheres by centrifugation and dry at room temperature (Scheme 12.8).

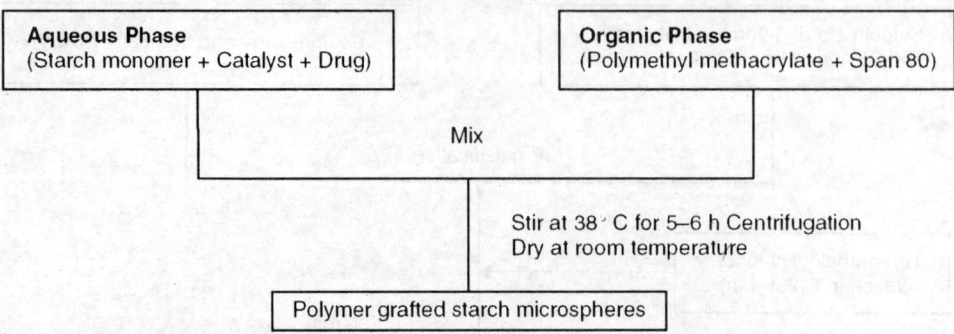

Scheme 12.8: *Preparation of polymer grafted starch microspheres for buccal administration*

PROTOCOL: 12.16

Preparation of Gelatin Microparticles by Complex Coacervation

Materials

Gelatin

EPA-EE

Acacia

Ethanol

Hydrochloric acid (HCl)

Procedure

- Dissolve 2.5 g gelatin in 100ml water at 50°C.

- Then, emulsify 5.0 g of oil phase (EPA-EE) in the gelatin solution by using an Ultraturrax (8000 rpm).

- Pour the emulsion into a beaker containing an aqueous solution of acacia (2.5%, w/v).

- Add 400 ml of water and adjust the pH to 4.0 with 1N HCl and cool the system to 4°C.

- After the sedimentation of the microparticles, decant the supernatant and add 2 × 150 ml ethanol to the sediment for hardening of particles.

- Finally, separate the microcapsules by filtration and dry overnight at room temperature (Scheme 12.9).

- Alternatively, after sedimentation, the sediment can be further processed by spray drying. For the spray-drying process. Apparatus parameters (aspiration: 20; pressure: 300 Nl/h; temperature at inlet: 140 °C, at outlet: 80 °C) are recommended alternatively they may be optimised as per desired specifications of the product especially in terms of size and surface morphology.

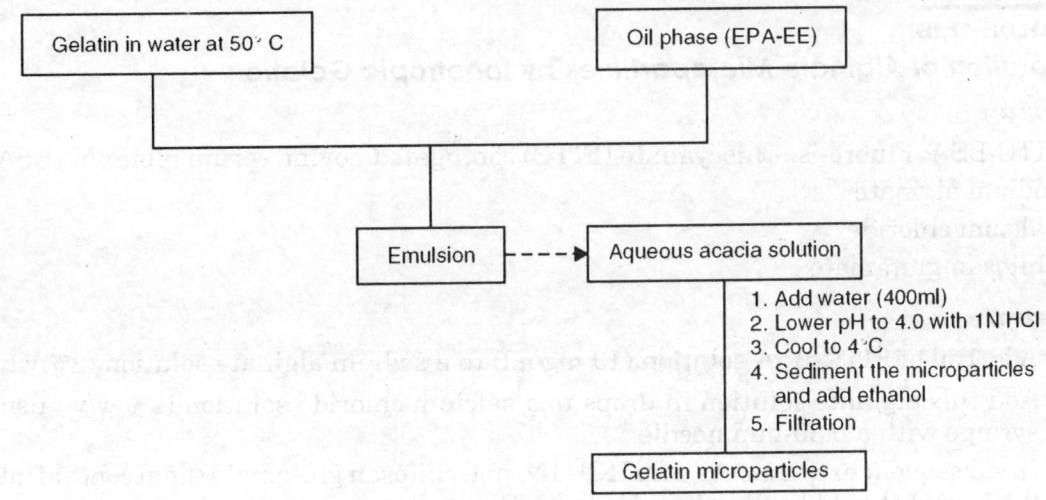

Scheme 12.9: *Preparation of Gelatin microparticles by complex coacervation method*

PROTOCOL: 12.17
Preparation of Fluorescent Microparticles by Double Emulsion Technique

Principle
The preparation of microparticles is based on water-in-oil-in-water emulsification-solvent evaporation method.

Materials
FITC-BSA: Fluoro-iso-thiocyanate (FITC) conjugated bovine serum albumin (BSA)

Polycaprolactone (PCL)

Polyvinyl alcohol (PVA)

Methylene chloride

Procedure
- Emulsify 1ml of a BSA-FITC containing aqueous solution (10 mg/ml) for 1 min by Ultraturrax into the polymer solution (800 mg of PCL) in methylene chloride (10ml). Pour this primary emulsion (W/O) into 300ml of PVA solution (0.25% w/w).

- A W/O/W-emulsion will be obtained on extensive stirring using a four-blade stirrer for 45 min at 1000 rpm.

- After decanting the supernatant, filter the microparticles (membrane filter pore size 0.45 micrometers), and wash 3 times with water (minimal volume 500 ml) and then dry overnight at room temperature.

PROTOCOL: 12.18

Preparation of Alginate Microparticles by Ionotropic Gelation

Materials

FITC-BSA: Fluoro-iso-thiocyanate (FITC) conjugated bovine serum albumin (BSA)
Sodium alginate
Calcium chloride
Chitosan glutamate

Procedure

- Add 1ml of FITC-BSA solution (10 mg/ml) to a sodium alginate solution (2% w/w).
- Add this alginate solution in drops to a calcium chloride solution (2% w/w) using a syringe with a 0.30-mm needle.
- In subsequent experiments, 1ml HCl (1N) and chitosan glutamate (final concentration: 0.1% w/w) should be dissolved in the CaCl$_2$ solution.
- When gelation occur, collect the particles by filtration, wash extensively with water, and dry overnight at room temperature.

PROTOCOL: 12.19

Bioerodible Polyanhydride Microspheres for Sustained Drug Delivery

Principle

Solvent removal technique from O/W emulsion

Materials

Sebacic acid (SA 99%)
p-carboxy benzoic acid (CPA, >99%)
1,6-dibromohexane (98%)
Poly (vinyl alcohol) (99–100% hydrolysed)
p-nitroaniline (PNA)
Sebacic acid
Acetic anhydride,
Chloroform,
Histo-Prep tissue embedding media
Methylene chloride
Deuterated chloroform
Petroleum ether (hexanes, 55% n-hexane)

Procedure

Polymer Synthesis

CPH diacid was synthesised by a method similar to that described by Conix for 1,3-bis (p-carboxyphenoxy) propane. CPH and SA diacids were acetylated to form the prepolymers.

Reflux the diacid in excess acetic anhydride for 30 min (SA) or 60 min (CPH) under dry nitrogen sweep. Remove the unreacted diacid by filtration while the mixture is still warm. Isolate the SA prepolymer by evaporating the solution to dryness at 50°C under vacuum and purify the prepolymers by dissolution in chloroform followed by filtration and subsequent precipitation in a 1:1 mixture of dry ethyl ether and dry petroleum ether. Filter the precipitate and dry overnight under vacuum. Crystallise the CPH prepolymer from the filtrate by evaporating the solution down to a volume of about 150 ml and store overnight under refrigeration. The crystals that are obtained by filtration are washed with ethyl ether and dried overnight.

Re-dissolve the crude CPH pre-polymer in chloroform and filter again to remove impurities. Evaporate the chloroform solution and dry overnight under vacuum. Use the ^{1}H NMR spectroscopy to determine the degree of polymerisation for each of the pre-polymers. Store the pre-polymers desiccated under dry argon to prevent hydrolysis and use the ^{1}H NMR spectroscopy periodically to monitor degree of hydrolysis.

Synthesise the homo-polymers and 50:50 co-polymers by melt poly-condensation of the pre-polymers at 180°C under vacuum (< 0.5 mmHg) for 90 min. Add approximately about 2ml of acetic anhydride to 4 g of prepolymer prior to polymerisation to ensure complete acetylation. Desiccate the polymers under dry argon to prevent degradation.

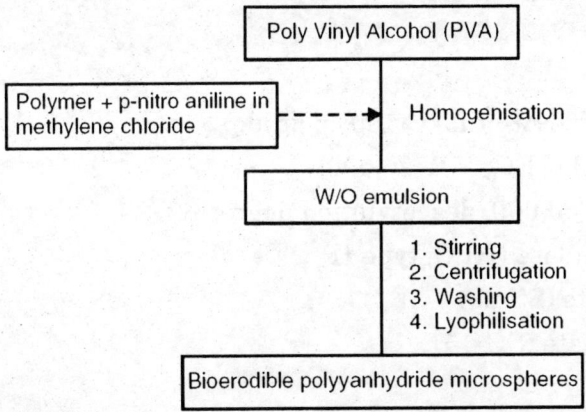

Scheme 12.10: *Preparation of bioerodible polyanhydride microspheres for sustained drug delivery*

Microspheres Preparation

- Bioerodible polyanhydride microspheres can be prepared by solvent removal technique employing an oil/water emulsion to fabricate microspheres. Choose an aqueous non-solvent phase to prevent hydrophobic drugs from diffusing out of the polymer solution during fabrication.

- Dissolve polymer (200 mg) and PNA (30 mg) in 2–4 ml methylene chloride. Add this solution to a 200 ml, 1% (w/v) aqueous solution of 99% hydrolysed PVA and immediately disperse by agitation at 20,000 rpm with a handheld homogeniser for 1 min.

- Stir the water/oil emulsion for 2 h at 300 rpm using mechanical overhead stirrer with a 3-blade impeller.
- Separate the microspheres by centrifugation for 5 min at 375 g.
- Decant off the PVA solution and add the fresh deionised water.
- Perform the centrifugation and decantation step at least 4 times to remove as much PVA and undissolved drug as possible.
- Re-suspend the microspheres in less than 20 ml of deionised water, flash frozen with dry ice and acetone, and lyophilise for overnight.
- Finally, sieve the microspheres to eliminate the particles that were larger than 53 mm in diameter (Scheme 12.10).
- Use the similar microsphere preparation technique for copolymers with slight modification, for the 50 : 50 copolymer, then perform the precipitation in an ice water bath, so that the precipitated polymer would be below its glass transition temperature of about 10°C.

PROTOCOL: 12.20

Chitosan-coated Microparticles

Materials

Drug

Ethylcellulose (EC; 49% ethoxy, 100 cp grade)

Polyethylene glycol (PEG; MW 20,000)

Chitosan H (MW 650,000, deacetylation degree 82)

Hydroxypropylcellulose (HPC; type H)

Sorbitan tristearate (SS-30)

Sorbitan sesquioleate (SO-15)

Procedure

Preparation of Fluorescein Isothiocyanate Labelled Chitosan (FITC-Chit)

- Dissolve 1.0 g chitosan in 1 litre of water and adjust the pH to 3.0 with 1 M HCl.
- After complete dissolution adjust the pH of chitosan to 6.5. Then, dissolve 30 mg FITC in 60 ml of water.
- Add FITC solution to the chitosan solution. Stir the mixture for 24 h at room temperature in the dark.
- Increase the pH of medium to 9.0 with the 1M NaOH to precipitate out the product and collect the precipitate by the centrifugation at 3000 rpm for 5 min.
- Wash the precipitate and dissolve in minimum amount of 1 M HCl and futher increase the pH of the medium with 1 N NaOH for subsequent precipitation.

- Wash again the precipitate with water, and lyophilise the aqueous suspension to obtain freeze dried FITC labelled chitosan (Scheme 12.11).
- Determine the content of FITC in FITC-Chi by dissolving FITC-Chit (0.6% w/w in 0.1 M acetate buffer, pH 5) by spectrophotometric (490 nm) measurement.

PROTOCOL: 12.21
Coated Ethylcellulose Microparticles

Principle: Dry-in-oil method

Procedure

- Dissolve 1.5 g polymer (ethyl-cellulose) and drug (1.5g) in 25 ml of acetone.
- Add this acetone solution drop-wise to 250 ml of liquid paraffin containing 2% w/v sorbitan tristearate-30 and stir the mixture at 600 rpm at 20°C.
- Then further stir the emulsion at room temperature for 1 h, followed by stirring at 35°C for 5 h and finally at 57°C for 1 h.

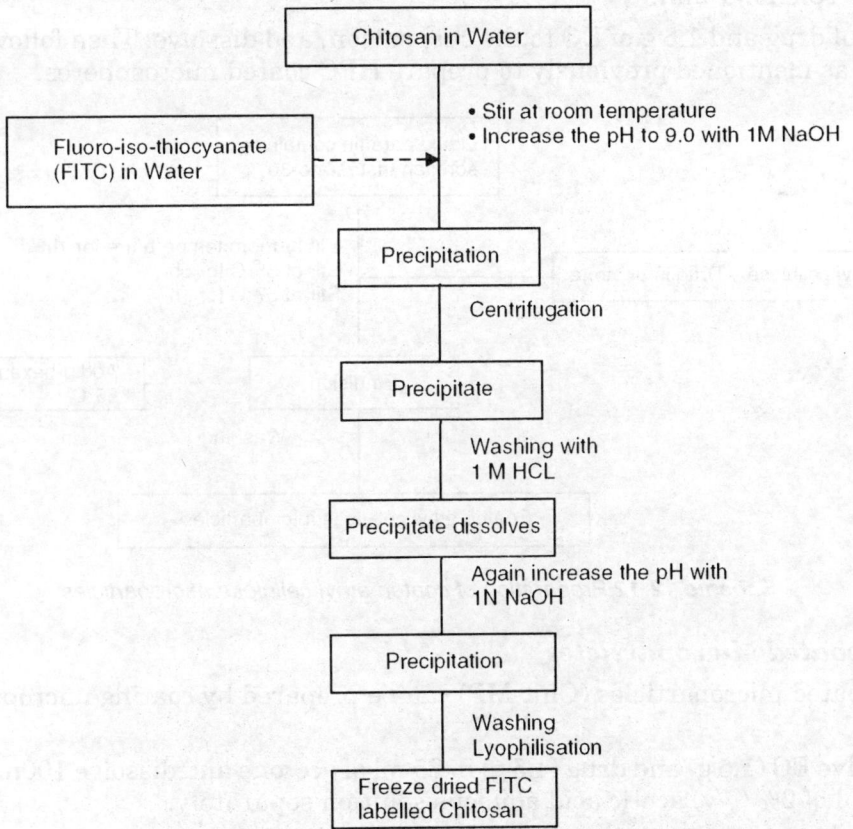

Scheme 12.11: Preparation of chitosan coated fluorescent microparticles

- Warm 100 ml of n-hexane at 55°C and add into the mixture and finally filter the mixture using a membrane filter with a pore diameter of 0.45 mm.
- Wash the residue with hot (55°C) n-hexane to yield ethyl cellulose microparticles (Scheme 12.12).

PEG-coated Ethyl Cellulose Microparticles

- To prepare microspheres with PEG dissolve PEG (0.15 g) in 25 ml of acetone and warm the solution at 35°C.
- After cooling the solution at 20°C, add 1.5 g of drug and 1.5 g polymer (ethyl cellulose) in acetone solution.
- Then follow the similar steps as mentioned previously to prepare PEG coated microspheres.

Hydroxypropylcellulose (HPC) Coated Microparticles

Ethyl cellulose microspheres coated with hydroxypropyl cellulose can be prepared as follows:

- Dissolve HPC (0.15 g) in 25 ml of acetone at 20°C, and stir the solution vigorously at 14000 rpm for 1 min.
- 1.5 g of drug and 1.5 g of EC to the suspension, and dissolve. Then follow the similar steps as mentioned previously to prepare HPC coated microspheres.

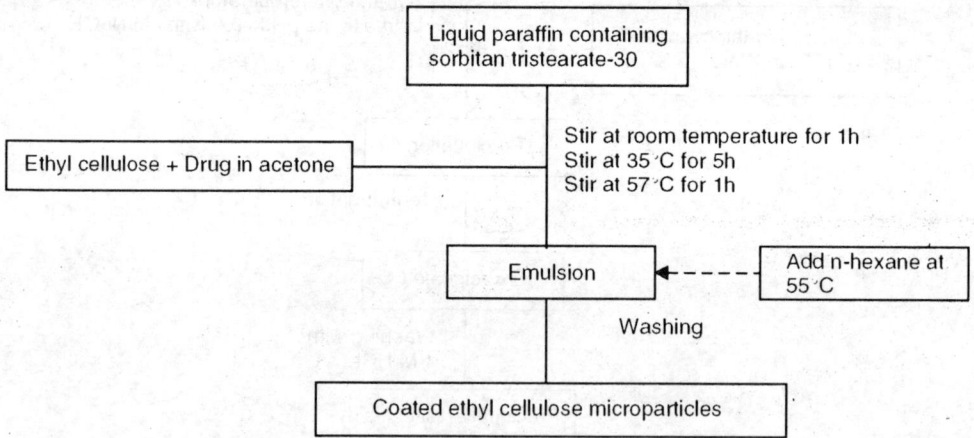

Scheme 12:12 *Preparation of coated ethyl cellulose microparticles*

Chitosan-coated Microparticles

Chitosan-coated microparticles (Chit-MP) can be prepared by coating microparticles with FITC-Chit.

- Dissolve EC (1.5 g) and drug (1.5 g) in 25 ml of acetone and dissolve 100mg FITC-Chit in 5 ml of 2% (v/v) acetic acid aqueous solution separately.
- Suspend the 100mg microparticles in the solution, and add 20 ml of liquid paraffin containing SO-15 at 1% (w/v) drop-wise and stir at 600 rpm.

- Add this suspension drop wise to 500 ml of double solvent layers of n-hexane/1 N NaOH (2:3, v/v) and stir at 300 rpm.
- One min later after the end of dropping, precipitate the particles in 1 N NaOH aqueous layer.
- Collect by filtration using mesh (opening 150 mm). Wash with 500ml of water, and dry in a desiccator in vacuum at room temperature to produce Chi-MP.

SUGGESTED READINGS

- Abdella, P.M. Smith, P.K. and Rover, G.P. (1979) Biochem. Biophys. Res. Commun. 87(3), 734.
- Evans, R.L, (1972) U.S. Patent 3,663,685.
- Evans, R.L. (1972) U.S. Patent 3,663,687.
- Kim, C.K. and Lee, E.J. (1992) Int. J. Pharm., 79. 11.
- Kramer, P.A. (1974) J. Pharm. Sci., 63, 1646
- Kreuter, J., (1983) Pharm. Acta Helv., 58, 242
- Lee, T.K. Sokolski, T.D. and Royer, G.P. (1981) Science, 213, 233.
- Levy, M.C. and Andry, M.C. (1990) Int. J. Pharm., 62, 27.
- Longo, W. Iwata, H. Lindheimer, T. and Goldberg, E.P. (1982) J. Pharm. Sci., 71, 1323.
- Margel S. and Offarim, M., (1983) Anal. Biochem.,128, 342.
- Margel S. and Weisel, E., (1984) J. Polym. Sci. 22, 145.
- Matt J. K., Elizabeth S., Amy D., Balaji N., (2002) Biomaterials 23, 4405.
- Miller, A.M. McMillan, L., Hannan, W.J. Emmett, P.C. and Aitken, R.J., (1982)Int. J. Appl. Radiat. Isot. 33, 1423.
- N. V. Larionova, N. F. Kazanskaya, N. I. Larionova1, G. Ponchel, and D. Duchene, (1999) Biochemistry (Moscow), Vol. 64, No. 8, pp. 857.
- O'Donnell PB, Mc Ginity, J.W., (1997). Advanced Drug Delivery Reviews, 28, 25.
- Przyborowski, M., Lachnik E., Wiza, J., and Licinska, I., (1982) Eur. J. Nucl. Med. 7, 71.
- Royer, G.P. (1982) U.S. Patent 4,349,530.
- Royer, G.P. and Lee, T.K. (1983) J. Parenter. Sci. Technol. 37(2), 34 .
- Widder, K., Flouret,G., and Senyei, A., (1979)J. Pharm. Sci., 68, 79 .
- Yapel, A.F. (1979) U.S. Patent 4, 147,767 .
- Zolle, (1976)U.S. Patent 3,937,668.

13

Nanoparticles, Nanospheres and Nanocapsules

The colloidal carriers based on biodegradable and biocompatible polymeric systems have largely influenced the controlled and targeted drug delivery concepts. It was realised that the nanoparticles loaded bioactives could not only deliver drug(s) to specific organs within the body but delivery rate in addition could be controlled as being bystanders, burst, controlled, pulsatile or modulated. The possibilities and potentials further prompted the work and as a result a great deal of related information covering preparation methodologies, characterisation, engineering, bio-fate and toxicology have been gathered. The understanding that relates to the biodistribution in particular has propelled and motivated the development of functionally designed nanoparticulates.

It is apparent that the polymers, the building blocks of nanoparticulate composites, belong to natural or synthetic origins. Some of them have already been exploited for their biomedical applications. Obviously, the literature is abound concerning their safety, toxicology and biodegradation consideration.

Nanoparticles are sub-nanosized colloidal structures composed of synthetic or semi synthetic polymers. The continual quest and manoeuvering towards physical stability improvement of liposomes resulted into development of solid core nanoparticles in eighties as an alternative drug carrier. The first reported nanoparticles were based on non-biodegradable polymeric systems (polyacrylamide, polymethyl-methacrylate, polystyrene, etc.) (Birrenbach and Speiser, 1976; Kreuter and Speiser, 1976). The possibilities of chronic toxicity due to tissue and immunological response towards non-degradable polymeric burden, their use for systemic administration however, could not be considered. Soon the biodegradable polymers were taken up and nano-particles based on poly(cyanoacrylate) were extensively studied (Couvreur *et al.,* 1982; Douglas *et al.,* 1987; Kreuter, 1991). The polymeric nanoparticles can carry drug(s) or proteinaceous substances, i.e. antigen(s). These bioactives are entrapped in the polymer matrix as particulates enmesh or solid solution or may be bound to the particle surface by physical adsorption or chemically. The drug(s) may be added during preparation of nanoparticles or to the previously prepared nanoparticles. The term particulate is suggestively general and does not account for morphological and structural organisation of the system. Thus they could be nanospheres, nanocapsules, nanocrystals or nanoparticulates. Nanospheres may be defined as solid core spherical particulates, which are nanometric in size. They contain drug embedded within the matrix or adsorbed onto surface; nanocapsules are vesicular system in which drug is essentially encapsulated within the central core surrounded by an embryonic continuous polymeric sheath. In the latre, drug(s) is mainly encapsulated in the solution system. The physical chemistry of these systems remains to be the same as of typical colloidal dispersions. The surface charges, dispersibility, density, hydrophobicity and hydrophilicity are some critical factors which ultimately determine the stability characteristics of a system vis-a-vis its *in vivo* disposition.

PREPARATION TECHNIQUES OF NANOPARTICLES

The selection of the appropriate method for the preparation of nanoparticles depends on the physicochemical characteristics of the polymer and the drug to be loaded. On the contrary, the preparation techniques largely determine the inner structure, *in vitro* release profile and the biological fate of these polymeric delivery systems (Kreuter *et al.*, 1991). Two types of systems with different inner structures are apparently possible including:

- A matrix type system consisting of an entanglement of oligomer or polymer units (nanoparticles/nanospheres)
- A reservoir type of system comprised of an oily core surrounded by an embryonic polymeric shell (nanocapsules).

The drug can either be entrapped within the reservoir or the matrix or otherwise be adsorbed on the surface of these particulate systems. The polymers are strictly structured to a nanometric size range using appropriate methodologies. These methodologies are conveniently classified as follows:

1. Amphiphilic macromolecule crosslinking
    a. Heat crosslinking
    b. Chemical crosslinking
2. Polymerisation based methods
    a. Polymerisation of monomers *in situ*
    b. Emulsion (micellar) polymerisation
    c. Dispersion polymerisation
    d. Interfacial condensation polymerisation
    e. Interfacial complexation
3. Polymer precipitation methods
    a. Solvent extraction/evaporation
    b. Solvent displacement (nanoprecipitation)
    c. Salting out

Nanoparticle(s) Preparation by Crosslinking of Amphiphilic Macromolecules

Nanoparticles can be prepared from amphiphilic macromolecules, proteins and polysaccharides (which have affinity for aqueous and lipid solvents). The technique of their preparation involves firstly, the aggregation of amphiphile(s) followed by further stabilisation either by heat denaturation (Gupta *et al.,* 1987a,b) or chemical crosslinking (Widder *et al.,* 1979). These processes may occur in a biphasic O/W or W/O type dispersed systems, which subdivide the amphiphile(s) prior to aggregative stabilisation. It may also take place in an aqueous amphiphilic solution where on removal, extraction, or diffusion of solvent, amphiphile(s) are aggregated as tiny particulates and subsequently rigidized via chemical crosslinking. The crosslinking is generally executed following dispersed phase solvent extraction, or depletion.

Crosslinking in W/O Emulsion

The crosslinking method is exhaustively used for the nano-encapsulation of drugs. The method involves the emulsification of bovine serum albumin (BSA)/human serum albumin (HSA) or protein aqueous solution in oil using high-pressure homogenisation (Kramer, 1974) or high frequency sonication (Sugibasayashi *et al.,* 1979). The water in oil emulsion so formed is then poured into preheated oil (temperature above 100°C). The suspension in preheated oil maintained above 100°C is held stirred for a specified time in order to denature and aggregate the protein contents of aqueous pool completely and to evaporate the water. Proteinaceous sub-nanoscopic particles are thus formed where the size of the internal phase globules mainly determines the ultimate size of particulates.

Emulsion Chemical Dehydration

Chemical dehydration has been reported for producing BSA nanoparticles with a narrow size distribution. Bhargava and Aindo, (1992) suggested a simplified chemical crosslinking method. Hydroxypropyl cellulose solution in chloroform was used as a continuous phase of emulsion while a chemical dehydrating agent, i.e. 2,2, di-methyl propane, was used to translate internal aqueous phase into a solid particulate suspension. The method reportedly avoids coalescence of droplets and could produce nanoparticles of smaller size (~300 nm), probably due to sonication used for comminution and to keep internal phase well dispersed is reduced considerably.

Phase Separation in Aqueous Medium (Desolvation)

The protein or polysaccharide from an aqueous phase can be desolvated by pH change, or change in temperature or by adding some appropriate counter ions. Crosslinking may be affected simultaneously or subsequent to the desolvation step (Marty *et al.,* 1978; Oppenheim *et al.,* 1982; Krause and Rohdewald, 1985; Oppenheim, 1986).

The method essentially proceeds involving three steps, i.e., protein dissolution, protein aggregation and protein deaggregation. In other words, using appropriate levels of desolvation, and resolvation, the aggregate size could be maintained and finally these aggregated nanoparticulates are cross-linked using glutaraldehyde.

Solvent competing agent, sodium sulphate, is mainly used as a desolvating agent while alcohol, i.e., ethanol and isopropanol are carefully added as desolvating or deaggregating solvents. The addition can be optimised turbidometrically using a Nephelometer. Only desolvation may give the final product as nanospheres. Desolvation deaggregates the protein and turns the suspension colloidal and hence milky in appearance.

Poly alkylcyanoacrylate (PACA) Nanoparticles

Poly(alkylcyanoacrylate) (PACA), a biodegradable polymer has created a great deal of interest in nanoparticulate carriers (Kreuter and Speiser, 1976; Kreuter, 1983; Chiannilkulchai *et al.*, 1989; De Verdiere *et al.*, 1997; Soma *et al.*, 2000). Polyalkylcynoacrylate (PACA) nanoparticles are prepared by an emulsion polymerisation technique. The polymerisation mechanism of PACA can be described as an anionic process initiated by OH⁻ ions resulting from the dissociation of the water. The mechanism of poly hexylcynoacrylate (PHCA) nanoparticles preparation is given in Fig.13.1. The hydroxyl ions induce polymerisation that proceeds very rapidly and can be influenced by pH. The polymerisation speed depends also on the molecular weight of the alkyl compound and decreases with the higher molecular weight. It is well established that the process of particle formation initiated in the aqueous phase and terminated by aggregation of polymeric chain and growing hydrophobicity, result in water insoluble colloids. For this reason pH is maintained below 2.5 and with some drugs even below pH 1, to enable controlled nanoparticle formation.

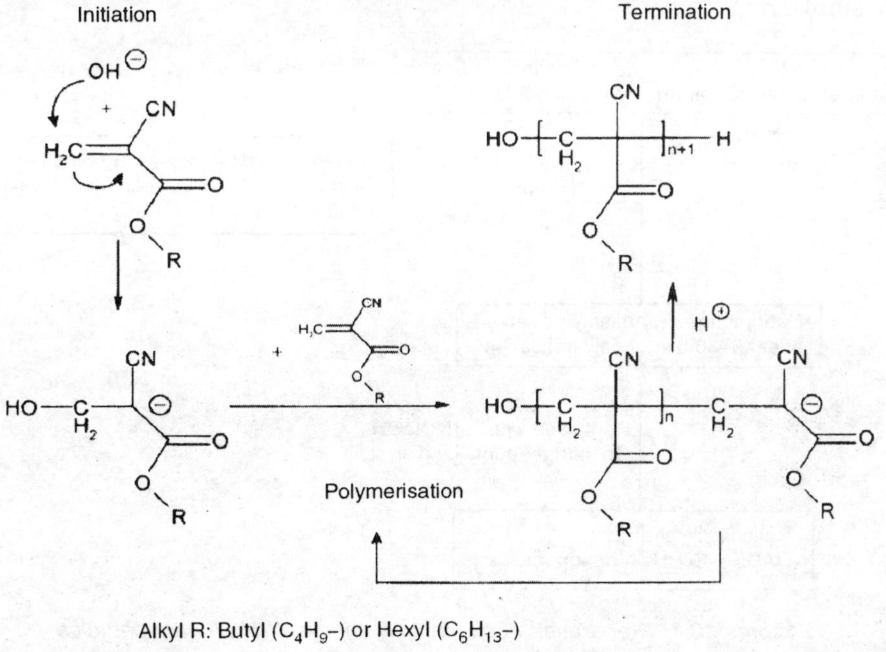

Alkyl R: Butyl (C_4H_9-) or Hexyl ($C_6H_{13}-$)

FIG. 13.1. *Anionic emulsion polymerisation of alkylcyanoacrylates. Initially the polymerisation starts in an aqueous medium with the addition of OH⁻ anions. The polymeristion is maintained unless the polymer remains soluble in the aqueous media. With growing chain length, the hydrophobicity increases and hence particle formation starts with the coagulation of hydrophobic polymer chains resulting into water-insoluble colloids*

Two different protocols are usually followed for the preparation of cationically or anionically charged PHCA nanoparticles.

PROTOCOL 13.1

Preparation of Cationically Charged PHCA Nanoparticles

Materials

DADE-Dextran (dextran derivatives)	0.2g
n-Hexylcyanoacrylate (PHCA) monomers	10% w/v solution
Dextran	0.3 gm
Hydrochloric acid	0.01N

Meth·ds

- To prepare cationically charged nanoparticles, take 10% w/v solution of n-Hexylcyanoacrylate monomers in organic solvent (chloroform and methanc' 3:1) and add drop-wise to the aqueous medium containing 0.2 g DADE-Dextran (M W 500,000) and 0.3 g Dextran 6000 in 50 ml of 0.01N HCl. Stir the mixture at room temperature for 24 hr. To initiate polymerisation carefully drip the monomer very slowly into a acidic solution.

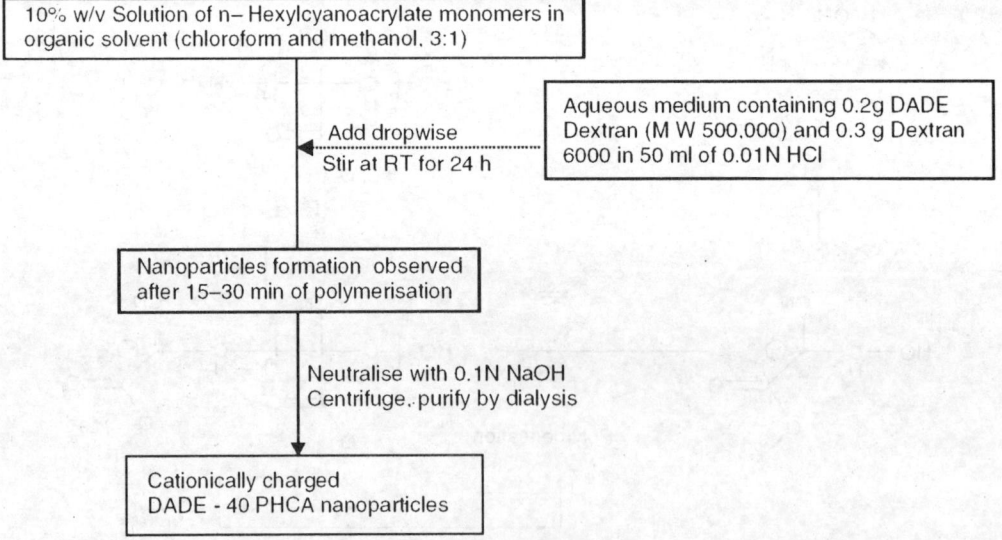

Scheme 13.1: Preparation of cationically charged PHCA nanoparticles

- Nanoparticles formation can be visually observed after 15–30 min of polymerisation as a milky appearance of the solution, which becomes more turbid as the polymerisation further proceeds. In general, the polymerisation is completed after a few hours. It is recommended that the solution be stirred for about 24 h.

- Subsequently, neutralise the nanoparticles suspension with 0.1N NaOH and remove larger aggregates by mild centrifugation. Additionally, purification by dialysis is a useful step to remove salts and other monomer as well as polymer residuals.

- Store the prepared nanoparticles at 4°C in suspension. Before dialysis, the unpurified suspension can also be freeze-dried if necessary.

- Finally, this protocol provides cationically charged nanoparticles (DADE-40 PHCA).

- The charge density of the particle surface can be modified by adjusting the ratio between DADE-dextran and normal dextran. A ratio of 40% DADE-dextran to 60% unmodified dextran is reported to be optimal for the nanoparticle preparation. If it is necessary to characterise the dextran/ PHCA ratio of the particles a NMR method can be used for rapid analysis (Scheme 13.1).

PROTOCOL 13.2

Preparation of Anionically Charged (PACA) Nanoparticles

Materials

Isohexylcyanoacrylate (PACA) monomers	10% w/v
Dextran (M W 70,000)	0.5g
Hydrochloric acid	0.001N
Phosphate buffer saline (pH 7.0)	0.1M

Procedure

Protocol 13.2 is very similar to protocol 13.1 except in step 3 where the excessive acid is neutralised with the phosphate buffer (pH 7.0). Instead of any cationic dextran just 1% unmodified dextran MW 70,000 is used as polymerisation stabiliser. If necessary, nanoparticles can be stored in the acid solution at 4°C or can be purified as mentioned before. This protocol results in negatively charged nanoparticles as described earlier.

PROTOCOL 13.3

Chitosan Nanoparticles

Materials

Chitosan hydrochloride salt MW 100kD
Acetic acid
Tripolyphosphate (TPP)

Procedure

- Dissolve chitosan at 0.25% w/v with 1% v/v acetic acid and then raise pH to 4.7–4.8 with 10 N NaOH.

- Add chitosan solution 500 μl to 100 μl of 0.3% w/v TPP solution prepared in water under magnetic stirring.

- It leads to the immediate formation of the nanoparticles (Scheme 13.2).

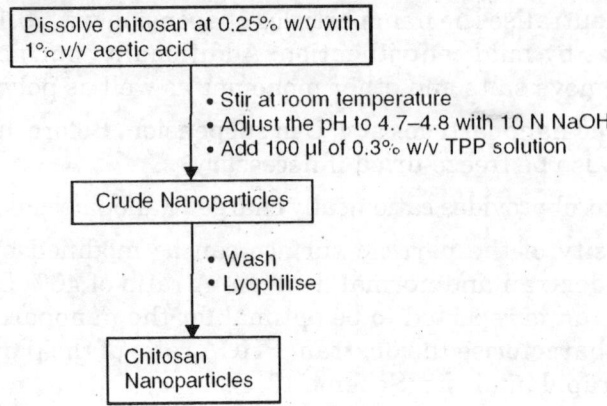

Scheme 13.2: *Preparation of Chitosan Nanoparticles*

PROTOCOL 13.4

Cyanoacrylate Nanoparticles

The method is used to prepare biodegradable polyacrylamide and polymethyl-methacrylate (PMMA) nanoparticles (Kreuter and Speiser, 1976). The acrylamide or methyl methacrylate monomer is dissolved in aqueous phase and polymerised by irradiation (Kreuter and Speiser, 1976) or by chemical initiation (ammonium or potassium peroxodisulphate) combined with heating to temperature above 65 °C (Kreuter *et al.*, 1986; Kreuter *et al.*, 1988). These nanoparticles are preferentially produced by emulsifier free polymerisation in aqueous media, because detergents may interact with and damage certain biological materials or change the immunological response.

Material and Methods

Purification of the Monomers

Extract 100 ml of methyl methacrylate three times with 20 ml solution of 5 g NaOH and 20 g NaCl in 100 ml distilled water twice.

1. *Polymerisation with gamma rays:* Take purified methyl methacrylate (between 0.1–1.5%) and dissolve in double distilled water and irradiated with 500 krad gamma rays using a ^{60}Co source. The resulting nanoparticles suspension can be used or stored as such or in lyophilised form. Instead of water, buffer can be used.

Drug Loading

Biologically active materials, as for instance antigens, can be entrapped within the particles by polymerisation of the monomer in the presence of the active material.

Alternatively, incubate the biologically entrapped material with preformed lyophilised nanoparticles, which is thereby loaded due to absorption on the surface of nanoparticles. The method is of choice especially for labile materials.

2. *Polymerisation with potassium peroxodisulfate:* The second method for the production of poly (methyl methacrylate) nanoparticles is the polymerisation by initiation with potassium peroxodisulfate at elevated temperatures (60 or 80°C). High initiator concentration (>5 mM) leads to precipitation and flocculation comparable to that observed with gamma irradiation. Lower initiator concentration lead to the formation of stable latex. The particle size increases significantly with increasing amounts of monomers.

Procedure

Add degassed double distilled water into a jacketed round or flat bottom flask that can be closed partially with a funnel in order to minimise the evaporation. Bubbles nitrogen through the water for 15 min and then add certain amount of monomer and dissolve in the water by stirring with a magnetic stirrer. Then raise the temperature gradually to 45°C. Subsequently add potassium peroxodisulfate dissolved in small amount of water (not exceeding 4% v/v of aqueous monomer solution) to the monomer solution and increase the temperature to 65°C or 85°C. Under stirring maintainng the temperature at this level for 2 hr. The resulting nanoparticles suspension can be treated by gamma rays (Scheme 13.3).

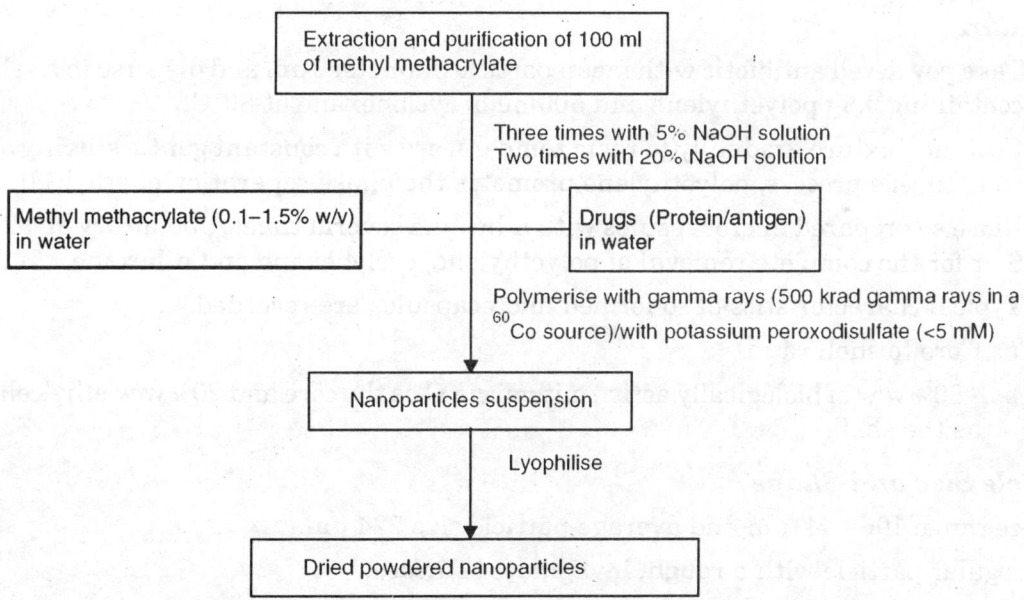

Scheme 13.3: *Preparation of a cyanoacrylate nanoparticles*

PROTOCOL 13.5

Ethylcellulose Microcapsules for Selective Drug Delivery

Microencapsulation is designed to protect, separate or change the diverse function of substances within a small particle of a diameter less than approximately 500 nm depending on the materials and structures of the shell, microcapsules can alter the physical properties of the encapsulated substances so that a desired availability is achieved while at the same time protecting the activity of the encapsulated substance.

Ethyl cellulose forms a stable, semipermeable membrane and is commonly used as an additive to foods and drugs because of its inert nature. It is soluble in an organic solvent in certain condition and could accumulate the water-soluble substances to make a semipermeable capsular membrane. Thus formed system can be explained mechanistically as coacervation or phase separation phenomenon.

Material

Ethyl cellulose

Prototype anticancer antibiotic such as mitomycin C

Polyethylene

Cyclohexane

Stirrer

Procedure

- Take powdered antibiotic with mean particle diameter 1μm and disperse in a solution containing 0.5g polyethylene and 500 ml of cyclohexane at 80°C.
- Cool the mixture gradually to room temperature with constant gentle stirring at 400 rpm. In this process, polyethylene promotes the phase separation of ethylcellulose.
- Rinse so prepared microcapsules with n-hexane several times, and airdry at 45°C for 6 hr for the complete removal of polyethylene, cyclohexane and n-hexane.
- Typical characteristics of so formed microcapsules are recorded.
  a. Core to shell ratio
  b. ~80% w/w of biologically active mitomycin C as the core and 20% w/w ethylcellulose as the shell.

Particle Size and Shape

Size range 106–441μm and average particle size 224 μm.

Irregular particle with a rough, invaginated surface.

Release Behaviour

In unstirred physiological saline at 37°C was 31% of the total encapsulated mitomycin C.

PROTOCOL 13.6

Polycynoacrylate Magnetic Nanoparticles

Principle

Solvent polymerisation method

Procedure

- Take an accurately weighed quantity of drug and dissolve in the monomer, methylmethacrylate solution in an organic phase.

- Add drug monomer solution drop-wise to the aqueous medium containing 0.5% w/v of Tween 80 (pH was maintained with 0.1N HCl) while continually stirring the medium.

- Add 1% hydrogen peroxide as an initiator, to start the polymerisation and stir continuously for 5–6 h at 55–60°C.

- Filter the nanoparticles through a G-4.0 sintered glass filter and wash with the warm distilled water to remove any trace of unpolymerised monomer.

- Redisperse the washed particles in distilled water and adjust the pH with phthalate buffer to 4–4.5 (Scheme 13.4).

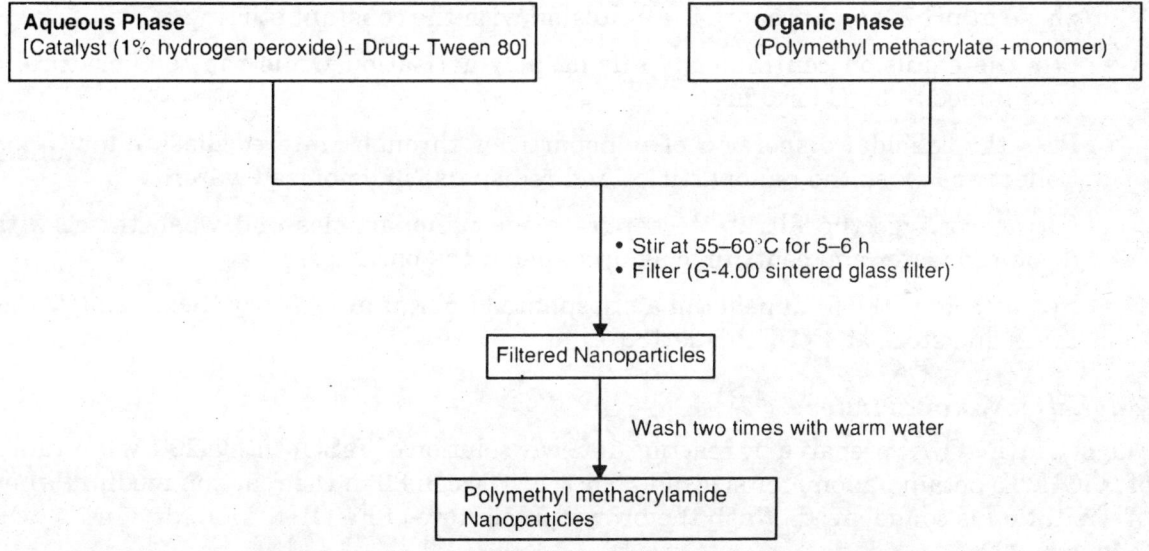

Scheme 13.4: *Preparation of polycynoacrylate nanoparticles*

PROTOCOL 13.7

Magnetite Nanoparticles

Principle

Emulsion Polymerisation

The emulsion polymerisation technique can be used to prepare nanoparticles entrapping magnetite. Suspend the magnetite in the monomeric methylmethacrylate phase containing the weighed quantity of the model drug. Then add the magnetic phase drop wise to the aqueous phase with the continuous stirring.

Materials

Methyl methacrylate

Magnetite (Fe_3O_4)

Model drug

Fanston's reagent

Tween 80

Procedure

- The internal phase of emulsion contain 2 mg of Fe_3O_4 (magnetite) of average particle size (30±6 nm) and 1 mg of model drug per 10ml of monomer methyl methacrylate.
- Take 0.5% w/w Tween and 0.02M 1% v/v Fanston's reagent (Fe^{2++} H_2O_2) in aqueous phase at pH 2.0 and prepare the emulsion with the constant stirring.
- Stir the emulsion continuously during polymerisation while the temperature is maintained at 55°C for 6 hr.
- Pass the colloidal dispersion of nanoparticles through sintered glass filter G-4.0. Collect and wash the nanoparticles and redisperse in deionised water.
- Ultracentrifuge the filtrate to separate the nanoparticles and wash thrice with deionised water and centrifuge again to pellet the particles.
- Re-suspended the final pellet in a phosphate buffer at pH 7.2, dry them using freeze dryer and store at 4°C (Scheme 13.5).

Magnetic Nanoparticles

Magnetite (Fe_3O_4) is prepared by reacting 10% w/v solution of $FeSO_4$ with a 20% w/v solution of NaOH. To obtain nanometer size, add 0.5% w/v Tween 80 in the reaction medium when precipitation is commenced. Wash the brown precipitate of $Fe(OH)_3$ well, dry and reheat to give Fe_3O_4.

Coating of Magnetite

Magnetite particles are higher in density and non-wettable in nature they have tendency to sediment. Coating of magnetite particles with silicone oil (polydimethylsiloxane) improves the wettability of magnetite particles in non-aqueous media and by reducing the density difference render them dispersible.

Magnetite is on the Whatman filter paper so add a 0.1% w/v solution of silicone oil in ether to percolate through the sample. The silicone coated magnetite is prepared after drying and then powdered and passed through a 300 mesh sieves. Test the retension of magnetic properties of the coated magnetite. The size of magnetite particles is determined using electron microscopy method or Malvern particle sizer. The average particle size should be 40± 5 nm preferably.

Characterisation of Magnetic Nanoparticles

Optimisation parameters: Concentration of magnetite, effect of monomer concentration, emulsifier concentration, transmission electron microscopy, drug concentration in monomer, pH of aqueous medium, drug release from magnetic nanoparticles, stirring rate, effect of process variables:

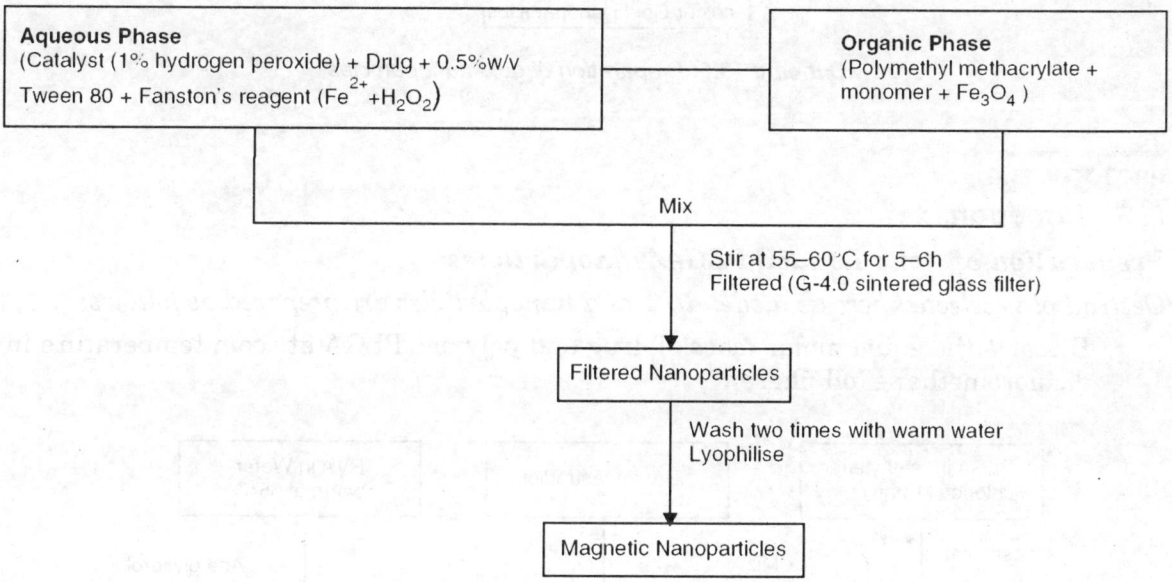

Aqueous Phase
(Catalyst (1% hydrogen peroxide) + Drug + 0.5%w/v Tween 80 + Fanston's reagent (Fe^{2+} +H_2O_2)

Organic Phase
(Polymethyl methacrylate + monomer + Fe_3O_4)

Mix

Stir at 55–60°C for 5–6h
Filtered (G-4.0 sintered glass filter)

Filtered Nanoparticles

Wash two times with warm water
Lyophilise

Magnetic Nanoparticles

Scheme 13. 5: *Preparation of magnetic nanoparticles*

PROTOCOL 13.8
Gold Nanoparticles

Preparation of Gold Nanoparticles

- Take 100ml solution of chlorauric acid and it allow to boil. Then add 5 ml of 1% (w/v) sodium citrate solution drop-wise with continuous stirring using magnetic stirrer.

- After the addition of sodium citrate, the solution starts to darken in colour and turn bluish-gray or purple.

- After approximately 5 min of completion, the reactions is confirmed by the final colour of the solution that is deep wine red.

- The colloids may then be viewed under the scanning electron microscope (SEM) and also subjected to laser light scattering analysis for particle size determination as well as tyndal effect (Scheme 13.6).

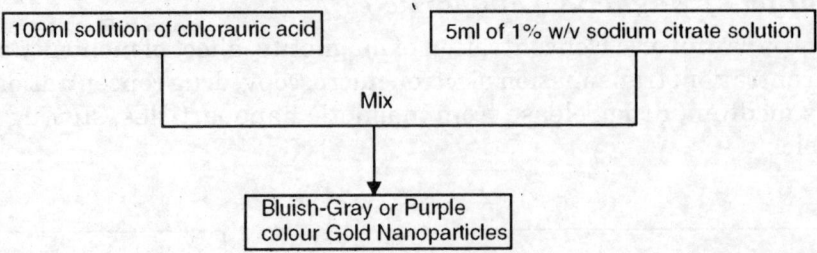

Scheme 13.6: *Preparation of gold nanoparticles*

PROTOCOL 13.9

PLGA Nanoparticle

Preparation of Drug Loaded PLGA Nanoparticles

Oestradiol is selected here as model drug and nanoparticles are prepared as follows:

- Dissolve the equal molar mass of drug and polymer PLGA at room temperature in dichloromethane (oil phase).

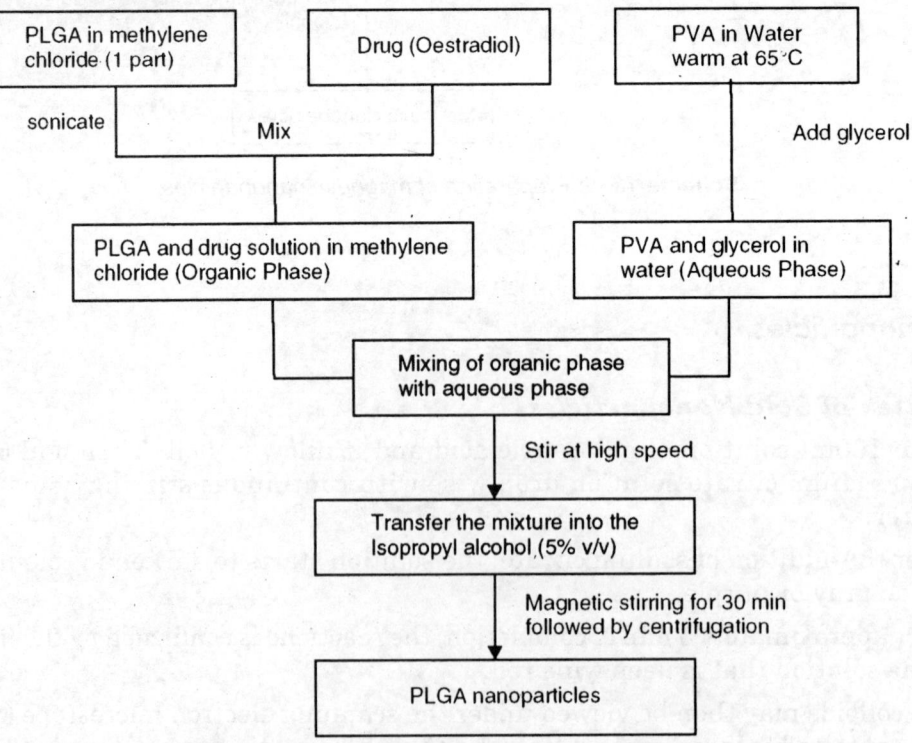

Scheme 13.7: *Preparation of PLGA nanoparticles*

- Prepare 2.5% w/v aqueous solution of the surfactant polyvinyl alcohol (PVA, MW 13,000–23,000, 87–89% hydrolysed; water phase)
- Slowly add the oil phase to the water phase under high speed blending (24,000 rpm) for two minutes, the mixtures form as a white cloudy emulsion.
- The emulsion is then allowed to stir in an uncovered beaker for several hours under vacuum to remove all traces of dichloromethane.
- Centrifuge the emulsion at 10,000 rpm for 30 min.
- Decant the supernatant and stored for analysis of drug concentration by spectrophometry.
- Re-suspend the white pellet of nanoparticles and wash twice with deionised water following centrifuge at 10000 rpm for 10 min.
- Finally, resuspend the nanoparticles pellet in a minimal amount of deionised water and freeze dry it overnight.
- The fine white powder of drug loaded PLGA nanoparticles is obtained and analyse using scanning electron microscopy (Scheme 13.7).

PROTOCOL 13.10
Preparation of Polymeric Nanoparticles

Materials

Polymers
Poloxamer 188 or
Polyacrylamide or
P(2-hydroxy ethyl methacrylate)
Insulin
Span 80 previously added to oil (0.5 to 1.5% v/v)

Procedure

- Dissolve the weighed amount of polymer and insulin in acidified methanol (pH 3.0).
- Emulsify the matrix phase in light paraffin oil containing an appropriate amount of Span 80.
- Stir the W/O emulsion so formed at room temperature till the complete evaporation of the internal phase.
- Filter the product through 6 no. sintered glass filter in order to filter off the particles above 1µ in size. Again filter the filtrate so obtained through Millipore filter (0.4µ).
- The nanoparticles will be retained over the filter.
- Wash them with solvent ether and dry at room temperature (Scheme 13.8).

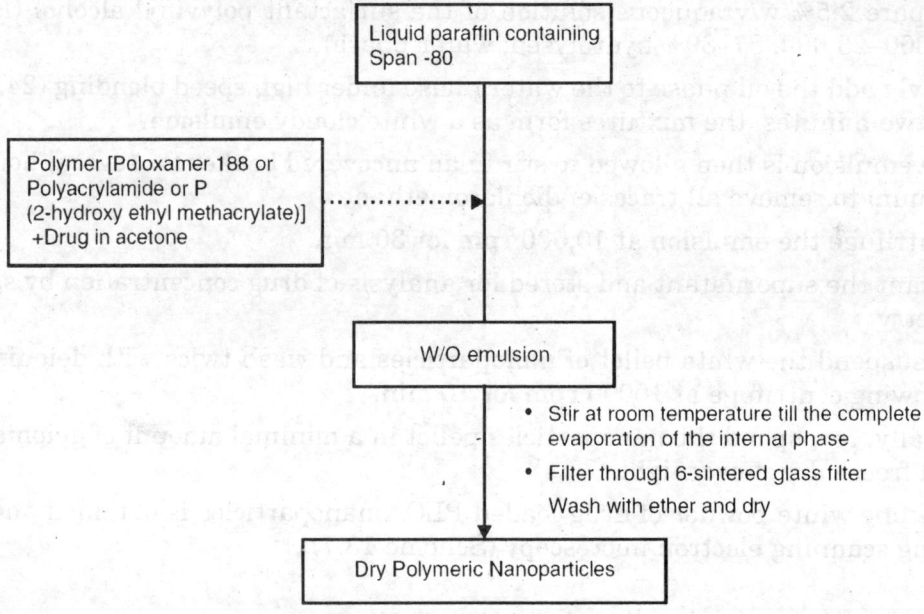

Scheme 13.8: Preparation of polymeric nanoparticles

PROTOCOL 13.11

Preparation of Surfactant-coated Nanoparticles

Principle

Acidic polymerisation using dextran 70,000 as stabiliser.

Materials

Dextran 70,000

Butyl cyanoacrylate

0.01 N NaOH

0.01 N HCl

Glucose

Magnetic stirrer

Lyophiliser

Procedure

- Dissolve 1% w/v dextran M/W 70,000 in 0.01 N HCl and butyl cyanoacrylate (1% w/v) under constant stirring using a magnetic stirrer at 500 rpm for 4 h. A milky white nanoparticle suspension is obtained after polymerisation.

- Neutralise the suspension with 0.1 N NaOH, to complete the polymerisation reaction, and filter through a sintered glass filter (pore size 10 µm).

- Add the anhydrous glucose (1%) to improve the ability of the nanoparticles to redisperse after lyophilisation.
- Then lyophilise the suspension of nanoparticles for 24 h, using a lyophiliser or a freeze drier.
- *Resuspend the lyophilized nanoparticles as follows:* Mix 100 mg amount of the freeze-dried nanoparticles with 0.5 ml of PBS under conditions of constant stirring, using a magnetic stirrer.
- Then dilute the resulting suspension to 5 ml by addition of 4.5 ml of PBS containing 5 mg of drug.
- Ultrasonicate the suspension for 5 min using a probe sonicator and allow the drug to adsorb onto the nanoparticles under constant stirring (300 rpm) for 3 h.
- Calculate the total amount of drug adsorbed by filtering the suspension through a membrane filter (10 nm pore size) and measuring the amount of unbound/unabsorbed drug in the filtrate by means of UV spectrophotometry.

PROTOCOL 13.12
Biodegradable Cyanoacrylate Nanosphere Preparation

Principle
Biodegradable PHDCA and stealthed PEG-PHDCA nanospheres are obtained by the method of nanoprecipitation (Fessi *et al.,* 1989).

Materials
Poly(hexadecylcyanoacrylate) (PHDCA)

Poly(MePEG2000 cyanoacrylate-co-hexadecylcyanoacrylate) (PEG-PHDCA)

Pluronic F68 (tensio-active agent)

Glucose 5%

Sucrose

Procedure
Control Nanospheres of PHDCA

- Typically, for the control nanospheres, take 300 mg PHDCA and dissolve in slightly warm 15 ml acetone.
- Pour organic phase rapidly through a syringe in 30 ml milliQ water under magnetic stirring. Nanospheres precipitation occurs instantaneously. Evaporate acetone under reduced pressure.
- Purify the colloidal suspension of nanospheres by ultracentrifugation (145,000 g, 1.5 h, 4°C), and suspend the resulting nanosphere pellet in a solution of 5% glucose (12 ml).
- Then filter the suspension using a sintered glass membrane (Millex AP 20; Millipore) (Scheme 13.9).

PEG Coated Stealth Nanospheres

For the PEG-coated nanospheres, only 50% (w/w) of the PEG-PHDCA copolymer is precipitated as nanospheres (the remaining fraction had a high PEG content and was thus soluble in the dispersion medium) (Brigger *et al.*, 2002).

- Take 460.0 mg of PEG-PHDCA and dissolve in 30 ml warm acetone. PEGylated nanospheres are obtained in the same way as discussed in control nanospheres under protocol 13.1.

- Pour the organic phase in 60 ml of milliQ water containing Pluronic F68 (1%, w/v).

- Purification and re-suspension steps are similar, as discussed for control nanospheres.

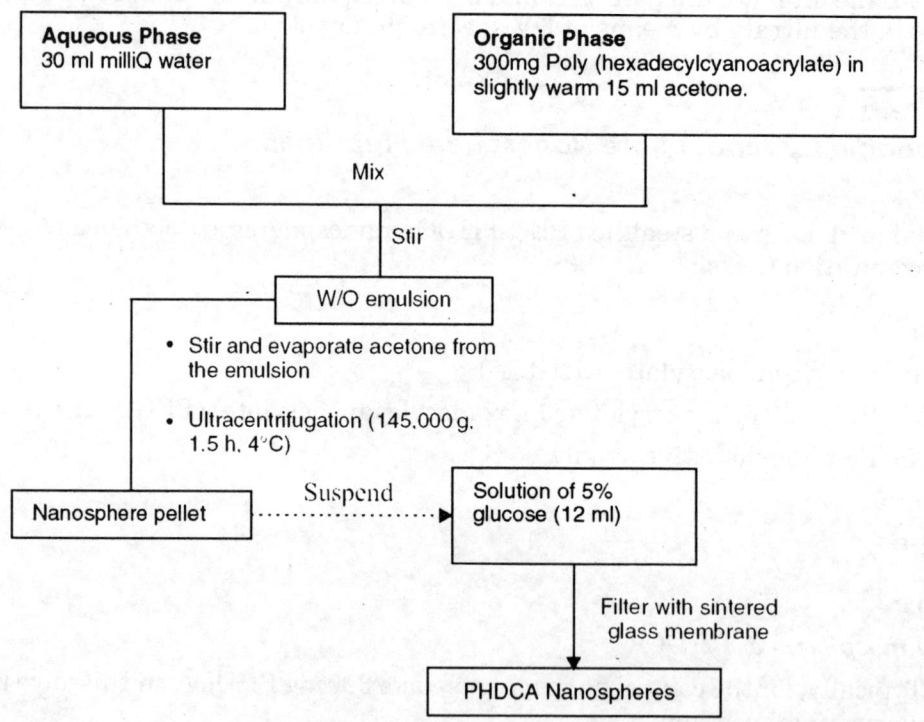

Scheme 13.9: *Preparation of cynoacrylate nanospheres*

PROTOCOL 13.13

Drug-loaded Acrylate Polymer Nanosuspensions for Ophthalmic Application

Principle

Quasi-Emulsion Solvent Diffusion (QESD) Method (Pignatello *et al.*, 2002)

Materials

Eudragit RS100

Eudragit RL100

FLU

Tween 80

Benzalkonium chloride (50% w/v)

Procedure

- The nanosuspensions can be prepared in the presence or absence of FLU, at different drug/polymer weight ratio and using different rates of agitation.

- Dissolve the drug and polymer in different weight concentration ratio at room temperature in ethanol (2 ml). Slowly inject the polymer solution (0.5 ml/min), with a syringe connected to a thin teflon tube, in 50 ml water containing Tween 80 (0.02% w/v) and benzalkonium chloride (0.1% w/v), and keep this mixture in an ice-water bath. During injection, the mixture is intimately mixed by an agitation at a speed of 20,000 rpm using a mechanical stirrer.

- The solution immediately turns into a pseudoemulsion of the drug and polymer ethanol solution in the external aqueous phase.

- Evaporate the organic solvent gradually that follows the precipitation *in situ* of the polymer and drug, with the formation of matrix-type nanoparticles.

- Then slowly agitate the ethanol residues to evaporate traces of solvent using a slow magnetic stirrer for 24 h at a slow speed to get the nanosuspension at room temperature. Centrifuge the nanosuspension and collect the pellets of nanoparticles. Wash the pellets with double distilled water.

- Centrifuge the 2.0 ml aliquots of the freshly prepared suspensions at 11,000 rpm and at 10°C for 15 min and the amount of unincorporated drug may be measured by UV analysis in the supernatant.

- Determine the particle size and zeta potential of nanosuspensions by photocorrelation spectroscopy techniques using Zetamaster sizer equipment.

- Determine the *in vitro* release by dialysis method using dialysis membrane.

SUGGESTED READINGS

- Bhargava, K and Aindo, H. Y. (1992) Pharm. Res., 9, 776.
- Birrenbach, G. and Speiser, R. (1976) J. Pharm. Sci., 65, 1763.
- Brigger, I. (2002) J. Pharmacol. Experiment. Ther., 928.
- Chiannilkulchai, N., Driouich, Z., Benoit, J. P., Parodi, A. L. and Couvreur, P. (1989) Sel. Cancer Ther,. 5, 1.
- Couvreur, P. and Vauthier, C. (1991) J. Control. Rel., 17, 187.

- Couvreur, P., Grislain L., Linaerts V., Brasseur P., Guiot P. and Biernacki A. (1986) In:Biodegradable polymeric nanoparticles as drug carriers for anti-tumour agents, Polymeric nanoparticles as drug carriers for antitumour agents, Guiot P. and Couvreur P. (Eds.), CRC Press, Boca Raton, FL, 27.
- Couvreur, P., Kante, B., Grislain, L., Roland, M. and Speiser, P. (1982) J. Pharm. Sci., 71, 790.
- Couvreur, P., Roblot-Treupel, L., Poupon, M. F., Brasseur, F. and Puisieux, F. (1990) Adv. Drug Deliv. Rev., 5, 209.
- de Verdiere, A.C., Dubernet, C., Nemati, F., Soma, E., Appel, M., Ferte, J., Bernard, S., Puisieux, F., Couvreur, P. (1997) Br J Cancer., 76, 198.
- Douglas, S. J., Davis, S. S. and Illum, L. (1986) Int. J. Pharm., 34, 145.
- Douglas, S. J., Davis, S. S. and Illum, L. (1987) CRC Crit Rev. Ther. Drug Carr. Syst., 3, 233
- Gupta, P. K., Gallo, J. M., Hung, C. T. and Perrier, D. G. (1987a) Drug Dev. Ind. Pharm., 13, 1471.
- Gupta, P.K., Hung, C.T., Lam, F.C. and Perrier, D.G. (1987b) Int. J. Pharm., 43, 167.
- Khouri N., Fessi, H., Roblot-Treupel, L., Devissaguet, J.P., Puisieux, F. (1986) Pharm Acta Helv. 61, 274.
- Kramer, P. A. (1974) J. Pharm. Sci. 63, 1647.
- Krause, H. J. and Rohdewald P. (1985) Pharm. Res. 5, 239.
- Kreuter, J. (1983) Int. J. Pharm. 14, 43.
- Kreuter, J. (1991) J. Control. Rel. 16, 169.
- Kreuter, J. (1994) Eur. J. Drug Metab. Pharmacokinet. 19, 253.
- Kreuter, J. (1994) In: Colloidal drug delivery systems, Kreuter J. (Ed.), Marcel Dekker, New York, 219.
- Kreuter, J. Alyautdin, R. N., Kharkevich, D. A. and Ivanov, A. A. (1995) Brain Res. 674, 171.
- Kreuter, J. And Haenzel I. (1978) Infect. Immun. 19, 667.
- Kreuter, J. and Speiser P. (1976) J. Pharm. Sci. 65, 1624.
- Kreuter, J., Berg, U., Liehl, E., Soiva, M. and Speiser, P. P. (1986) Vaccine 4, 125.
- Kreuter, J., Liehl, E., Berg, U., Soiva, M. and Speiser, P. P. (1988) Vaccine 6, 253.
- Kreuter, J., Stieneker, F. and Lower, J. (1991) Poc. Int. Symp. Controlled Release Bioact. Mater., 18, 277.
- Marty, J. J., Oppenheim, R. C. and Speiser, P. (1978) Pharm Acta Helv, 53, 17.
- Nakagawa, Y., Takayama, K., Ueda, H., Machida, Y. and Nagai, T. (1987) Drug Des Deliv., 2, 99.
- Oppenheim, R. C. (1986) In: Nanoparticulate drug delivery systems based on gelatin and albumin, Polymeric nanoparticles as drug carriers for antitumour agents. Guiot P. and Couvreur P. (Eds.), CRC Press, Boca Raton, FL, 27.
- Oppenheim, R. C., Stewart, N. F., Gordon, L. and Patel, H. M. (1982) Drug Dev. Ind. Phar., 8, 531.
- Pignatello, R., Bucolo, C., Spedalieri, G., Maltese, A. and Puglisi G. (2002) Biomaterials, 23, 3247.
- Roger, M. and Kissel, T. (1993) Eur. J. Pharmacol. Biopharm., 39, 8.
- Soma, C.E., Dubernet, C., Bentolila, D., Benita S., Couvreur P. (2000) Biomaterials, 21, 1.
- Sugibasayashi, K., Morimotot, Y., Nada, T., Kato Y., Hasegawa, A. and Arita T. (1979) Chem. Pharm. Bull., 27, 204.
- Widder, K., Flouret, G. and Senyei, A. (1979) J. Pharm. Sci., 68, 79.

14

Resealed Erythrocytes

Red blood cells (RBCs), by their sheer numbers, 5 million/microlitre in the circulation totalling 30 trillion in humans, and their long lifetimes of 120 days, are uniquely positioned to modulate the properties of blood-borne and vascular components. The breadth and diversity of vascular traffic afford a multitude of opportunities, with a vast clinical potential, for intervening in pathologies involving cellular or humoral components. The idea of using red cells as storage containers (erythrocyte encapsulation), whereby biologically active entities can be packaged within the cell and later released, continues to be pursued as a means of drug delivery and targeting. Various other cellular carriers proposed are: (a) lymphocytes, (b) leukocytes, (c) platelets, and (d) granulocytes (Krantz 1997).

COMPOSITION OF ERYTHROCYTES

The blood contains about 55% of fluid portion (plasma) and nearly 45% of corpuscles or formed elements. The fluid portion contains a large number of organic and inorganic substances in solution, which may be diffusible (electrolytes, anabolic and catabolic substances formed during metabolism) and non-diffusible (proteins). The formed element or cellular portion of the blood consists of erythrocytes (red blood cells), leukocytes (white blood cells) and thrombocytes (platelets). The plasma constituents help in maintaining the isotonicity and the morphology of the red blood cells. Manipulation in plasma compositions *ex vivo* could be used to design various delivery systems. Normal blood cells have extensile, elastic, biconcave and non-nucleated configuration with a diameter ranging from 6–9 µm with a mean diameter of 7.5 µm. The thickness is nearly 1 µ in the centre with an increased thickness (~2µm) near the periphery. They have a lifespan of about 100–120 days. The erythrocytes being non-nucleated do not have the machinery to synthesise new carbohydrates, proteins and lipids and replace them with plasma components to rebuild its membrane constituents. Erythrocytes have a solid content of about 35% (rest 65% being water) most of which is haemoglobin, which remains tightly bound to the stroma of the cell membrane.

Haemoglobin is determined spectrophotometrically at 540 nm, either directly or after the conversion of haemoglobin to cyanomethyl-haemoglobin using Drabkin's reagent. Most of the remaining solid is represented by proteins and lipids, which form the stroma or framework which concentrate on the cell surface as limiting membrane (cell wall). The phosphate content (50–100 mg/100 gm) of the erythrocytes is higher than that found in the plasma, most of which is organic in nature, i.e., triphosphate, hexosephosphate, ATP and traces of NAD and NADP. The lipid content of the erythrocytes essentially includes cholesterol, lecithin and cephaelins.

Electrolyte Composition of Erythrocytes

The electrolyte composition of the erythrocytes is although qualitatively similar to that of plasma however, quantitatively it differs from that of plasma. The concentration of K^+ and Na^+ differ in that the former is more in erythrocytes and the latter in plasma. The osmotic pressure of the interior of the erythrocytes is equal to that of plasma and termed as isotonic (normally equivalent to the osmotic pressure of 0.9% NaCl, commonly known as normal or physiological saline). Changes in the osmotic pressure of the medium surrounding the red blood cells (either *in vivo* or *in vitro*) change and manipulate the morphology and tonicity of the cells. If the medium is hypotonic, water diffuses into the cells and they get swelled and eventually loose all their haemoglobin content and may burst. On the other hand, if the medium is hypertonic, (i.e., one having a higher osmotic pressure than 0.9% NaCl) they will shrink and become irregular (crenated) in appearance. However, 0.9% saline solution lack necessary ions for the functionality of the cells. Balanced ion solutions like Ringer's, Ringer-Loche and Tyrode's solution, which are not only isotonic but also contain ions in proper quantity, are used in erythrocyte related experiments.

The flexibility of red blood cells (erythrocytes, RBC) retains its shape and morphology when placed in isotonic saline after being challenged with altered tonicity environments. These properties lend them suitable carriers for drugs and enzymes.

METHODS OF DRUG LOADING

Hypotonic Haemolysis and Isotonic Resealing Methods

This method is based upon hypotonic lysis of cells in a solution containing the drug/enzyme to be entrapped followed by restoration of tonicity to reseal them. Four variations of the procedure have been described based upon modes, by which hypotonicity is produced. The ghost populations so obtained are heterogenous. Three types of ghosts can be distinguished: type I ghosts which reseal immediately after haemolysis; type II ghosts which reseal after reversal of haemolysis by addition of alkali ions; and type III ghosts which remain leaky under different experimental conditions. The ratio of three fractions depends on temperature at which haemolysis is affected and on time interval between haemolysis and restoration of tonicity.

Loading by "Red Cell Loader"

Magnani and coworkers, (1998) developed a novel method for the entrapment of non-diffusible drugs into human erythrocytes. The equipment designed for this method was termed as "red cell loader". The method requires as little as 50 ml of blood. By using a new apparatus, it is possible to entrap a variety of biological compounds into erythrocytes in as little time as 2 h at room temperature under blood banking conditions. The method is based on two sequential and controlled hypotonic dilutions of washed red blood cells followed by concentration with a haemofilter. Subsequent isotonic resealing of erythrocytes allow a 35–50% cell recovery and approximate 30% entrapment of added drug.

Dilutional Haemolysis

Population of erythrocytes when exposed to hypotonic saline solution (0.4% NaCl), swells until it reaches a critical value of volume or pressure where membrane ruptures and becomes permeable to macromolecules and ions, therefore permitting the escape of cellular components (Ihler *et al.*, 1973; Ihler and Tsang, 1987). One volume of washed erythrocytes could be treated with 2–20 volumes of materials to be loaded in a hypotonic buffer at 0 °C for 5 min. Further incubation at 25°C in an isotonic solution (0.9% NaCl) reseal them again. In general, the method is rapid and simplest especially for low molecular weight drugs, however the entrapment efficiency remains to be low (1–8%).

Preswell Dilutional Haemolysis

The technique is based upon initial controlled swelling of erythrocytes without lysis by placing them in slightly hypotonic solution followed by centrifugation at low 'g' to take them up to point of lysis (Ihler and Tsang, 1987). Finally, the addition of small volume of drug solution to attain drug loaded resealed erythrocytes.

Isotonic Osmotic Lysis

In order to avoid the potential disadvantages associated with hypotonic haemolysis, efforts were made to prepare resealed erythrocytes under isotonic (and/or isoionic) conditions. Haemolysis in isotonic solutions can be achieved both by chemical and physical means. If erythrocytes are incubated in solutions of a substance with high transerythrocytic membrane permeability (i.e., small reflection coefficient as defined by the thermodynamics of irreversible processes) the solute will diffuse into the cells due to inwardly directed chemical potential gradient. This will be followed by water uptake until osmotic equilibrium is restored. Various methods are based on this mechanism including

- Conventional (classical) haemolysis in isotonic urea solutions
- Polyethylene induced haemolysis
- Ammonium chloride induced haemolysis.

Dialysis

The major limitation of dilution procedure is low entrapment efficiency. It can be overcome by carrying out lysis and resealing within a dialysis tube. Several methods for dialysis based loading of erythrocytes are reported but all take advantage of the common principle that the semipermeable dialysis membrane maximises the intracellular: extracellular volume ratio for macromolecules during lysis and resealing, but also allows for free flow of small ions, responsible for lysis and resealing of the erythrocytes. It is this intracellular: extracellular volume ratio during the time that the erythrocyte membrane tends to be permeable that determines the percentage entrapment of bioactives. It considerably reduces the extracellular solution volume that equilibrates with intracellular spaces of erythrocytes during lysis.

Electro-insertion or Electro-encapsulation

Kinsota and Tsong, (1977; 1978) have suggested the use of transient electrolysis to generate desirable membrane permeability for drug loading into red blood cells. The erythrocyte membrane could be opened by dielectric breakdown and subsequently the pores can be resealed by incubation at 37°C in an osmotically balanced medium. The method is based on creating electrically induced permeability changes at high membrane potential differences. Electric-breakdown is evident when the membrane is polarised for microseconds using varied voltage values. The components can be entrapped when an electric pulse of greater than a threshold voltage of 2 kV/cm is applied for 20μ sec (Teissie *et al.*, 1982).

Loading by Electric Cell Fusion

In this method, the molecules are first loaded into erythrocyte ghosts. These ghosts are then caused to adhere to target cells. Electric pulses are applied to induce fusion of ghost with target cells with subsequent release of the encapsulated molecule. This loading can be exemplified with the loading of cell specific monoclonal antibody to erythrocyte ghosts. An antibody against a specific surface protein of the target cells can be chemically crosslinked to drug loaded ghosts. The antibody will direct these ghosts to target cell for adhesion. Electric cell fusion then allows injection of these drugs into the target cells.

Entrapment by Endocytosis

Schrier and co-workers, (1975) described drug entrapment in erythrocyte ghosts by endocytosis. The vesicle membrane separates the endocytosed substance from the cytoplasm, which may shelter drugs prone to inactivation in erythrocytes or alternatively protect the erythrocytes from drug. The resulting erythrocytes contain vacuoles and probably have different *in vivo* survival characteristics from resealed cells, prepared using other methods. The swollen ghosts so prepared exhibit larger (>0.5 μ diameter) endocytic vacuoles. The drug substances are trapped in these endocytic vacuoles.

Loading by Chemical Perturbation of Membrane (Drug Mediated Loading)

This method is based upon the observation that the permeability of the erythrocytic membrane is increased, when it is exposed to some chemical agents. This allows the low molecular weight substances to get entrapped. A haemolysis technique in isotonic solution developed by Lin and co-workers, (1975) is based on the use of an anaesthetic; halothane, which changes the permeability and selectivity of the membrane (colloid osmotic haemolysis).

Amphotericin B, a polyene antifungal antibiotic, damages microorganism by increasing permeability of their membranes to metabolites and ions. Kitao and Hattori, (1980) utilised this feature for the entrapment of daunomycin in human and mouse erythrocytes. The *in vivo* survival of loaded erythrocytes by this technique however was found to be poor. Due to residual membrane defects they are sequestered from circulation by RES predominant organs.

In vitro characterisation

Resealed erythrocytes after loading are characterised for following parameters. These *in vitro* characterisations are pivotal to ensure their *in vivo* performance and therapeutic benefits. Some of the routine characterisation parameters used to evaluate resealed erythrocytes are described in brief.

Drug Content

Packed loaded erythrocytes (0.5 ml) are first deproteinised with acetonitrile (2.0 ml) and subjected to centrifugation at 2500 rpm for 10 min. The clear supernatant is analysed for the drug content using specified estimation methodology for entrapped drug (Vyas and Jain, 1994). In case, the resealed erythrocytes are loaded with magnetite to make them magnoresponsive (Vyas and Jain, 1994), a horseshoe magnet (1200 G) is placed adjacent to the base of the centrifuge tube in order to retain the entrapped magnetite. The magnetite concentration in drug-loaded erythrocytes could be determined using atomic absorption spectroscopy or some other appropriate procedures (Vyas and Jain, 1994). ·

In vitro Drug and Haemoglobin Release

Normal and loaded erythrocytes are incubated at $37\pm2°C$ in phosphate buffer saline (pH 7.4) at 50% haematocrit in a metabolic rotating wheel incubator bath. Periodically, the samples are withdrawn with the help of a hypodermic syringe fitted with a 0.8 µm Spectropore membrane filter. The samples are then deproteinised with acetonitrile and can be estimated for the amount of drug released. Per cent haemoglobin can similarly be calculated at various time intervals at 540 nm spectrophotometrically (Vyas and Jain, 1994). The cumulative percentage release profile as function of time can be calculated. Per cent haemolysis can also be determined by comparing the absorbance of supernatant with the absorbance obtained after complete hydrolysis of same number of cells in distilled water (Vyas and Jain, 1994). Laser light scattering may also be used to evaluate haemoglobin content of individual resealed erythrocytes.

Another parameter, which evaluates the haemoglobin disposition after the resealing, is the mean corpuscular haemoglobin. It is the mean concentration of haemoglobin per 100 ml of cells, and is an index, which is independent of the size of the red cell and therefore, it is a true expression of their haemoglobin content.

Osmotic Fragility

It is the parameter, which simulates and mimics the bioenvironmental conditions that are encountered following *in vivo* administration, *in vitro* handling and the effect of loaded contents on the survival rates of the erythrocytes. When red blood cells are exposed to solutions of varying tonicities their shape changes (swell in hypotonic and shrink in hypertonic environments) due to osmotic imbalance (Sprandel and Zollner, 1985). To evaluate the effects of varying tonicities, drug loaded erythrocytes are incubated with saline solutions of different tonicities (from isotonic to hypotonic, i.e. 0.9 % w/v to 0.1% w/v) at 37 ± 2 °C for 10 min. The suspension after centrifugation at 300 g for 15 min is assayed for drug and/or haemoglobin release, which should be in the acceptable range for a system to be therapeutically effective.

Osmotic Shock

Osmotic shock describes a sudden (and not tapering) exposure of drug-loaded erythrocytes to an environment, which is far from isotonic to evaluate the ability of resealed erythrocytes to withstand the stress and maintain their integrity as well as appearance (Ingrosso *et al.,* 1997). Incubating the resealed erythrocytes (1 ml, 10–50% haematocrit) with distilled water (5 ml) for 15 min followed by centrifugation at 3000 rpm for 15 min, may cause the release of haemoglobin to varying degrees, which could be estimated spectrophotometrically.

Turbulence Shock

The parameter indicates the effects of shear force and pressure by which resealed erythrocytes formulations are injected, on the integrity of the loaded cells. Loaded erythrocytes (10% haematocrit, 5 ml) are passed through a 23-gauge hypodermic needle at a flow rate of 10 ml/min (Vyas and Jain, 1994). After every pass, aliquot of the suspension is withdrawn and centrifuged at 300 g for 15 min, and haemoglobin content, leached out are estimated spectrophotometrically. Resealing of the erythrocytes makes them sensitive towards turbulence or mechanical agitation and hence an estimation of turbulence shock provides their expected performance *in vivo.*

Morphology and Percent Cellular Recovery

Phase-contrast optical microscopy, transmission electron microscopy and scanning electron microscopy are the microscopic methods used to evaluate the shape, size and the surface features of the loaded erythrocytes. Per cent cell recovery (after loading) can be determined by assessing the number of intact erythrocytes remaining per cubic mm with the help of a haemocytometer.

PROTOCOL: 14.1

Magnetically Responsive Drug Loaded Erythrocytes Carrier

Materials

Drug (Ibuprofen)

Magnetite

Buffers

1. Reversed Hank's balanced salt solution (reversed HBSS)

    Composition

KCl	10.18 g/l
KH_2PO_4	0.1 g/l
$NaHCO_3$	1.276 g/l
NaCl	0.316 g/l
$Na_2HPO_4.H_2O$	0.1 g/l
Glucose	2.0 g/l

2. Phosphate buffered saline (PBS); pH 7.4

    Composition

$Na_2HPO_4.H_2O$	1.38 g/l
KH_2PO_4	0.19 g/l
NaCl	8 g/l
NaOH	0.1N to pH 7.4.

Procedure

Step 1. Isolation of Erythrocytes

- Dampen the ear tips with xylol and collect the blood from the auricular vein into a heparinised syringe. Collect the blood from ear veins of white male rabbits (avg. wt. 3–4 Kg).
- Centrifuge the whole blood at 2500 rpm for 5 min at 4°C in a refrigerated centrifuge.
- Carefully remove the serum and buffy coat and wash the packed cells three times with PBS (pH 7.4). Dilute the washed cells with phosphate buffered saline (pH 7.4) and stored at 4°C until used.

Step 2. Loading of Drug and Magnetite

- Load the isolated erythrocytes with drug and magnetite by the pre-swell dilution technique.
- In this method, transfer 1ml of packed erythrocytes to a glass centrifuge tube and add 4 ml of reversed HBSS medium. The reversed HBSS medium used here with some modification that is concentration used for Na⁺ and K⁺ ions were equal for intracellular concentrations during encapsulation. Maintain the isotonicity for reversed HBSS medium, to 0.65 of the normal value. Recover the swollen cells by centrifugation at 600g for 5 min and remove the supernatant.

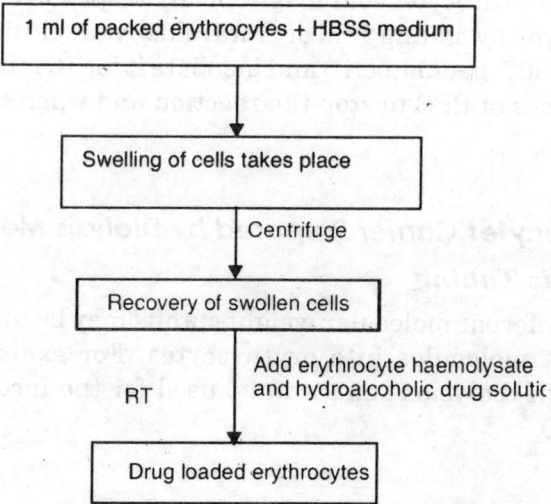

Scheme 14.1: *Preparation of drug-loaded erythrocytes*

- Cover the swollen cells with a layer of 200μl erythrocyte haemolysate (prepare haemolysate by adding 1 ml of water to 1 ml of packed cells). Without disturbing the layer haemolysate, add 200μl of hydroalchoholic solution (1:1) of ibuprofen (drug; 2

mg/ml) and 100µl of magnetite (2% w/v) on the top of the mixture and mix the contents of the tube gently by occasional inversion. The purpose of haemolysate layer is to provide an osmotic barrier against the hypotonic drug solution. The addition of 200µl of drug and magnetite solution (100µl) is sufficient to bring the swollen cells to the point of lysis; further addition of drug solution can cause complete lysis.

- Reseal the cells by adding a calculated amount of 10 times hypertonic HBSS required to restore the tonicity of the erythrocytes suspension.

- Incubate the erythrocytes for 30 min at 37±2°C and recover the loaded cells by centrifugation followed by three times washing with normal HBSS to remove any adhered drug (Scheme 14.1).

- Remove the magnetite particles that had not been entrapped from the cell suspension, with the help of a horseshoe magnet (1200G). Following the same procedures plain ibuprofen-loaded erythrocytes can be prepared.

Effect of Various Process Variables for Preparation of Drug Loaded Erythrocytes

   (i) Drug concentration

  (ii) Magnetite concentration

 (iii) Sonication speed and time

Glutaraldehyde Treatment of Loaded Erythrocytes

Treat the drug loaded erythrocytes and magnetically responsive drug loaded erythrocytes with 0.5% glutaraldehyde by adding 1 ml of glutaraldehyde solution in PBS (pH 7.4) to 1 ml of loaded erythrocytes (50% haematocrit) and incubate it for 10 min. After incubation, dilute the cells with 20 volumes of PBS to stop the reaction and wash three times with PBS.

PROTOCOL: 14.2
Drug Loaded Erythrocytes Carrier Prepared by Dialysis Method

Treatment of Dialysis Tubing

Dialysis tubing with different molecular weight cutoffs may be utilised when incorporating low molecular weight molecules into erythrocytes. For example, Spectra/Por 61,000 molecular weight cutoff dialysis tubing can be used for the incorporation of drug having molecular weight 1200.

Lysis Time

Lysis time is dependent on haematocrit present in the dialysis bag. 45 min gives total lysis with a 50% haematocrit, whereas 75 min is required with an 80 % haematocrit.

Lysis Temperature

The 0−4 °C temperature is utilised for lysis, however 0°C gives higher entrapment compared to 4 °C.

Addition of Exogenous Material

Two procedures can be followed according to the molecular weight of the compound to be encapsulated.

For protein and large molecular weight substances, the material is added to the RBC before dialysis. Since the final encapsulation efficiency is ultimately dependent on the hematocrit of the RBC; dilution of the packed RBC should be as little as possible. Concentration of protein to RBC should be above 1:5 v/v. Avoid addition of lyophilised protein to packed RBC as clumping of protein can occur leading to adherence to the RBC thus reducing the encapsulation efficiency.

For the entrapment of small molecules, the addition to RBC is always carried out after dialysis because the dialysis process will result in a significant loss of the smaller dialyzable molecules.

It is limited to the packed volume of the RBC in the haematocrit. In operational terms, the maximum encapsulation per cent is further limited by the loss of RBC in the dialysis process. The loss of RBC is due to intrinsic properties of the different RBC and typically cell recovery is 50 to 90%.

$$\text{Percentage encapsulation} \frac{\text{amount encapsulated} \times 100}{\text{amount added to RBC}}$$

PROTOCOL 14.3:

Preparation of White Resealable Erythrocytes by Column Method

Material

> Agarose 50–100 mesh
>
> Sodium acetate (1M, –1°C)
>
> *Erythrocyte wash medium:* 146 mM NaCl and 20 mM HEPES pH 7.6, room temperature. Any buffer may be used providing the pK near to 7.5.
>
> Column haemolysis buffer 5 mM $MgSO_4$, 5 mM KCl, 5mM PIPES, pH 6.5, 0°C.
>
> Stock ionic strength reversing medium
>
> 3 M KCl, 0°C.
>
> Column preserving medium
>
> 146 mm NaCl, 20 mM Tris-HCl, 0.02 % sodium azide, pH 7.5, room temperature.
>
> Enzymes or any other agents should be kept as concentrated stock solution (10-20X, 0°C)

Procedure

Column Preparation

- Pack a short-jacketed column (Diameter 2.5 to 10 cm, Table 14.1) and use sodium acetate (1M, –1°C) as medium to be run in outer jacket of column as a coolant.

- Replace standard nylon mesh in the flow adapter to 25 μ which allow free passage of the membranes.
- Equilibrate the column overnight with either pH 6.5 column haemolysing buffer B or C, under gravity flow.
- Conduct haemolysis at 0°C.
- Shortly before the addition of the washed cells, an isotonic wash buffer (solution A, 0°C) step of about a one tenth bed volume is applied to the top of the column.
- Apply about a one eighth bed volume of 10 % cell suspension to the top of the column and elute with wash buffer (solution A) at a moderate flow rate (Scheme 14.2).

Table 14.1: *Nominal column volumes required for white ghost preparation*

Parameter	Preparation		
	1	2	3
Column diameter (cm)	2.5	5.0	10
Gel bed length (cm)	30	30	25
Gel volume (L)	0.15	0.6	2.0
Nominal void volume (L)	0.04	0.2	0.5
Elute with solution B or C pH 6.5 buffer	0.4	1.8	5.0
Elute with Solution A; pH 7.6 buffer (ml)	15	60	200
Maximum expected ghost pellet (ml)	2.0	7.5	25
After first appearance of membranes (ml)	20.0	75.0	250.0
Restore isotonicity with solution E (ml)	1.06	3.98	13.25

Gel: Agarose A-50m, 50-100 mesh, Bio-Rad.

Erythrosomes

Erythrosomes are novel class of cellular carriers in which chemically crosslinked human erythrocyte cytoskeletons are used as a support upon which a lipid bilayer is coated. The lipid coating is affected by the reverse phase evaporation procedure normally used in REV preparation. These proteoliposomes, which we term erythrosomes, are of large size (an average diameter of 3μm) and extremely uniform in size distribution. They are mechanically stable and easily prepared in large quantities. The protein content of erythrosomes is well defined essentially being that of the erythrocyte cytoskeleton. The erythrosomes can be made from well-defined exogenous lipids. They contain less than 4% of erythrocyte lipids. The encapsulation efficiency of the erythrosomes is at least 4 times greater than that of typical REV and 200 times greater than that of SUVs. The erythrosomes possess a diffusion barrier to many ions and non-charged molecules as tight as those of SUV and REV. These carrier systems may serve as a useful encapsulation system for drug delivery.

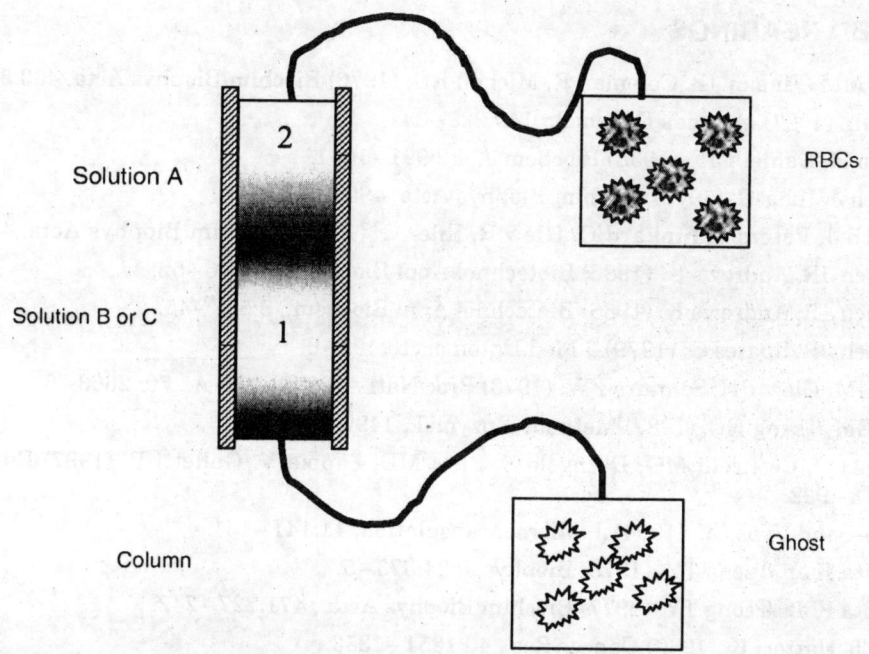

Scheme 14.2: *Preparation of white resealable erythrocytes by column methods*

Preparation of Erythrosomes

Crosslinked Erythrocyte Cytoskeletons

- Prepare human erythrocyte membranes (ghosts) 99.9% free of haemoglobin from erythrocytes of freshly outdated whole banked blood after depletion of white cells and platelets.

- Pack the ghosts in 20mM sodium phosphate buffer (pH 7.4) and treat with 100mM glutaraldehyde for 5min at room temperature. Then add and mix this solution with sufficient volume of 5% Triton-X-100 in balanced salt solution (BSS) consisting of 125 mM Na^+ 5 mM K^+, 3.75 mM Ca^{2+}, 2.5mM Mg^{2+}, all as chlorides and 10mM Tris-HCl (pH 7.4) to give 50mg Triton per ml of packed ghost.

- Extract with detergent at room temperature for 30 min. Then layer the mixture over an equal volume of 20% (w/v) sucrose in BSS (pH 7.4) and wash the cytoskeletons and pellet by centrifugation at 4000g for 5 min.

- Aspirate the supernatant and part of the sucrose cushion and collect the pellet. Again layer the crosslinked cytoskeletons thus, pelleted over 10 volumes of 10% sucrose cushion in BSS and repeat the washing step.

- Mix the packed cytoskeletons with an equal volume of 5% w/v PEG 6000 in BSS (pH 7.4). At this stage the residual detergent associated with the packed cytoskeletons is less than 0.02mg/mg protein, as estimated with tritiated Triton X-100.

SUGGESTED READINGS

- Billah MM, Finean JB, Coleman R, Michell RH. (1976) Biochim Biophys Acta, 433:54–62.
- Dale GL. (1987) Methods Enzymol., 149:229–34.
- Davson H, Danielli JF. (1938) Biochem J., 32:991–1001.
- Deloach J, Ihler G. (1977) Biochim Biophys Acta. 496:136–45.
- Deloach J, Peters S, Pinkard O, Glew R, Ihler G. (1977) Biochim Biophys Acta.,496:507–15.
- DeLoach JR, Andrews K. (1986) Biotechnol Appl Biochem., 8: 546–52.
- DeLoach JR, Andrews K. (1986) Biotechnol Appl Biochem., 8:537–45.
- DeLoach JR, Spates G. (1979) J Med Entomol.,16:493–6.
- Ihler GM, Glew RH, Schnure FW. (1973) Proc Natl Acad Sci U S A., 70: 2663–6.
- Ihler GM, Tsang HC. (1987) Methods Enzymol., 149:221–9.
- Ingrosso D, Cotticelli MG, D'Angelo S, Buro MD, Zappia V, Galletti P. (1997) Eur J Biochem., 244:918–922.
- Jain SK and Vyas SP. (1994) J. Microencapsulation, 11:141–151.
- Kinosita K Jr, Tsong TY. (1978) Biophys J. 24:373–5.
- Kinosita K Jr, Tsong TY. (1977) Biochim Biophys Acta., 471:227–242.
- Kitao T, Hattori K. (1980) Cancer Res., 40:1351–1353.
- Krantz A. (1997) Blood Cells, Molecules and Diseases, 23: 58–68.
- Rossi L, Magnani M. (1998) Methods Mol Biol., 108:245–256.
- Schrier SL. (1987) Methods Enzymol., 149:260–270.
- Sprandel U, Zollner N. (1985) Res Exp Med (Berl)., 185:77–85.
- Teissie J, Knutson VP, Tsong TY, Lane MD. (1982) Science., 216: 537–8.
- Vyas SP and Jain SK. (1994) J. Microencapsulation, 11: 9–29.

15

Transfersomes and Ethosomes

Transfersomes are complex, most often, vesicular aggregate optimised to attain extremely flexible and self-regulating membrane; this makes the vesicle very deformable. Transfersome vesicle therefore can cross microporous barrier very efficiently, even when available passage are much smaller than the average aggregate size. A transfersome crossing the skin thus mimics the behaviour of a parasite during its invasion of the host body (Cevc *et al.*, 1998). Transfersome consist of natural amphipathic compound suspended in a water-based solution, sometimes containing biocompatible surfactant. Similar to liposome transfersome have a lipid bilayer that surrounds an aqueous core however in contrast to liposome, transfersome contain at least one component that soften the membrane and makes skin more flexible. This allows an easy and rapid change of transfersome shape.

Mechanism of Transfersomes Penetration

The efficacy of transpore movement of transfersomes is quite high, a suspension of transfersomes with an average diameter of 500nm can be transported through the pore 5 times smaller nearly as rapidly and efficiently as pure water. Such a high penetration capability is seen, when the stress suffered by transfersomes (e.g. the flow-driving pressure) is sufficiently high. This is a key characteristic of transfersomes, with roots in the self-optimising capability of transfersomes body or membrane. The passage of transfersomes through pores that are "too small" is nearly perfect even when their size exceeds the pore diameter by a factor of approximately 4 or even 10 (Fig. 15.1).

One naturally occurring transdermal gradient is osmotic gradient. Such a gradient is created by the difference in the total water concentration between the skin surface and the skin interior. When a lipid suspension is placed on the skin surface and partly dehydrated by water evaporation loss, the lipid vesicles feel this gradient and try to escape complete drying by moving along this gradient. They can only achieve this if they are sufficiently deformable to pass through the narrow pores in the skin. Less deformable vesicle like standard liposomes, are confined to the skin surface where they dehydrate completely and fuse (Cevc *et al*, 1995).

Lipid hydrophilicity leads to xenophobia, the tendency to avoid dry surrounding and causes carriers sitting near or at the skin surface to resist to dehydration in order to remain maximally swollen. Transfersomes near the skin surface thus try to follow the local hydration gradient and thereby get into deeper and better-hydrated skin strata. This causes transfersomes carrier to retract from the relatively dry skin surface and to get into more humid region in the deeper skin layers (Cevc & Blume, 1992).

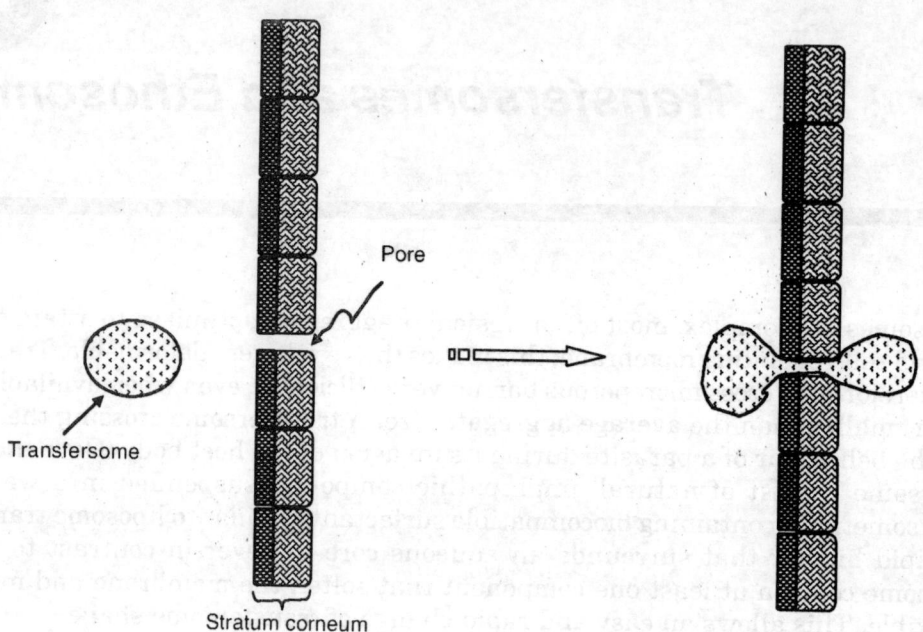

Fig. 15.1: *Penetration of transfersome through the pore in stratum corneum*

An important difference between transfersomes and liposomes is the much higher hydrophilicity of the former. This forces transfersome membrane to swell more than conventional lipid vesicle bilayer. Higher membrane hydrophilicity and flexibility both help transfersome to avoid aggregation and thus fusion, which is observed with liposome exposed to an osmotic stress. Transfersome fulfill basic criteria for efficient skin permeation and thus can be used as a potential carrier system for the proteins, interleukin, analgesic and anaesthetic agent, nonsteroidal anti-inflammatory drug, corticosteroids, etc.

Elasticity (Deformability) Measurement

Deformability is the unique characteristics of transfersomes. Different component in the transfersomes are chosen so as to be able to accommodate to particle shape changes. Transfersomes constituent with strongly divergent packing characteristics. At least one of these components tends to destabilise the membrane under certain conditions.

Comparative measurement of elasticity of the bilayer of transfersomes, niosomes and liposomes was carried out by extrusion measurement (Bergh *et al*, 2001). Briefly, the vesicles were extruded through polycarbonate filter with a pore size of 50 nm at constant pressure. The elasticity of vesicle was expressed in terms of deformability index which is proportional to $j(rv/rp)2$ where, j is the weight of suspension, which was extruded in definite time interval through a polycarbonate filter of 50 nm pore size, rv the size of vesicle and rp the pore size of membrane.

ETHOSOMES

Ethosomes are lipid vesicle with high content of ethanol. They can penetrate the skin and enhance compound delivery both to deep skin strata and systemically because ethanol fluidises both lipid bilayers of the stratum corneum and intercellular lipid. The soft, malleable vesicles then penetrate the disorganised lipid bilayers (Berry, 2001).

The ethosomal system consists of phospholipids, ethanol and water. Ethosomal system is much more efficient at delivering a fluorescent probe to the skin in terms of quantity and depth than either liposomes or hydroalcoholic solution. Ethosomes have a high entrapment capacity for molecule of various lyophilicities (Touitou *et al*, 2000).

In comparison to liposomes prepared in the absence of ethanol, the phospholipid in ethosomes is packed less tightly and the membrane has permeability for cations (Dayan and Touitou, 2000). Permeation enhancement from ethosomes is greater than ethanol alone and this indicates that there may be some kind of synergistic mechanism between ethanol, vesicles and skin lipids. The ethosomal lipids are in a more fluid state than liposomes from the same components without ethanol.

Mechanism of Penetration

When ethosomal carriers are applied to the skin a number of concomitant processes may take place, involving the stratum corneum and pilosebaceous pathways. Ethanol in the ethosome disturbs the organisation of the stratum corneum lipid bilayer and enhances its lipid fluidity. The flexible ethosome vesicle can then penetrate the disturbed stratum corneum bilayers and can even forge a pathway through the skin by virtue of their particulate nature. The release of entrapped molecule in the deeper layers of the skin and its transdermal absorption may be the result of fusion of ethosome with skin lipids and drug release at various points along the penetration pathways. Ethosomal penetration may also involve pilosebaceous pathways as they may be trapped in follicles (Touitou *et al*, 2000).

PROTOCOL 15.1

Transfersomes

Formula

Soya phosphatidylcholine

Surfactant (sodium deoxycholate)

Drug/antigen

Procedure

- Transfersomes may be prepared by combining an ethanolic solution of SPC with sodium deoxycholate.
- Add required amount of antigen/ drug in PBS to the above mixture.

- Push resulting suspension through a series of filters (pore size 0.45, 0.22, 0.11 and 0.05µm). This results in Transfersomes in the size range 170–200 nm (Scheme 15.1 and Fig. 15.2).

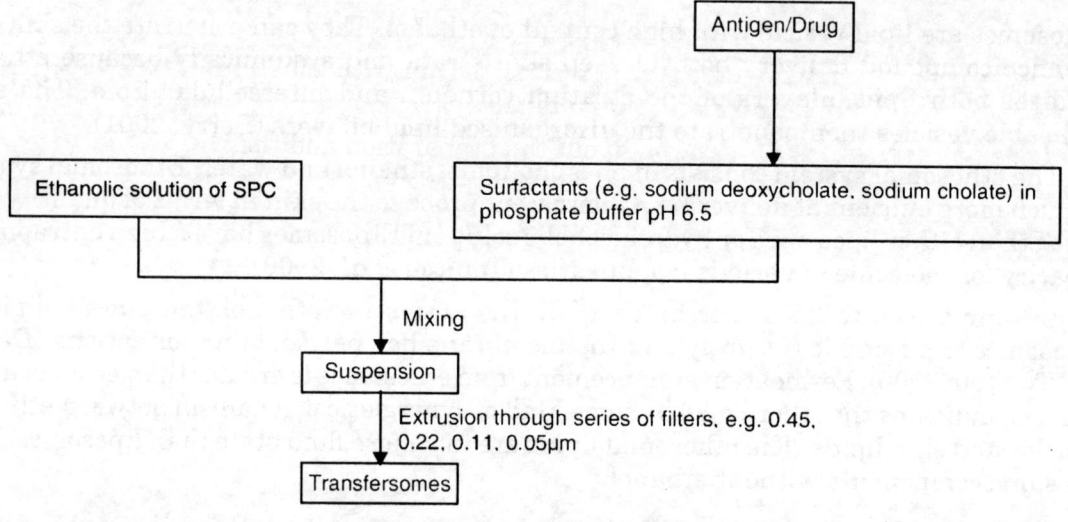

Scheme 15.1: *Preparation of transfersomes*

PROTOCOL 15.2

Ethosomes

Phospholipid

Ethanol

Water

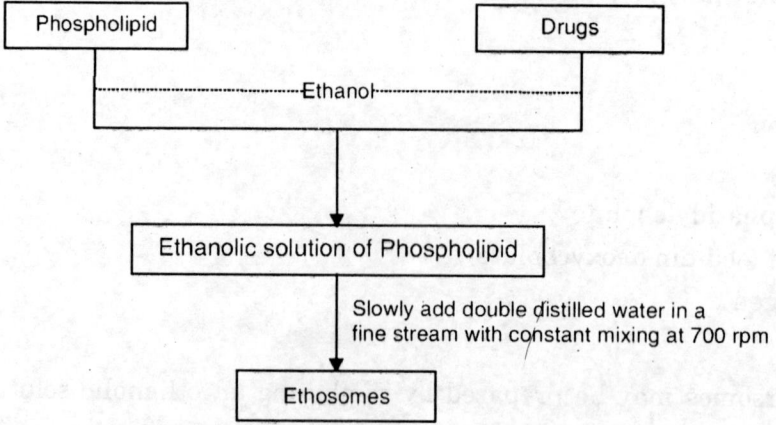

Scheme 15.2: *Preparation of ethosomes*

Procedure

- The ethosomal system may constitute of 2–5% phospholipid, 20–50% ethanol and water to 100%.
- Dissolve phospholipid and drug in ethanol.
- Add double distilled water slowly in fine stream with constant mixing at 700 rpm. Continue mixing for an additional 5 min.
- Keep the system at 30°C through out the preparation and then leave to cool at room temperature (Scheme 15.2).

PROTOCOL 15.3
Preparation of Ultraadaptable Vesicles
Procedure

- Take 8.7 w% Soya phosphatidylcholine, 1.3 w% cholate and approximately 8.5 v/v% ethanol.
- Combine lipid mixture with triethanolamine-HCl buffer to yield 10 w% total lipid concentration.
- The resulting suspension may be sonicated, freezed and thawed and brought to the desired size (as measured by means of photon correlation specroscopy) by ultrasonication or intermediate pressure homogenisation.
- Sterilise the vesicle suspension by filtration through a 0.2µm microporous filter. The final vesicle size may be checked by dynamic light scattering.

PROTOCOL 15.4
Ethosomes as a Carriers for Skin Delivery

Materials

Soya phosphatidylcholine (Phospholipon 90)

Ethanol

THP (trihexylphenidyl hydrochloride)

Procedure

- Dissolve phospholipon 90 (PL), and THP in ethanol.
- For the preparation of THP ethosomes containing 0.03% fluorescent probe D-289 (4-(4-diethyl amino) styryl-N methylpyridinium iodide) (A Molecular Probes), dissolve PL, THP and D-289 in ethanol.
- Add water in small quantities.
- Mix the preparation at 700 rpm for 5 min at room temperature (RT).

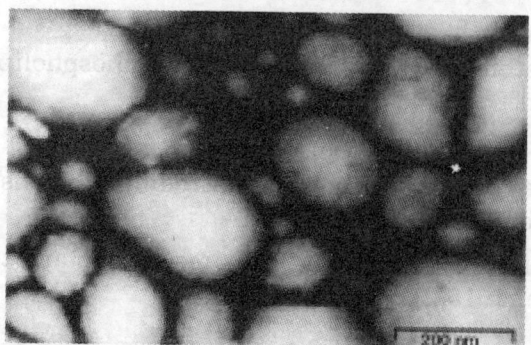

Fig 15.2: TEM image of transferosomes

The Entrapment Capacity

The entrapment capacity of THP by ethosomes may measure by ultracentrifugation method. Keep the vesicular preparations containing 1% THP overnight at 43°C and centrifuge in a ultracentrifuge at 43°C, at 40,000 rpm for 2 h. Assay, THP both in the sediment and in the supernatant. The presence of vesicles or PL in the supernatant can be analysed by TEM, DLS and by the Bartlett assay for phospholipid determination.

Skin Permeation of THP from Vesicles

Use side-by-side diffusion cells for 18 h at 37°C through the dorsal skin of male nude mice, 5–7 week old. Before the experiments, pass the systems through a 0.2 μm filter. Keep the receiver content 30%w/w hydroethanolic solution, in order to ensure pseudo-sink conditions. Withdraw samples of 200–400 μl at predetermined intervals. Remove each sample from the receiver, and replace an equal volume of receiver medium to keep a constant volume. At the end of the experiment, remove the skin, clean and extract in 30% hydroethanolic solution.

SUGGESTED READINGS

- Bergh, B.A.I., Wertz, P.W., Junginger, H.E., Bouwstra, J.A., (2001) Int. J. Pharm. 217: 13.
- Berry B W, (2001) Drug Discovery Today, 6: 967.
- Cevc G and Blume G, (1992) Biochim Biophys Acta, 1104: 226.
- Cevc, G., Gebauer, D., Stieber, J., Schaltzein, A., Blume, G., (1998) Biochim. Biophys. Acta 1368:201.
- Cevc, G., Schatzlein, A., Blume, G., (1995) J. Control. Rel. 36:3.
- Dayan N and Touitou E, (2000). Biomaterials, 21: 1879.
- Paul, A., Cevc, G., Bachhawat, B.K., (1998) Vaccine, 16: 188.
- Touitou E., Dayan N., Bergelson L., Godin B., Eliaz M., (2000) J Control Rel, 65: 403.

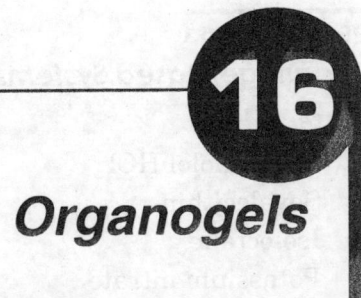

Organogels

ORGANOGELS

Organogels are highly self-structured systems, which are isotropic, thermoreversible, semirigid systems formed by peculiar kinds of small organic molecules (Fig. 16.1). They are efficiently self assembled into a 3-dimensional network of nanoscale measurement thereby turning a liquid into a gel (e.g. lecithin, gelatin, or sorbitan ester based gels). Hence the movement of the dispersing medium is restricted by interlacing 3-dimensional scaffold structure of particle of solvated macromolecules of dispersed phase (Klech, 1994).

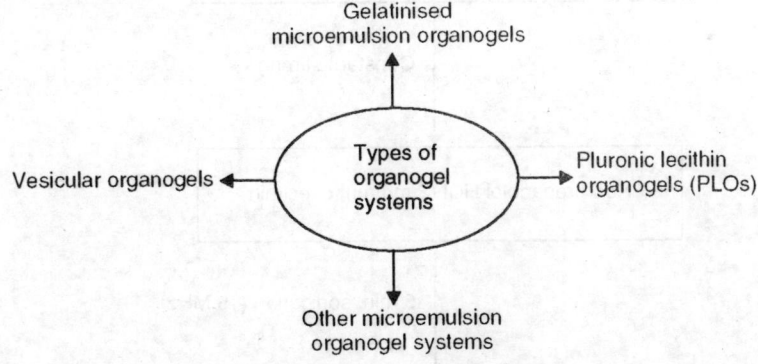

Fig. 16.1: Various organogels

Pluronic Lecithin Organogels (PLOs)

PLOs are the modified form of lecithin organogels.

Lecithin + organic solvents

↓　　Stirring at room temperature

Clear + cloudy solutions

↓　　Minimal amounts of water

Gel

PROTOCOL: 16.1

Organogel Based Systems for Transdermal Delivery of Propranolol

Materials

Propranolol HCl
Soyalecithin
Iso-octane
Potassium nitrate

Procedure

- Dissolve a preparation of water in oil microemulsion: soya lecithin (200mM) in 30ml iso-octane under constant stirring.
- Add an aqueous solution of propanolol HCl (2 mg/ml) in required amount to the lecithin solution and sonicate at a frequency of 15,000 kHz for 5 min in order to obtain the microemulsion.
- Centrifuge the dispersed phase at 1000 rpm for 5 min.
- Discard the supernatant and redisperse the pellet to a suitable dilution (Scheme 16.1).

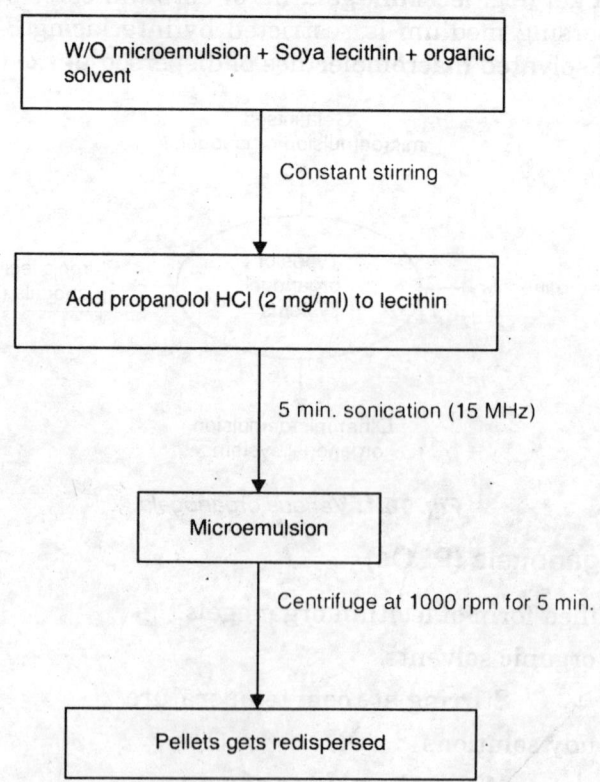

Scheme16.1: Organogel-based system for transdermal delivery

Characterisation of Organogel

Determination of Solubilised Water

Estimate the content of solubilised water in the polar core of lecithin reverse micelle by spectroscopic methods. Use the potassium nitrate solution as polar probe. Determine the λ_{max} of potassium nitrate solution by scanning the aqueous solution in the UV range using a Shimadzu spectrophotometer.

Add the probing agent solution in varying amounts to the lecithin/iso-octane system and record the gradual shifts or variations in λ_{max} on each addition. The shift in λ_{max} on each addition on increment of aqueous phase is plotted against the molar fraction of aqueous solution added.

Effect of Added Water on Viscosity

The viscosity of the lecithin /iso-octane/water system depends on the amount of water inclusion in the micelles. Therefore the effect of molar ratio of added water and soya-lecithin on the viscosity of the system should also be studied. Measure the viscosity after each addition using a Brookfield's viscometer.

Drug Micelle Interaction

Determine the capacity to solubilise a water-soluble drug, propranolol HCl in the micelle core of the gel by studying the UV absorption of the drug. The spectrum corresponds to the pure drug solution and the drug entrapped in the micellar phase of lecithin gel will be determined. The shift in the λ_{max} of propranolol HCl accounts for the difference in the microenvironment of the drug, which in turn will be used as an autosending /probing in the determination of the nature of the aqueous phase in organic solvent, viz. whether it is bulk water or solubilised water.

PROTOCOL: 16.2

Water in Oil Organogels

Materials

Sorbitan monostearate
Polysorbate 20
Hexadecane
Isopropyl myristate
5, 6-Carboxyfluorescein

Procedure

- Weigh accurate quantities in a vial to prepare a sorbitan monostearate (10% w/v) and polysorbate 20 (2% w/v) and add organic solvent (hexadecane or isopropyl myristate) to dissolve the contents.
- Heat the mixture to 60°C in a water bath until it becomes a transparent organic solution.

- Cool the solution at room temperature. It produces an opaque, thermo-reversible semisolid gel (Scheme 16.2).

- *Preparation of W/O gel*

   Add the aqueous phase drop-wise to the oil phase (the gel prepared as above) while vortexing, keeping temperature at 60°C on a water bath. A W/O emulsion will be produced. The gel will be converted in an opaque thermo-reversible semisolid on cooling at room temperature.

- *Preparation of O/W gel*

   Add aqueous phase drop-wise to the oil phase (10% w/v sorbitan monooleate + 2% w/v isopropyl myristate) while vortexing and keeping the temperature at 60°C. Water in oil emulsion will be obtained.

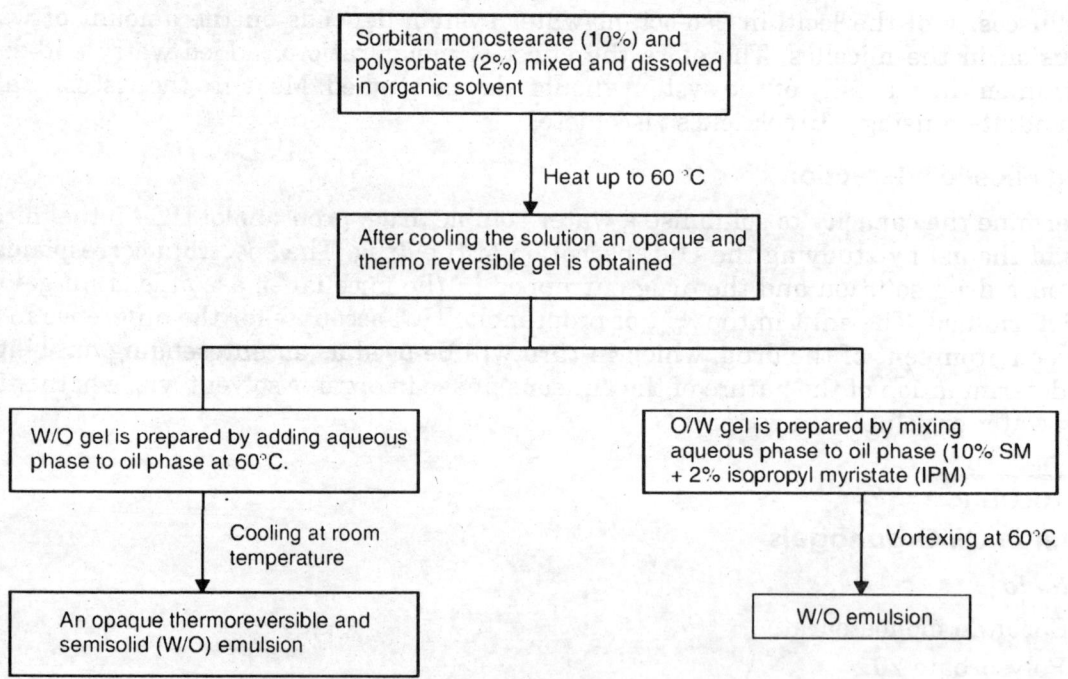

Scheme16.2: *Preparation of water in oil organogels*

PROTOCOL: 16.3

Microemulsion-based Organogels

Materials

Sodium salicylate

Surfactant: Sodium salt of AOT (HLB: 10.2, MW 444.6)

Miglyol 812N [a medium chain triglyceride]

Polyoxyethylene (20) sorbitan monolaurate (Tween 20, HLB: 16.7, RMM 1128)

Polyoxyethylene (4) sorbitan monolaurate (Tween 21, HLB: 13.3, MW 523)

Polyoxyethylene (20) sorbitan monooleate (Tween 80, HLB: 15.0, MW 1310), polyoxyethylene (5) sorbitan monooleate (Tween 81, HLB: 10.0, MW 645), polyoxyethylene (20) sorbitan trioleate (Tween 85, HLB: 11.0, MW 1839),

Sorbitan trioleate (Span 85, HLB: 1.8, MW 958)

Sorbitan monooleate (Span 80, HLB: 4.3, MW 429),

Sorbitan monolaurate (Span 20, HLB: 8.6, MW 346),

Polyoxyethylene (4) lauryl ether (C12E4, HLB: 9.7, MW 363)

Polyoxyethylene (10) lauryl ether (C12E10, HLB: 14.0, MW 626)

Polyoxyethylene (10) oleyl ether (C18: 1E10, HLB: 12.4, MW 708)

Polyoxyethylene (20) oleyl ether (C18: 1E20, HLB: 15.3, MW 1148)

Polyethoxyethylene (25) glycerol trioleate (Tagat TO, HLB: 11.3, MW 1982)

Polyoxyethylene (6) lauryl ether (C12E6, HLB: 10.6, MW 451)

The HLB of the various surfactant mixtures examined was determined using weight fractions of the surfactants.

Triglyceride and fatty acid esters

Acid-hydrolysed pig-skin gelatin (Bloom Number 300)

Triply distilled water was used throughout.

Procedure

- Take 1.5 g powdered gelatin (Bloom number 300) to 10 g of a mixture comprising of 25% w/w surfactant, 20% w/w aqueous phase (Drug + Tween) and 50% w/w oil at 25°C, leading to a final sample composition of 13% w/w gelatin, 21.7% w/w surfactant and 17.4% water.

- Then increase the temperature of the mixture up to 55°C with constant stirring and allow the mixture to stand for solubilisation of the gelatin. Then stop the agitation and the temperature of the sample returned to ambient yielding clear, homogeneous, nonbirefringent gels.

PROTOCOL: 16.4

Microemulsion Based Organogels Using Isopropylmyristate

Materials

Sodium salicylate

Surfactant sodium salt of Bis-2-(ethylhexyl) sulphosuccinate (AOT)

Polyoxyethylenesorbitan monolaurate (Tween 2)

Polyoxyethylenesorbitan monooleate (Tween 80)

Polyoxyethylenesorbitan trioleate (Tween 85)

Isopropyl myristate (IPM)

Acid-hydrolysed pig-skin gelatin (Bloom 300)

Procedure

- Prepare the W/O microemulsions containing the model drug by injection of an aqueous stock solution of sodium salicylate to a reverse micellar surfactant solution. A clear solution forms after brief shaking.

- Add solid gelatin (up to 0.14 g/g) to a previously prepared W/O microemulsion containing 25% w/w surfactant, 25%w/w water and 50% w/w IPM. Then increase the temperature to 55°C with constant stirring until solubilisation of the gelatin complete.

- Stop the agitation and allow the sample to cool at room temperature. Formulations yield clear, homogeneous, non-birefringent microemulsion based organogel systems (Scheme 16.3).

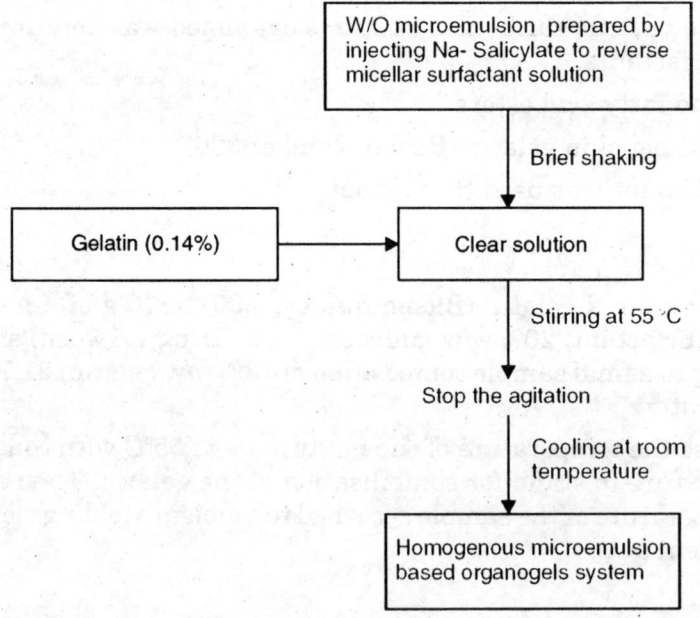

Scheme 16.3: *Preparation of microemulsion based organogels*

Topical Liposome Gels

Principle

Topical liposome gels are prepared by incorporation of lyophilised liposomes into a structured vehicle (1%, w/w, chitosan gel base). Liposomes embedded into a structured vehicle of chitosan show significantly slower release than hydrogels.

Materials

Phospholipon 90H–gel state

Cholesterol

5-fluorouracil

Chitosan

Saccharose

Preparation and Characterisation of Liposomes

- Prepare the lipid phase by dissolving different quantities of lipid components, PL 90H and CH, in chloroform (series L1, L2, L3). Afterwards, remove the organic solvent by evaporation under vacuum at 65 °C to obtain a dry lipid mixture.

- Hydrate the lipid film and gently shake with different quantities of the aqueous phase bearing total drug, 5-FU, in phosphate buffer pH 7.4 (formulations marked a, b, c; drug/lipid phase mass ratio 1:3.2). The final lipid/aqueous phase mass ratio could vary from 1:31.3 to 1:12.5.

- After 24 h, in order to remove the unentrapped portion of the drug, wash liposome dispersions with phosphate buffer pH 7.4 and centrifuge twice at 20000 rpm for 45 min.

- Lyophilise the resulting liposome dispersions (temperature – 40 °C, pressure 200 Pa) using saccharose as a cryoprotector, incorporated in the internal and external aqueous phase of liposomes (lipid phase/saccharose mass ratio = 1:1.3). Determine the mean particle diameter of liposome vesicles by the laser diffraction technique. Quantify the percentage of 5-FU encapsulated into liposomes by spectrophotometry at 266 nm after dissolving the liposomes in a chloroform/methanol mixture.

Preparation of Topical Gel Formulations

- First prepare the structured vehicle of chitosan (1%, w/w) by continuous mixing of chitosan with a 1% (m/v) solution of lactic acid. Incorporate lyophilised liposomes into a structured vehicle of chitosan in a 1:3 ratio (series LG1, LG2, LG3).

- For the comparative purpose, prepare hydrogels (HG1, HG2, HG3) containing different concentrations of 5-FU (0.2, 0.5 and 0.8%, respectively) in 1% (w/w) chitosan gel base (Scheme 16.4).

In vitro Dissolution Studies

In vitro dialysing method is used for the release rate determination. A weighed amount of prepared liposome gel or hydrogel formulation is poured into the glass cell and dialysed against phosphate buffer pH 7.4 as a dialysing medium. Dialysing medium is kept at 37°C while stirring at 100 rpm. Use the samples within a period of 8 h.

Take the aliquots at regular intervals and analyse spectrophotometrically.

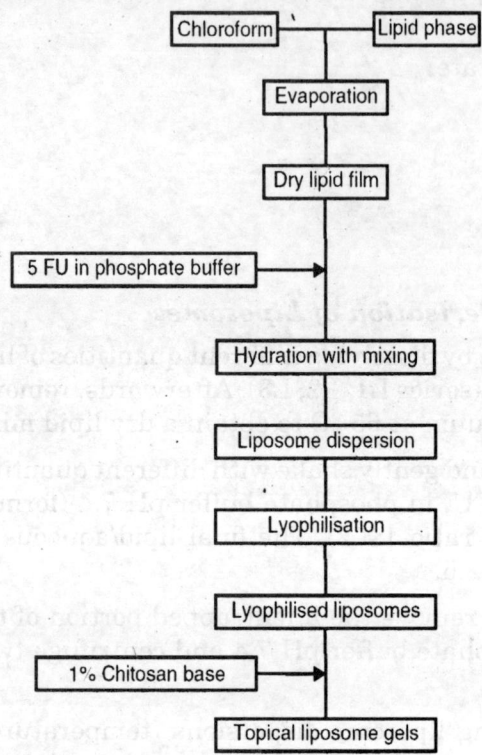

Scheme 16.4: *Preparation of topical liposome gel*

PROTOCOL 16.5

Hydroxypropylmethylcellulose Based Organogels

Materials

Hydroxypropyl methyl cellulose (HPMC)

H_3PO_4–NaH_2PO_4–Na_2HPO_4 (pH 1.68–8.0) Buffer

$Na_2B_4O_7$–NaOH (pH 9.0–10.01) buffer solutions

0.02 M CH_3COOH–NaOH buffer system.

Solvents ($CHCl_3$, CCl_4, C_2H_5OH, CH_3OH)

Cellulase enzyme C-0901, from *Penicillium funiculosum*.

Procedure

- Prepare the homogenous mixture of HPMC with water to give certain concentration, which is varying from 0.5–60 wt %. Keep the mixture of dispersed materials for a few days at room temperature to ensure complete dissolution and uniform distribution of polymer chains. Higher concentration solutions ($\geq$ 30 wt %) were very thick gels almost like solid.

- After few days, pour the HPMC solutions between two PTFE sheets to form film using IKEDA Cold Press and then place the prepared film into polyvinylidene chloride bag to avoid the penetration of oxygen during irradiation, after removal of the air by a vacuum pump.
- Irradiate the HPMC samples with an electron beam (EB) generated from a Cockcroft-Walton type accelerator (maximum voltage and current are 2 MV and 30 mA, respectively). The irradiation was carried out 1 mA beam current and acceleration energy of 1 MV, an apparent average dose rate of 1.4 Gy/s (Scheme 16.5).
- Use the thin film thickness of 0.5 mm and the thickness of samples with covering sheet and package was less than 1 mm for EB irradiation, which guaranteed the uniform penetration of beam and distribution of energy throughout the entire material.

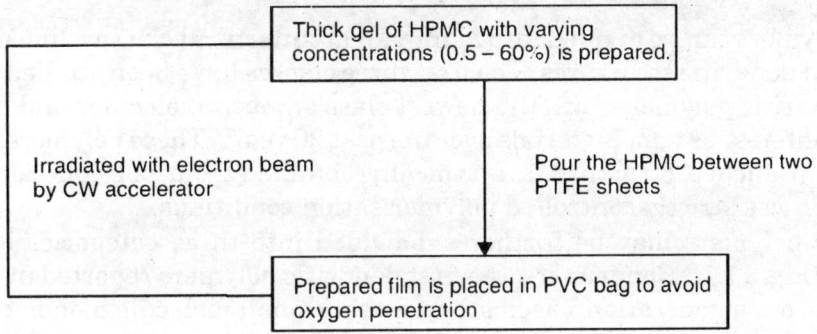

Scheme 16.5: *Preparation of hydroxy propylmethyl cellulose based organogels*

SUGGESTED READINGS:

- Ajayaghosh A., Praveen VK. Acc Chem Res. 2007 40(8), 644.
- Dominguez MP, Xenakis A., Stamatis H., Sinisterra JV. Biotechnology Letters 26, 19, 2004.
- Goto S., Kawata M., Suzuki T., Kim NS, Ito C. J. Pharm. Sci. 1991, 80 (10): 958.
- Jenta TRJ., Batts G., Rees GD., Robinson BH. (2000) Biotechnology and Bioengineering. 53 (2) 121–131.
- Kantaria S., Rees GD., Lawrence MJMJ. Control. Rel. (1999) 2:355.
- Luisi P.L., scartazzini R., Haering G., Schurtenberger P. (1990)Colloid & Polymer Science.(4) 268.
- Motulsky A., Lafleur M., Couffin-Hoarau AC., Hoarau D., Boury F., Benoit JP., Leroux JC. (2005) Biomaterials. : 31 6242
- Murdan S. (2005) Organogels in drug delivery. 3: 489.
- Murdan S., Bergh VDB., Gregoriadis G., Florence AT. (1999) J-Pharm-Sci 88 (6): 615–9.
- Murdan S., Bergh VDB., Gregoriadis G., Florence AT. (2000)J-Pharm-Sci 88 (6): 615–9.
- Murdan, Sudaxshina. (2005) Exp Opinion Drug Del. 3: 489.
- Naagayama K., Tada K., Naoe K., Imai M. (2003) Biocatalysis and Biotransformation. 6: 321.
- Nasseria AA., Aboofazeli R., Zia H., Needham TE. (2003) Iranian Pharmaceutic Res 117.
- Pisal S., Shelke V., Mahadik K., Kadam S. (2004)AAPS PharmSciTech 5 (4) 63.

Synthetic polymers can be divided into four main architectural classes: linear, crosslinked, branched, and dendritic structures. The first three classes have been studied extensively in the past. Dendritic polymers form the newest class of macromolecules and have attracted considerable interest as nanomaterials over the past 20 years. These polymers, characterised by a cascade-branched structure, are typically obtained from polyfunctional monomers under more or less strictly controlled polymerisation conditions.

Dendritic polymers may be further subdivided into three categories based on their architecture (Fig. 17.1). Dendrimers, the first dendritic polymers reported in the literature, are obtained from a generation-based scheme using small molecule monomers as building blocks. Their synthesis is performed either in a core first (divergent) or core last (convergent) manner, using cycles of protection, condensation, and deprotection of ABn-type monomers. Since strict control is attained over molecular architecture in this approach, dendrimers can have extremely narrow molecular weight distributions (M_w/M_n, <1.01) and exactly predictable molecular weights. However, since small molecule building blocks are used, many reaction cycles are necessary to synthesise high molecular weight dendrimers. These complex reaction sequences are avoided in the synthesis of hyper-branched polymers, the second family of dendritic polymers. High molecular weight hyper-branched polymers are obtained in onspot self-condensation reactions of ABn monomers, albeit with limited control over structure. The random nature of the condensation reaction results in polymers with many structural flaws, and a molecular weight distribution (MWD) corresponding to a Flory distribution ($M_w/M_n \approx 2$) is obtained only at low levels of conversion. The molecular weight and MWD observed at higher conversions are expected to tend towards infinity with increasing conversion, according to statistical derivations. The third class of dendritic polymers is the dendrigraft systems, introduced simultaneously in 1991 as Comb-burst® polymers by Tomalia *et al*. Dendrigraft polymers typically obtained by ionic polymerisation and grafting, combine features of dendrimers and hyperbranched polymers. Dendrigraft polymer synthesis follows a generation based growth scheme similar to dendrimers, but use polymeric chains as building blocks. This leads to a very rapid increase in molecular weight per generation, and high molecular weight branched polymers can be produced in a few steps. Since the grafting reaction is a random process, the branched structure bears similarities to hyperbranched polymers. Even though the architecture of dendrigraft polymers is not as strictly defined as for dendrimers, the MWD achieved for these materials typically remain quite narrow (M_w/M_n <1.1)

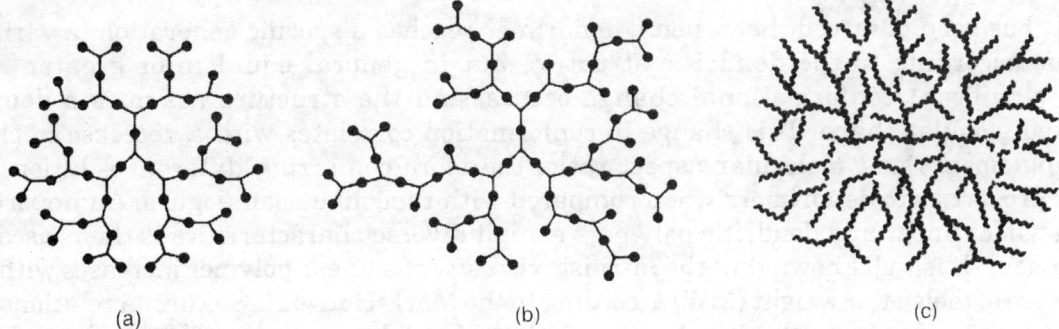

(a)   (b)   (c)

Fig. 17.1. *Comparison of the structures of (a) dendrimers, (b) hyperbranched, and (c) dendrigraft polymer*

A typical dendrimer (Fig. 17.1) consists of three main structural components: a multifunctional central core (C), branched units (B) and surface groups (S). The branched units are organised in layers called "generations", and represent the repeating monomer unit of these macromolecules. Dendrimers are characterised by an ideally branched structure and the presence of a high number of functional groups, which can have a significant effect upon the physical properties both in the solid state and in solution. Furthermore, the macromolecular dimensions can be controlled, since the synthesis involves a repetitive sequence of steps. Dendrimers are synthesised from monomers of the ABx type (xP2) through a step-growth polymerisation process. There are two general synthetic approaches used to generate dendrimers: (i) divergent, and (ii) convergent. Both synthetic strategies possess relative advantages and disadvantages and the appropriate route depends mainly on the kind of monomer employed and the target polymer structure.

Although Flory first reported the potential role of highly branched structures in macromolecular systems in 1952, the first synthetic examples of branched macromolecules obtained by the divergent approach was only described in the late seventies by Vogtle and coworkers, who referred to the synthesis as a cascade approach. In 1984, Tomalia *et al.* published the synthesis and full characterisation of a novel class of poly(amidoamine) (PAMAM) macromolecules, and referred to these hyperbranched polymers as dendrimers. This divergent type synthesis commenced with a Michael addition of a molecule of ammonia (the dendritic core) to three molecules of methyl acrylate, followed by exhaustive amidation of the esters by an excess of ethylenediamine, generating a macromolecule with six amine protons. The exhaustive Michael addition-amidation reaction sequence was then repeated in a reiterative fashion to achieve an almost monodispersed dendritic structure with a molecular weight of over 25,000 Da and dendrimers of this type are now commercially available under the trade name Starburst Dendrimers.

Hawker and coworkers first reported the convergent growth approach in 1989. In contrast to the divergent growth approach, dendrimer construction begins at what will eventually become the outer surface shell of the ideally branched macromolecule and proceeds inward, by a step-addition of branching monomers, followed by the final attachment of each branched dendritic sub-unit (or dendron) to a poly-functional core.

It has been observed that when a dendrimer reaches a specific generation (a variable factor according to the dendritic structure but in general equal to or greater than 4) a significant conformational change occurs, and the structure assumes a densely packed globular shape. This change in conformation correlates with a decrease in chain entanglements and molecular aspect ratio, therefore conferring different solution and bulk properties to dendrimers when compared with their linear analogues. An important area where linear and dendritic polymers exhibit diverse characteristics is their viscosity behaviour. It is well known that the intrinsic viscosity of a linear polymer increases with the increase of molecular weight (MW) according to the Mark-Houwink-Sakurada relationship. However, dendrimers exhibit a linear relationship at lower generation numbers and a maximum that corresponds to the change in shape, followed by a smooth decrease in intrinsic viscosity at higher molecular weight. Another important characteristic of dendritic molecules is their high solubility in a large number of organic solvents, potentially offering better processability characteristics and rapid dissolution. These distinguishing features of dendritic macromolecules render these novel materials a reliable alternative to traditional polymers in a wide range of applications.

The unique properties of dendrimers, primarily their controlled branched architecture, nanometric size, monodispersity and host– guest chemistry (Patri *et al.* 2002; Tomalia *et al.* 1990) have spurred impetus in the dendrimer based drug delivery research. Dendrimers can be used to deliver drugs either by encapsulating them in the internal cavities or by conjugating to the surface functionalities (Esfand *et al.* 2001; Aulanta *et al.* 2003; Lee *et al.* 2005).

Polyamidoamine (PAMAM) dendrimer with an ellipsoidal or spheroidal shape is one of the most studied starburst macromolecules. Due to specific synthesis, PAMAM dendrimers have some interesting properties, which distinguish them from classical linear polymers, e.g. PAMAM has a much higher amino group density comparing with the conventional macromolecules, a third generation PAMAM prepared from ammonia core has 1.24×10^{-4} amine moieties per unit volume (cubic Angstrom units) in contrast to the 1.58×10^{-6} amine moieties per unit volume of a conventional star polymer (Tomalia *et al.* 1990). The high density of functional groups ($-NH_2$, $-COOH$, $-OH$) in PAMAM dendrimers may be expected to have potential applications in enhancing the solubility of low aqueous solubility drugs and delivery systems for bioactive materials (Newkome *et al.* 1991). Also, these functional groups on the outer shell are responsible for high reactivity which means dendrimers can be modified or conjugated with a list of interesting guest molecules. Furthermore, PAMAM dendrimers possess empty internal cavities, which are able to encapsulate hydrophobic guest molecules in the macromolecule interior. Drugs or other molecules can either be attached to dendrimers' end groups or encapsulated in the macromolecule interior (Naylor *et al.* 1989). These specific properties make dendrimers suitable for drug delivery systems (Svenson *et al.* 2005; Roseita *et al.* 2001; Anil *et al.* 2002; Elizabeth and Frechet, 2005).

PROTOCOL 17.1
Preparation of PAMAM Dendrimers

PAMAM dendrimers are novel class of synthetic nanosised carriers having large number of surface functionalities depending upon its generation. PAMAM dendrimers are generally composed of ethylenediamine core with the repetitive unit of methylacrylate monomers. PAMAM dendrimers have specific features including controlled structure, nanosised, branched structures having terminal functional groups. There are various dendrimers which have been synthesised so far depending upon various core and monomer used.

The general scheme for PAMAM dendrimer synthesis using ethylenediamine core and methyl acrylate monomer is shown in scheme 17.1.

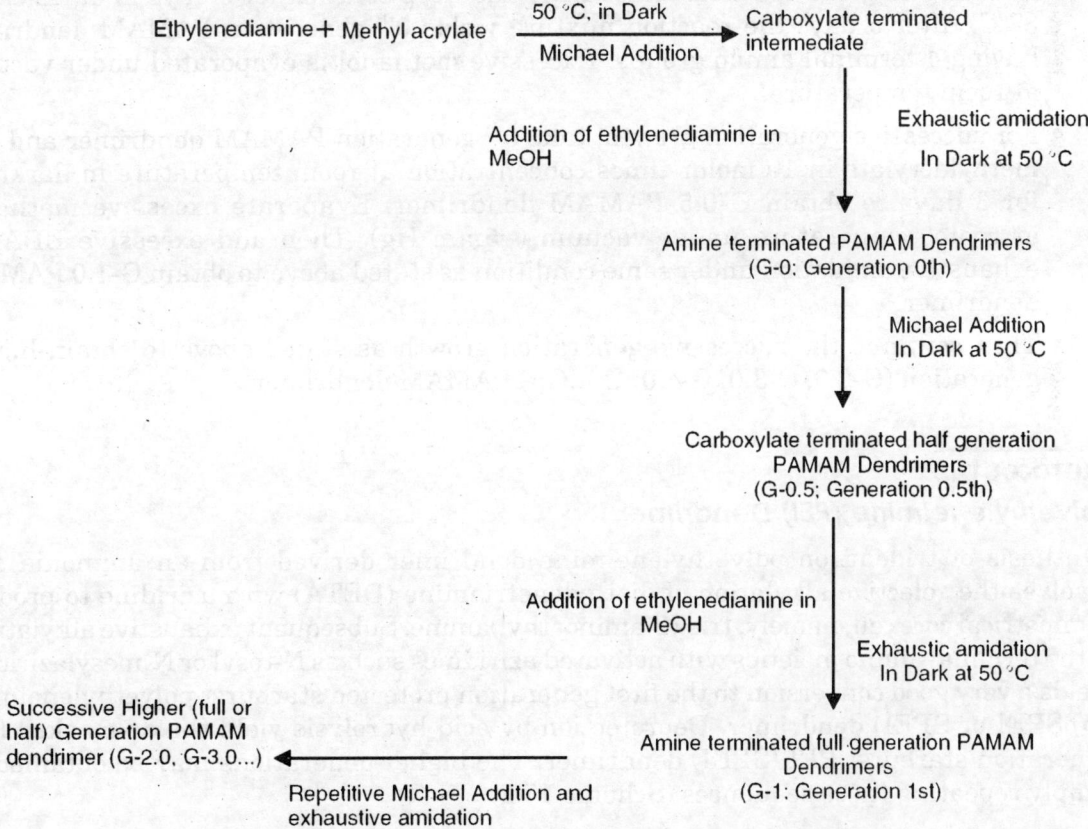

Scheme 17.1:Presentation of PAMAM dendrimer synthesis

Materials

Ethylenediamine (EDA)　　　　　　　1 mole

Methylacrylate   10–20 % molar excess of EDA
Methanol   10–20 molar times of EDA

Procedure

- All material used for PAMAM dendrimer must be of analytical grade. Redistill methylacrylate and ethylenediamine with Mg.
- Calculate the quantities of materials used for PAMAM dendrimer synthesis according to stoichiometric calculation.
- Add 1 M EDA in black paper covered round bottom flask containing 30 ml methanol and then add methylacrylate (10% molar excess) to this solution. Keep the reaction mixture in dark at 50°C for 3 days. Then evaporate the excessive methanol in dark condition and add 10 molar times EDA and keep solution for 5 days in darkness at 37°C. After 5 days the reaction mixture yields 0th generation PAMAM dendrimer having 4 terminal amino groups. Excessive methanol is evaporated under vacuum at room temperature.
- For successive generation growth, take 0th generation PAMAM dendrimer and add methylacrylate in 10 molar times concentration at room temperature in darkness for 3 days to obtain G-0.5 PAMAM dendrimer. Evaporate excessive methanol at room temperature under vacuum (~5mm Hg). Then add excessive EDA for exhaustive amidation under same condition as stated above to obtain G-1.0 PAMAM dendrimer.
- Then continue the successive generation growth as stated above to obtain higher generation (G-2.0, G-3.0, G-4.0........Gn) PAMAM dendrimer.

PROTOCOL 17.2

Polyethyleneimine (PEI) Dendrimer

Synthesis of tridendron polyethyleneimine dendrimer derived from an ammonia core involves the selective alkylation of diethylenetriamine (DETA) with aziridine to produce symmetrical core cell, namely, tris-(2-aminoethyl)amine. Subsequent exhaustive alkylations of the terminal amino moieties with activated aziridines such as N-tosyl or N-mesylaziridine yields a very good conversion to the first generation protected starburst polyethyleneimine (proSPEI or SPEI) dendrimer. Deprotection by acid hydrolysis yield the de-masked first generation starburst PEI (SPEI) dendrimer. The higher generations may be obtained by simply repeating these sequences (Scheme 17.2).

Material Used in PEI Dendrimer Synthesis

Diethylenetriamine (DETA)   1 mol
Aziridine
N-mesylaziridine
H_2SO_4 0.1N

Procedure

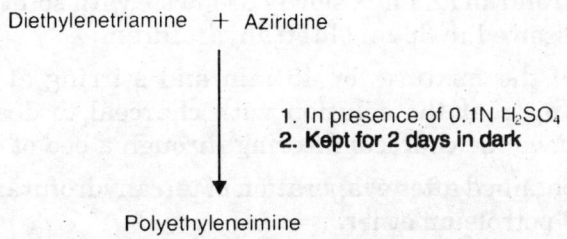

Scheme 17.2: *Synthesis of PEI dendrimer*

Bulk-polymerisation of EI and HEEI.

- Place the freshly distilled ethyleneimine (2 ml, 1.664 g, 38.63 mmol) under nitrogen atmosphere in a dry 25 ml flask fitted with a magnetic stirring bar. Cool the monomer bulk to −70 °C, and initiate the polymerisation by adding 100 µl of a 32 % v/v hydrochloric acid (116 mg, 1.02 mmol) under stirring.

- Allow the mixture to warm up slowly to room temperature, and continue the stirring for 5 days. Finally, heat the substance up to 100 °C for 6 h.

- Collect the resulting highly viscous, slightly yellowish polymer and determine the quantitative yield.

PROTOCOL 17.3
Branched Poly (L-glutamic Acid) as Biodegradable Drug Carrier

Materials

L-glutamic acid g-benzyl ester

Poly (L-glutamic acid)

Triphosgene

2,4, 6, -trinitrobenzenesulfonic acid (TNBS)

5,5-dithio-bis(2-nitrobenzoic acid) (Ellman's Reagent)

PAMAM dendrimer G-1.0

PAMAM dendrimer G-2.0

PEI

ICG

Procedure

Synthesis of branched PG

Step 1. *Conversion of L-Glutamic acid g-benzyl ester to the corresponding N-carboxyanhydride (NCA):*

- Suspend 6.0g (0.025 mol) of L-glutamic acid g-benzyl ester in 60 ml of freshly distilled tetrahydrofuran and mix slowly dropwise with solution of 3.8g (0.0125 mol) of triphosgene dissolved in 30 ml of tetrahydrofuran.
- After refluxing of the mixture for 45 min and stirring at room temperature for an additional 12h, treat the solution with charcoal to deactivate the remaining triphosgene. Remove the charcoal filtering through a bed of celite.
- Collect the solid obtained after evaporation of tetrahydrofuran and recrystallize from ethyl acetate and petroleum ether.
- Determine the yield, melting point, and elemental compositions of the product.

Step 2. *Polymerisation of Glutamic derivatised NCA (intermediate product).*

- Polymerise the Glu(OBz)-NCA in 1,2-dichloroethane (DCE) using G-1.0 PAMAM, G-2.0 PAMAM, or PEI as the initiator.
- Add the solution of Glu(OBz)-NCA, in 100 ml of dichloroethane, into an aliquot of G-1.0 PAMAM, G-2.0 PAMAM, or PEI in 5 ml of dimethylsulfoxide.
- Stir the reaction mixture at room temperature for 3 days. Wash the organic solution with water and dry over anhydrous Na_2SO_4.
- Bubble the dry hydrogen bromide gas (HBr) into the solution for 30 min and allow the solution to stand overnight.
- Collect the polymer precipitate and dissolve in 1.0 M $NaHCO_3$, and then extract with dichloroethane to remove benzyl bromide.
- Dialyse the aqueous solution extensively (molecular weight cut-off 10 K) against deionised water using dialysis tubing and filter through a 0.45 µm filter, and lyophilise to yield a white solid.
- Characterise the prepared compound by UV spectroscopy, proton NMR spectroscopy and ESI mass spectroscopy.

PROTOCOL 17.4

Synthesis of Pegylated Dendrimer

Materials

Amine terminated diaminobutane poly(propylene imine) dendrimer with 64 primary amino groups in the periphery (DAB- 64)

Methoxypoly(ethyleneglycol)-isocyanate (MW 5000)

Betamethasone valerate

Betamethasone dipropionate

Procedure

- Add 0.004 or 0.008 mol of methoxypoly(ethyleneglycol)-isocyanate (PEG-isocyanate) dissolved in aqueous trimethylamine solution of pH 13 to 0.001 mol of DAB-64 dissolved in water.

- Allow the mixture to react for about 1h, followed by dialysing with a 12,400 cut-off membrane for removing unreacted dendrimer and PEG-isocyanate.
- Finally lyophilise and dry the product.
- Perform the PEGylation of n-propylamine in an analogous manner and subject the product to dialysis with a 1200 cut-off membrane. The formation of PEGylated dendrimers may be established by ^{13}C-NMR. Specifically the chemical shifts of α and β carbons, in the vicinity of primary amino groups of the parent dendrimer may be observed at 40 and 31 ppm and shifted to 44 and 28 ppm respectively for the PEGylated derivatives due to the introduction of the urea moiety. In addition the carbonyl group of the urea moiety may be observed at 159 ppm.

PROTOCOL 17.5

Dendrimers of Citric Acid and Poly (Ethylene Glycol)

Materials

Poly (ethylene glycol) 600 diacid dried over Na_2SO_4.

Citric acid and pyridine (purified with refluxing over NaOH for 2 h and subsequent distillation)

Thionylchloride was purified by refluxing a mixture of 10 wt% linseed oil in thionylchloride for 2 h and subsequent distillation.

Dicyclohexyl carbodiimide (DCC)

5-Amino salicylic acid (recrystallised from water)

Diclofenac and mefenamic acid.

Procedure

Step 1: *Preparation of Gn(n = 1–3) Pyridine Complex*

- For the preparation of Gn(n = 1–3)pyridine complex, first dissolve the dendrimers with stirring in pyridine at room temperature for 2h, then precipitate the product in diethylether or n-hexane.
- Again dissolve the obtained product in water or ethanol/ water (1:4 v/v) at 80°C and stir for 30–50 min then filter off and remove the water under vacuum at 80°C.
- Dissolve the complex in methanol, filter it and precipitate in cyclohexane and then again wash with acetone and toluene to yield the yellow solid compound. The important absorption bonds in IR spectra for Gn(n = 1–3)pyridine complex are: COOH (broad and weak, 3520–2670cm^{-1}), C=O (1750–1730 cm^{-1}), C=C (1620, 1480cm^{-1}), C–O (1117,1202cm^{-1}).

Step 2: *Preparation of Gn(n=1–3) Diclofenac and Mefenamic Acid Complexes*

- For the preparation of complexes of Gn(n=1–3) diclofenac and mefenamic acid, dissolve the dendrimers in 20ml THF. Add these solutions to a round-bottom flask equipped with reflux condenser and magnetic stirrer containing a solution of drugs in 20ml THF. Then stir the solutions for 2h at 30°C.

- Precipitate the complexes in n-hexane and then dissolve in dichloromethane and again precipitate in diethylether to yield yellow (mefenamic acid) and green (diclofenac) compounds. The absorption bands in IR spectra for Gn(n=1–3) diclofenac and mefenamic acid complexes are: COOH (broad and weak, 3505–2840 cm^{-1}), C=O (1748 cm^{-1}), C=C (1610, 1475 cm^{-1}), C–O (1125, 1204 cm^{-1}) and COOH (broad and weak, 3490–2862 cm^{-1}), C=O (1740–1645 cm^{-1}), C=C (1655, 1580 cm^{-1}), and C–O (1112, 1190 cm^{-1}), respectively.

Step 2a: *Preparation of the Gn(n=1–3)/5-ASA (5-Amino Salicylic Acid) Complexes*

- Add a solution of dendrimers in 20 ml ethanol/DMF (3:1 v/v) to a solution of excess 5-ASA and stir the solutions for 2 h at 30–50°C. Then precipitate the complexes in diethylether and dissolve in dichloromethane and reprecipitate in diethylether for several times to yield the red-brown (5-ASA) compounds. The important bonds in IR spectra for Gn(n=1–3)/5-ASA complexes are: COOH (broad and weak, 3520–2650 cm^{-1}), C=O (1749, 1732 cm^{-1}), C=C (1620, 1490 cm^{-1}), and C–O (1120, 1210 cm^{-1}).

PROTOCOL 17.6

Synthesis of Peptide Dendrimers

Materials

Di-tertiary butyl pyrocarbonate (di-BOC)

1-hydroxybenzotriazole (HoBt)

n,n-dicyclohexyl carbodiimide (DCC)

Dimethylaminopyridine (DMAP)

Dimethyl formamide (DMF)

Triflouroacetic acid (TFA)

Procedure

Step 1: Protection and Characterisation of Amino Acid (L-lysine) by Di-BOC

- Preparation of homogeneous dendrimers may be initiated with the protection of the functional groups on amino acid, L-lysine. Protection of L-lysine with di-BOC should be accomplished under basic conditions.

- Dissolve L-lysine (410 mg) in a mixture of solvents containing 2.5mL of dioxane, 2.5mL of distilled water and 2.5mL of 1M sodium hydroxide. Add di-tertiary butyl pyrocarbonate (4.8 g, 22mM) to the lysine mixture with constant stirring (room temp., 30 min).

- Concentrate the solution on a rotary evaporator to about 10–15 mL, and cool the solution in an ice water bath.

- Cover the mixture with a layer of ethyl acetate (30 mL) and acidify with dilute aqueous potassium hydrogen sulfate (KHSO$_4$) solution to pH 2–3.

- Extract the aqueous phase with ethyl acetate (2×15 mL) cool the extract, wash with water (2×30 mL) and dry over anhydrous Na$_2$SO$_4$ and evaporate in vacuum.

- Subject the di-BOC protected lysine to IR spectroscopy using KBr pellet method and 1H-NMR.
- Perform a qualitative analysis to confirm the protection of L-lysine by di-BOC. Mix aqueous solution of di-BOC protected lysine with two drops of Kaiser A (0.5mL of aqueous KCN solution 0.065% w/v, with 24.5mL of dry pyridine and 2.5mL of 400% w/v, phenol/ethanol mixture) and Kaiser B (5% w/v, ethanolic ninhydrin solution) and observe colour (Scheme 17.3).

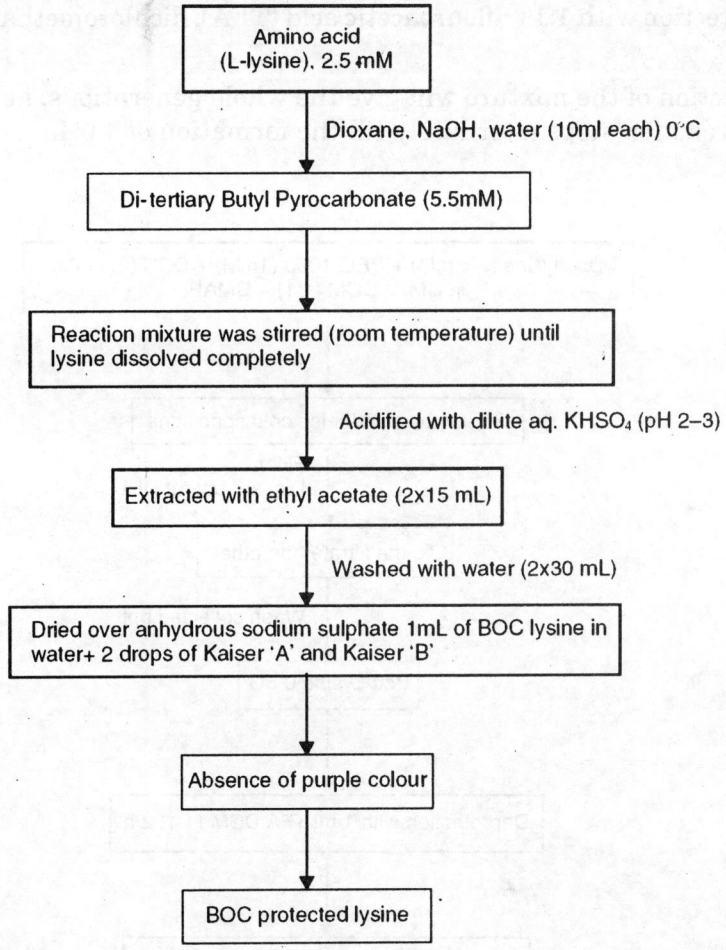

Scheme 17.3. *Presentation showing protection of L-lysine by di-BOC*

Step 2: *Synthesis and Characterisation of Poly-L-lysine Dendrimer (Scheme 17.4)*

- Dissolve di-BOC–lysine (2.5mM; 0.865 g), PEG-1000 (1mM; 1.0 g), dicyclohexyl carbodiimide (DCC) (2.5mM; 0.515 g) in a flat bottom flask containing 10mL of 1:1 solution of dichloromethane (DCM) and dimethyl formamide (DMF) and 10% of dimethylamino pyridine (DMAP) and 1-hydroxybenzotriazole (HoBt) acting as a catalyst.

- Allow the mixture to stir under perfect ice-cold conditions for 24 h using magnetic stirrer. After 24 h, filter the precipitate, and again stir the reaction mixture.

- Add the concentrate mixture in quantity 6 times the volume of the reaction mixture and allows precipitation by keeping it in deep-freezer for one day.

- Collect the precipitate thus obtained (0.5G) and subject for further reaction preceded by its deprotection with 1:1 triflouroacetic acid (TFA): dichloromethane (DCM) (1 mL) (usually 2 h).

- The deprotection of the mixture will give the whole generations, i.e. 1.0G, 2.0G, etc. Repeat the reaction steps alternately till the formation of 4.0G.

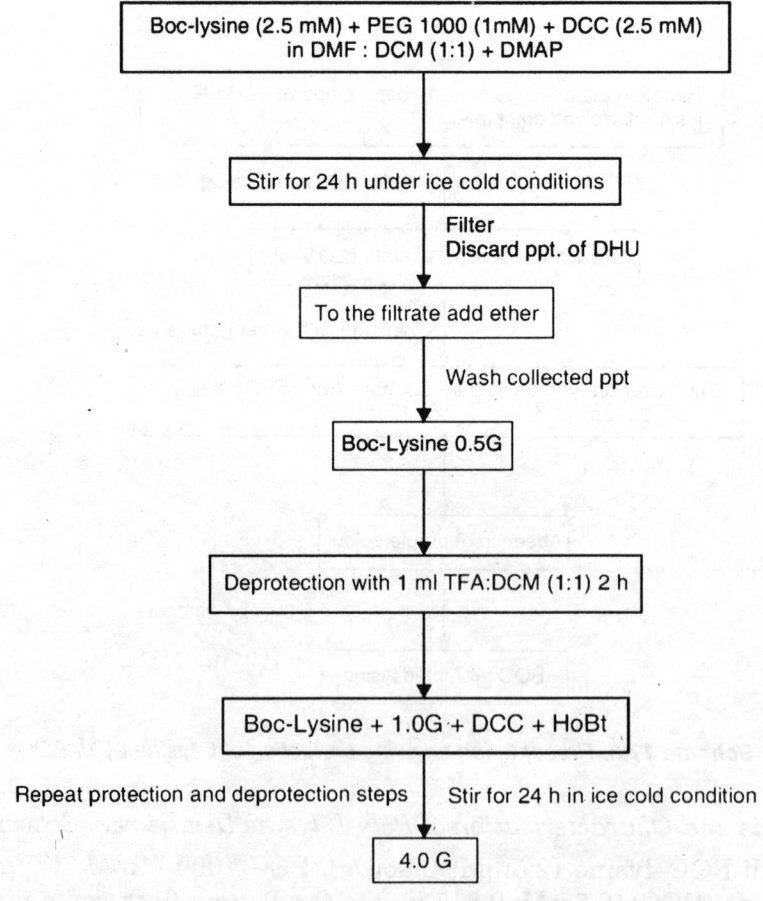

Scheme 17.4: *Synthesis of 4.0 G Poly-L-Lysine Dendrimers*

SUGGESTED READINGS

- Agrawal P, Gupta U, Jain NK. (2007) Biomaterials; 28: 3349.
- Anil KP, Majoros IJ, Baker JR. (2002) Current Opinion in Chemical Biology 6: 466.
- Aulenta F, Hayes W, Rannard S. (2003) Eur Polym J 39: 1741.
- Elizabeth RG, Frechet JMJ. (2005) Drug Discovery Today; 10: 35.
- Esfand R, Tomalia DA. (2001) Drug Discov Today 6:427.
- Lee CC, MacKay JA, Frechet JMJ, Szoka FC. (2005) Nat Biotech 23:1517.
- Namazi H, Adeli M. (2005) Biomaterials 26:1175.
- Naylor AM, Goddard WA, Kiefer GE, Tomalia DA, (1989) J American Cheml Society; 111:2339.
- Newkome GR, Moorefield CN, Baker GR. (1991) Angewandte Chemie (International ed. in English) 30:1178.
- Patri AK, Majoros IJ, Baker Jr JR. (2002) Curr Opin Chem Biol 6: 466.
- Roseita E, Tomalia DA. (2001) Drug Discovery Today 6: 427.
- Sideratou Z, Tsiourvas D, Paleos CM. (2001) J Colloid and Interface Science; 242:272.
- Svenson S, Tomalia DA. (2005) Advanced Drug Delivery Reviews; 57: 2106.
- Tomalia DA, Baker H, Dewald JR. (1985) Polymer Journal 17: 117.
- Tomalia DA, Baker H, Dewald JR. (1986) Macromolecules; 19: 2466.
- Tomalia DA, Dewald JR. U.S. Patent 4587329, 1986.
- Tomalia DA, Naylor AM, Goddard WA. (1990) Angewandte Chemie (International ed. in English) 29:138.

18

Niosomes and Discomes

Niosomes are essentially non-ionic surfactant based multilamellar or unilamellar vesicles in which an aqueous solution of solute(s) is entirely enclosed by a membrane resulted from the organisation of surfactant macromolecules as layers. Similar to liposomes, niosomes are formed on hydration of non-ionic surfactant film, which eventually hydrates imbibing or encapsulating the hydrating aqueous solution (Baillie *et al* 1985). One alternative of phospholipids is the hydrated mixture of cholesterol and non-ionic surfactants such as alkyl ethers, alkyl esters or alkyl amides non-ionic surfactants. This type of vesicle formed from the above mixture has been known as niosomes or non-ionic surfactant vesicles. The structure and properties of niosomes are similar to those of liposomes. Both hydrophobic and hydrophilic substances can be embedded in niosomal vesicles. The chemical stability as well as the relatively low cost of the materials used to prepare niosomes make these vesicles more attractive than liposomes for industrial productions both in pharmaceutical and cosmetic applications.

Furthermore, there are large numbers of non-ionic surfactants available for the design of vesicles on demand. These vesicle has been reported to decrease side effects, give sustain release and enhance penetration of the trapped substances through skin. Several mechanisms has been used to explain the ability of niosomes to modulate drug transfer through skin, e.g. (1) adsorption and fusion of niosomes on the surface of skin leading to high thermodynamic activity gradient of drug at the interface, which is the driving force for permeation of lipophilic drug, (2) reduction of the barrier properties of stratum corneum resulting from the property of vesicles as a penetration enhancer.

Many drugs such as oestradiol, tretinoin, dithranol and enoxacin have been successfully encapsulated in niosomes for topical application. Niosomes as delivery devices have also been studied with anticancer, anti-tubercular, anti-leishmanial, anti-inflammatory, hormonal drugs and oral vaccine. The encapsulation of drugs in niosomes can decrease drug toxicity, increase drug absorption and retard removal of drug from the circulation due to slow drug release. However, characteristics of vesicles prepared with non-ionic surfactants such as dispersion stability, particle size and microfluidity have not yet been made clear. Most of the technical researches in this area pay attention to the formulations of drugs in this vesicle as a delivery system.

Niosome Preparation and Drug Loading

The more commonly used laboratory methods of niosome preparation and drug loading identified in the literature are listed below.

- The injection of an organic solution of surfactants: lipids in an aqueous solution of the drug to be encapsulated, which is heated above the boiling point of the organic solvent (ether injection) (Baillie *et al.*, 1985).

- The formation of a surfactant: lipid film by the evaporation of an organic solution of surfactants: lipids. This film is then hydrated with a solution of the drug (hand shaking) (Azmin *et al.*, 1985; Baillie *et al.*, 1985). This method was previously described by Bangham and others (Bangham *et al.*, 1965) for the preparation of liposomes.

- The formation of an oil in water (O/W) emulsion from an organic solution of surfactants: lipids and an aqueous solution of the drug.

- The organic solvent is then evaporated to leave niosomes dispersed in the aqueous phase. In some cases, a gel results which must be further hydrated to yield niosomes. (Reverse phase evaporation) (Kiwada *et al.*, 1985a), previously described by Szoka and Papahadjopoulos (Szoka and Paphadjopoulos, 1978) for the preparation of liposomes.

- The injection of melted lipids surfactants into a highly agitated heated aqueous phase in which presumably the drug is dissolved or the addition of a warmed aqueous phase dissolving the drug to a mixture of melted lipids and hydrophobic drug (Niemec *et al.*, 1994).

- The addition of the warmed aqueous phase to a mixture of the solid lipids: surfactants (Handjani- Vila *et al.*, 1979).

- Niosomes may also be formed from a mixed micellar solution by the use of enzymes (Chopineau *et al.*, 1994). A mixed micellar solution of $C_{16}G_2$, DCP, polyoxyethylene cholesteryl sebacetate diester (PCSD) converts to niosome dispersion when incubated with esterases. PCSD is cleaved by the esterases to yield polyoxyethylene, sebacic acid and cholesterol. Cholesterol in combination with $C_{16}G_2$ and DCP then yields $C_{16}G_2$ niosomes.

- The homogenisation of a surfactant: lipid mixture followed by the bubbling of nitrogen gas through this mixture.

- Apparently the homogenisation step may be omitted from the procedure without affecting particle size, although a longer 'bubbling' time is required.

Size Reduction of Niosomes

A reduction in vesicle size may be achieved by a number of methods.

- Probe sonication (Azmin *et al.*, 1985; Baillie *et al.*, 1985), which yields $C_{16}G_3$ niosomes in the 100–140 nm size range.

- Extrusion through 100 nm nucleopore filters (Stafford *et al.*, 1988) which yields sodium stibogluconate $C_{16}G_3$ niosomes in the 140 nm size range.

- In some instances the combination of sonication and filtration (220 nm Millipore® filter) can be used to achieve 200 nm size range (Uchegbu *et al.*, 1995).
- High-pressure homogenisation also yields vesicles of below 100 nm in diameter although drug loading is ultimately sacrificed to achieve this small size.

Removal of Unentrapped Material

The methods that have been used for the removal of unentrapped material include:

- Exhaustive dialysis (Baillie *et al.*, 1985, 1986).
- Separation by gel filtration (Sephadex G50) (Yoshioka and Florence, 1994).
- Centrifugation (7000g for 30 min) for DOX $C_{16}G_3$ niosomes prepared by hand shaking and ether injection methods.
- Ultracentrifugation (150000g for 1.5 h) for PK1 niosomes.

PROTOCOL: 18.1

Preparation of Niosomal Vesicles by Conventional Chloroform Film Method

Materials

Brij 30 (polyoxyethylene 4 laurylether)

Brij 72 (polyoxyethylene 2 stearylether)

Span 60 (sorbitan monostearate)

Tween 60 (polyoxyethylene sorbitan monostearate)

Cholesterol

Diglyceryl monolaurate

Glyceryl distearate

Glyceryl monostearate

Span 80 (sorbitan monooleate)

Tetraglyceryl monolaurate

Note: Molecular formulae of these non-ionic surfactants are shown in Table 18.1

Diphenyl- 1,3,5-hexatriene (DPH) and calcein.

Procedure

- Dissolve the non-ionic surfactants and cholesterol in chloroform. Evaporate at 60–80°C under vacuum by rotary-evaporator.
- Dry the resulting surfactant film over night in desiccators under vacuum at room temperature (25–28°C).
- Hydrate the obtained film with PBS (phosphate buffered saline) under mechanical agitation for about 1 h at 60–80°C.

Table 18.1: *Vesicle formation ability, HLB values, phase transition temperature of various non-ionic surfactants*

Name and chemical structures of surfactants	HLB	Tc (°C)	Vesicles formation without cholesterol	Minimum amount of cholesterol for vesicle formation (mol%)
Sorbitan monostearate (Span 60)	4.7	45	Yes	–
Glyceryl monostearate (GMS)	3.8	>65	Yes	–
Polyoxyethylene 4 laurylether (Brij 30)	9.7	<10	No	30
Diglyceryl monolaurate (DGL)	6.7	34	No	10
Tetraglyceryl monolaurate (TGL)	10.0	40	No	30

- Confirm the bilayer vesicle formation by maltase cross formation under a LPM (type IMT2-NIC2, Olympus Optical Co., Ltd, Japan) and the ability of the vesicles to entrap water-soluble substance.
- The shape of vesicles may be observed by using a differential interference optical microscope (Scheme 18.1).

Determination of Entrapment Efficiency

- The entrapment efficiency of a water-soluble fluorescent marker (calcein) in niosomal vesicles may be determined by spectrofluorophotometer. Calcein concentration used to prepare niosomes may 0.1 mM.
- Dilute the niosomal dispersions to 1:50 with PBS, measure the total fluorescence intensity (I_{total}).
- Quench calcein in the bulk aqueous phase by complexation with cobalt ions using cobalt chloride.
- Then, measure the fluorescent intensity (I_{in}). Subsequently, rupture the niosomal membrane by Triton X-100.
- The excitation and emission wavelengths are 490 and 520 nm, respectively.
- Calculate the entrapment efficacy of calcein according to the following equation:

Entrapment Efficiency (%)

$$\frac{I_{in} - I_{tx}xr}{I_{total} - I_{tx}r} \times 100$$

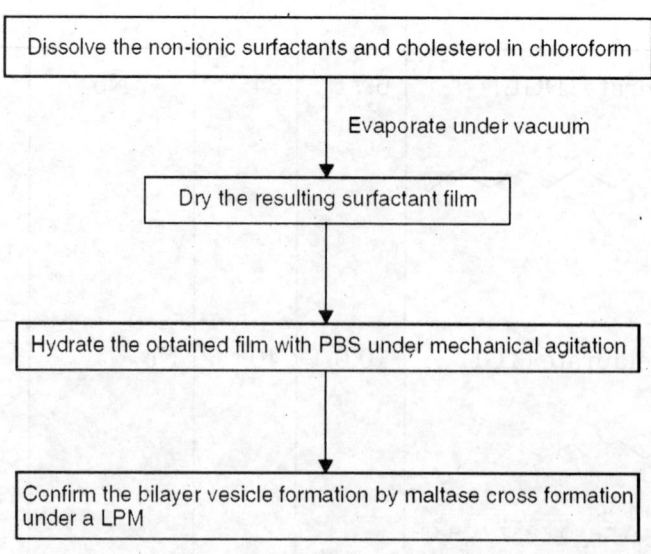

Scheme 18.1: *Preparation of niosomal vesicles by conventional chloroform film method*

PROTOCOL: 18.2
Niosomes as Carriers for Tretinoin

Material

Tretinoin-loaded niosomes may be prepared from—

Polyoxyethylene (4) lauryl ether (Brij® 30),

Sorbitan esters (Span® 40 and Span® 60)

Commercial mixture of octyl/decyl polyglucosides (Triton® CG110).

Enriched soy phosphatidylcholine (Phospholipon® 90, P90)

Hydrogenated soy phosphatidylcholine (Phospholipon® 90H, P90H)

Triton® CG110 (TrCG110)

Cholesterol

DCP

Sorbitan esters (Span® 40 and Span® 60)

Procedure

- Dissolve the phospholipids or surfactants, cholesterol, DCP and tretinoin (4 mg/ml) in chloroform.
- Evaporate the organic solvent and dry resulting lipid film under a nitrogen stream for 30 min.
- Hydrate the obtained lipid film under mechanical stirring with distilled water (pH 5). Adjust the final pH of the prepared formulations ranged between 5.3 and 5.8.
- For the preparation of large unilamellar niosomal vesicles (LUVs) by the extrusion technique transfer the MLV dispersion into a Liposofast® (Avestin) extrusion device and for LUVs niosomes extrude the preparation (21 times for each preparation) through a polycarbonate filter of definite pore size (Nucleopore®, 400 nm).
- To achieve sonicated unilamellar vesicles (SUVs) sonicate (10 times for 1 min each) the MLV dispersion using a probe sonicator.
- In order to prepare vesicles at a temperature above the gel–liquid transition temperature (Tc) of the amphiphiles used, work at 80°C (P90H) or 60°C (sorbitan esters) or at room temperature (Triton® CG110, Tc < 2°C).
- Prepare all suspensions under yellow light and then store in the dark at all times.
- Purify the vesicle dispersions by gel chromatography on a Sephadex G-50 or G-75 column.
- Finally dilute all formulations with distilled water in order to achieve the same TRA concentration (i.e. 0.2 or 0.4 mg/ml).

PROTOCOL: 18.3
Hand Shaking Method

- Take 150 µmol of Span-85 and cholesterol (in different molar ratio) and dissolve in 10 ml of diethyl ether in a 50 ml round bottomed flask.
- Remove ether at ambient temperature (28°C) under reduced pressure in a rotary flash evaporator (Buchi, yorko india).
- Hydrate the dried film of surfactant with occasional shaking for 45 min at 45°C with 5 ml of aqueous phase (0.1N HCl) containing 25mg of drug rifampicin.

PROTOCOL: 18.4
Ether Injection Method

- Dissolve 150µmol of Span-85 and cholesterol in different molar ratio in 20 ml of diethyl ether.
- Inject this ether solution slowly through a 14-gauge needle into 5 ml aqueous phase consisting of 25 mg rifampicin in 0.1N HCl, maintained at 60±2°C.
- Dialyse the resultant dispersion of rifampicin-loaded niosomes exhaustively in cuprophan dialysis tubing against 0.1N HCl.

PROTOCOL: 18.5
Reverse Phase Evaporation Method

- Dissolve surface-active agents in chloroform and emulsify 0.25 volume of phosphate saline buffer to get W/O emulsion.
- Sonicate the mixture and subsequently evaporate chloroform under reduced pressure.
- The lipid or surfactant forms a gel first and subsequently hydrates to form vesicles.
- Remove free drug (unentrapped) by dialysis (Kiwada *et al.*, 1985; Kiwada *et al.*, 1988).

PROTOCOL: 18.6
Proniosomes as Novel Carrier
Materials

The nonionic surfactant sorbitan monostearate (Span 60)
Cholesterol (CH)
Sorbitol
Dicetyl phosphate (DCP)
Ibuprofen
5(6)-carboxyfluorescein (CF)
Chloroform
Ethanol
Ultrapure water,

Procedure

- Attach a 100 ml round-bottom flask containing 1 g of sorbitol to the rotary evaporator.
- A surfactant mixture 500 mM solution of Span 60 (in chloroform-ethanol, 5:1, V: V), and 500 mM solution of cholesterol (in chloroform), and a 50 mM dicetyl phosphate solution (in chloroform), and take desired ratio of Span 60, cholesterol, and dicetyl phosphate in a total concentration of 100 mM.
- Introduce the surfactant solution into the round-bottom flask on the rotary evaporator by sequential spraying of aliquots onto the surface of sorbitol powder.
- During the spraying period, control the rate of application so that the powder bed of sorbitol should not become overly wet (such that slurry would form).
- Evacuate the evaporator and lower the rotating flask into a water bath at 65–70°C. Rotate the flask in the water bath under vacuum for 15– 20 min or until sorbitol appear to be dry, and then introduce another aliquot of surfactant solution.
- Repeat this process until all of the surfactant solution has been applied. After addition of the final aliquot, continue evaporation until the powder gets completely dry (about 20–30 min).
- Dry the material further in a desiccator under vacuum at room temperature for overnight.
- This dry preparation is referred to as 'proniosomes'.
- Hydrate the proniosome preparation with 80°C distilled water and vortex mixing for 2 min to get proniosome-derived niosome dispersions.
- Determine the resulting niosome dispersion for the entrapment efficiency, particle size analysis, and morphological studies.

PROTOCOL: 18.7

Polymer-coated Niosomes

Principle

Artificial pH induced polymerisation method

Meterials

Span 60
Cholesterol
Dicetyl phosphate (DCP)
Acrylonitrile
Diclofenac sodium (model drug)

Procedure

- Take the niosomes forming constituents, i.e. span 60, cholesterol, and dicetylphosphate, in different per cent mole fraction and dissolve in the minimum quantity of diethyl ether, then add 5 ml an equimolar quantity of polymer coat forming monomer, i.e. acrylonitrile.

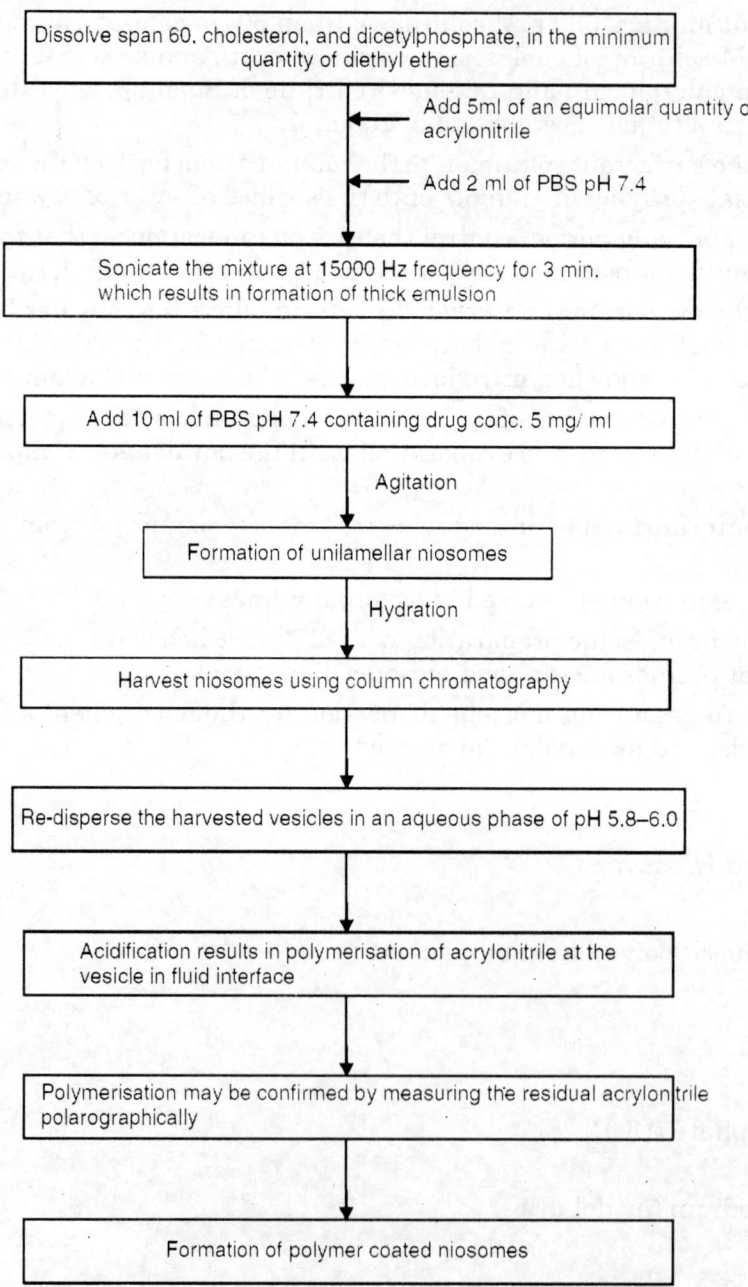

Scheme 18.2: *Formation of polymer coated niosomes*

- To this solution, add 2 ml of phosphate buffer saline PBS pH 7.4 and sonicate the resultant biphasic mixture at 15,000 Hz frequency for 3 minutes, which results in a thick emulsion. Finally, add 10 ml of PBS pH 7.4 containing the drug concentration 5 mg/ml at 50°C to bring about phase inversion. Under constant agitation, unilamellar niosomes of uniform size will form.

- After 2 h, complete the hydration and harvest the niosomes using column chromatography. Re-disperse the harvested vesicles in an aqueous phase of pH 5.8–6.0.

- Acidification results in spontaneous polymerisation of acrylonitrile at the vesicle in fluid interface.

- Polymerisation will complete in one hour, which may be confirmed by measuring the residual acrylonitrile polarographically.

- Prepare the uncoated or plain niosomes similarly using all of the constituents listed above except acrylonitrile.

- Separate the unentrapped drug or solute from the vesicles by gel chromatography.

- Apply 2 ml aliquot of the vesicle suspension to a sephadex G-50 column and fractionate vesicles using PBS, pH 7.4 as eluent (Scheme 18.2).

PROTOCOL: 18.8

Poly (Phthaloyl-l-lysine) Coated Multilamellar Vesicles (Multilamellar Coated Niosomes)

Materials

Span 60
Cholesterol
Dicetyl phosphate (DCP)
L-lysine
Model drug (diclofenac sodium)
Diethyl ether
p-Phthaloyldichloride

Procedure

- Dissolve Span 60, cholesterol and dicetyl phosphate (DCP) in 10 ml of diethyl ether in a 250 ml round bottom flask.

- Remove ether under reduced pressure to form a thin film of lipid over the wall of the flask.

- Hydrate the dry film at 50°C over a water bath using 5 ml of phosphate buffer saline (PBS pH 7.4), containing 10 mg/ml of diclofenac sodium (model drug), until the hydration will complete.

- To coat polymer poly (phthaloyl-L-lysine) on the surface of multilamellar vesicles, take the constant monomer ratio, i.e. p-phtaloyldichloride: L-lysine in 1:1 molar ratio.

- Add p-phtaloyldichloride in the lipid mixture during the film preparation and induce the interfacial polymerisation by the addition of the aqueous phase PBS (pH 7.4) containing drug with L-lysine.

Characterisation of Niosomes

1. Size and Shape

Determine the mean vesicle diameter of the prepared plain and polymer-coated vesicles using an optical microscope at 100 × magnifications with the help of a stage micrometer (Leitz Biomed, Germany). Visualise the shape of the vesicles using the optical microscope.

2. Lamellarity

- Immobilise the prepared polymer-coated vesicles in alginate gel and dry the resultant beads using reduced pressure under vacuum.
- Disperse the prepared alginate beads in polystyrene solution and further dry under vacuum and microtome them using ultramicrotome.
- Collect the microtome section of beads and treat them with absolute alcohol for 5 min
- Dry the samples and impregnate with 1% osmium oxide for 1 h. Dry excessive water using blotting paper. Place the samples on proper grid and observe under transmission electron microscope.

3. Encapsulation Efficiency

- Add 1 ml of the vesicle dispersion to a 1% n-propanol phosphate saline buffer mixture, and allowing it to stand for a few minutes in order to facilitate disruption of the vesicles.
- Measure drug content in niosomal suspension after making up the volume with PBS pH 7.4 and analyse at 284 nm using a spectrophotometer.
- Determine the encapsulation efficiency of the polymer-coated vesicles by estimating the amount of free drug and deducting it from the total drug added.
- Separate the unentrapped drug from the prepared multilamellar vesicles by gel filtration using sephadex G-50 minicolumn.
- Place the vesicular suspension on the top of the column and allow flowing through the column at 1 ml/min. Fractionate the vesicles using PBS (pH 7.4) as eluent.

4. Osmotic Shock

- The effect of osmotic shock on vesicle size and structural integrity is investigated by monitoring the reduction or expansion of vesicular mean diameter following the gradual addition of small volumes of hypertonic solution, normal saline and hypotonic solution to the vesicular suspension.

5. In vitro Release Rate may be Determined by Using Dialysis Bags

- Take 1 ml of the prepared plain/polymer coated vesicle, tie both ends of the dialysis bag, suspend it in 50 ml of double distilled water of PBS pH 7.4.
- Place the bag in a beaker containing 250 ml PBS pH 7.4, placed over a magnetic stirrer and stir contents at 37° C at a constant speed. Withdraw aliquots of samples at regular intervals of 1 h for 10 h and thereafter at 24 h.

- After each sampling time, replace the volume 5ml of receptor compartment with an equal volume of fresh PBS pH 7.4.
- Calculate the drug content in the sample and plot against time.

DISCOMES

Discomes are large (16–20µm) sized vesicular structures capable of entrapping water-soluble solutes, formed by solubilisation of niosomes with a nonionic surfactant-Solulan C-24. They act as drug reservoirs in the field of drug delivery. Progressive incorporation of Solulan C-24 into the vesicular dispersion leads to partitioning of this soluble surfactant between the bilayer and the aqueous phase with the net result that vesicular structure is no longer favoured and the large flattened disc-like structure-discomes are formed in its place.

Discomes (disc shaped vesicles) are formed as intermediate structures in the vesicles-micelle transition by nonionic surfactant-solulan C-24 (SC-24). These are prepared by two general methods as (i) solubilisation of niosomes with SC24 (ii) incorporation of SC24 in the bilayer itself. The detailed discussion of method of preparation of discomes are given below:

(i) *Preparation of discomes by solubilisation of niosomes with SC24:* In this method discomes are prepared in two steps- (a) preparation of niosomes, and (b) solubilisation of niosomes.

(a) *Preparation of niosomes:* Various methods have been used for preparation of niosomes, i.e. cast film method, reverse phase evaporation, ether injection method, and sonication method. Cast film method is more convenient and easier method for discomes preparation in which large micron size discomes formed that can easily be identified and seen in simple microscope.

Preparation of Niosomes by Cast Film Methods

- Accurately weigh total lipid of 0.3mM consisting of span 40 and cholesterol in molar ratio of 1:1 and dissolve in 20 ml diethyl ether, in a round bottom flask.
- Cast the lipid film onto the bottom of flask by evaporation of ether utilising a rotary flash evaporator.
- Allow the dried surfactant film to dry so as to ensure complete removal of organic solvent.
- Hydrate subsequently with 5ml of ATS (pH 7.4, freshly prepared) at 55°C over a water bath for one hour in order to facilitate hydration.

Solubilisation of niosomes with Solulan C-24: Incubate niosomal dispersion of various compositions obtained from above step with various proportion of 2% Solulan C-24 in a water bath shaker at 55–85 °C for 1 hour. Allow the mixtures to cool, this results in dispersion with total lipid: SC-24 in the molar ratio of 11:1 to 1:1. The molar ratio and the temperature at which discomes form may be determined by using turbidity measurements.

Preparation of Drug Loaded Discomes

Previous studies report that discomes are formed at lipid: SC-24 ratio between 9.15:1 and 3.0:1. Hydrate the dry lipid film of 0.3mM total lipid with span 40: Cholesterol in the molar ratio of 2.5:1 obtained by cast film method as described earlier, with 5ml of ATS (pH 7.4) containing 12.5 mg of timolol maleate (filtered through 0.2µm filter) in order to form drug loaded niosomes.

Further incubate 2.5ml of this niosomal dispersion (0.15mM) with SC-24 at 75°C for 1 hr (0.0167mM, 0.0188mM, 0.0214mM, 0.025mM, 0.03mM, 0.0375mM and 0.05mM) to obtain various formulations of discomes. Prepare all these formulations under aseptic conditions.

PROTOCOL: 18.9

Preparation of Discomes by Incorporation of SC24 in the Lipid Layer

- Discomes may be prepared using lipids (Span 40 and Cholestrol) and SC-24 in the molar ratio of 9:1 to 3:1 to observe the differences with their respective counterparts prepared by solubilisation process.
- Dissolve total lipid of various molar proportions (Lipid: SC-24 ratio) each in 20ml diethyl ether and cast the film utilising rotary flash evaporator.
- Hydrate the film with 5ml ATS containing 12.5mg of drug timolol maleate at 75°C for 1hr.
- The preparations may then be utilised for characterisation.

Characterisation of Discomes

Characterise the formulations for various parameters like shape, size, entrapment volume, % drug entrapment and *in vitro* drug release.

Shape of discomes: multi-lamellar, oval shape discs with asymmetric structures.

Size: By optical microscopy method

Enumeration: Naubar's chamber method (same as haemocytometric method).

Entrapment efficiency: via dialysis method.

PROTOCOL: 18.10

Preparation of Discoidal Niosomes

Principle: Film casting and then niosome solubilisation.

Materials

Span 40

Cholesterol

Solulan C24 (SC24)

Procedure

Step 1. Preparation of Niosome Suspension

- Weigh accurately 0.3 mM film forming constituents (Span 40, cholesterol and SC24) in different molar ratio (cholesterol: SC24 ratio from 9:1 to 3:1) and dissolve in 20 ml diethyl ether in a round bottom flask and cast a thin and uniform film by using a rotary flash evaporator.
- Hydrate the dried lipid film with the 5 ml of PBS (pH 7.4) containing drug at 55°C using a covered water bath for 1 h to facilitate complete hydration.

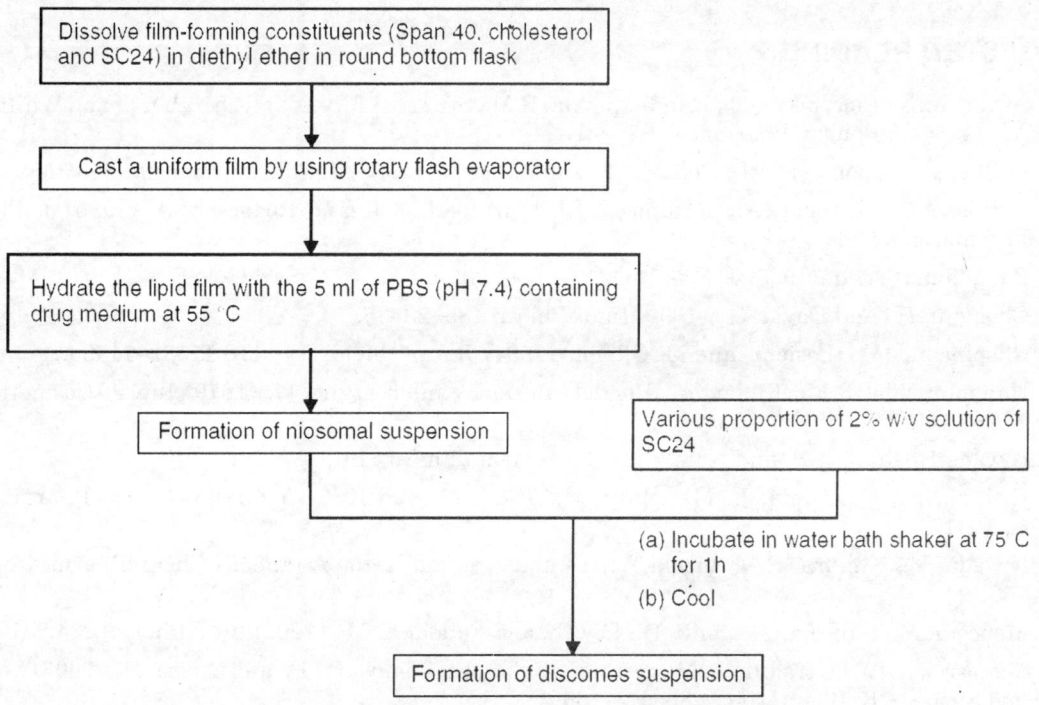

Scheme 18.3: *Preparation of discoidal niosomes*

Step 2: Transition of Niosomes to Discomes

- Take niosomal suspension of various lipid compositions and incubate with various proportions of 2% w/v solution of SC24 in a water bath shaker at 75°C for 1h.
- Cool the mixture. After cooling, turbid suspension of discomes will be obtained (Scheme 18.3).

Characterisation of Discomes

- *Size and shape:* By optical microscopy
- *Entrapment efficiency:* By dialysis method
- Active drug loading by pH gradient hydration method
- *In vitro* release study

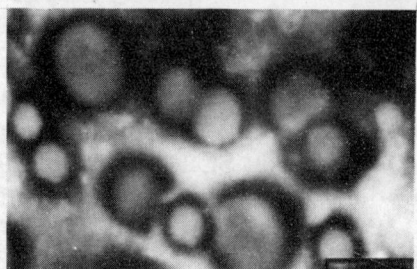

Fig 18.1: *TEM image of niosomes*

SUGGESTED READINGS

- Azmin, M.N., Florence, A.T., Handjani-Vila, R.M., Stuart, J.F.B., Vanlerberghe, G. and Whittaker, J.S. (1985) J. Pharm. Pharmacol. 37: 237–242.

- Baillie, A.J., Coombs, G.H., Dolan, T.F. and Laurie, J. (1986) J. Pharm. Pharmacol. 38:502–505.

- Baillie, A.J., Florence, A.T., Hume, L.R., Murihead, G.T. and Rogerson, A. (1985) J. Pharm. Pharmacol. 37:863.

- Bangham, A., *et al* (1965) J. Mol. Biol. 13: 238–252.

- Chengjiu, H., and David, G., (1999) Int J Pharm 185: 23–35.

- Chopineau, J., S. Lesieur, and M. Ollivon. (1994) J. Am. Chem. Soc. 116:11582–11583.

- Handjani-Vila, R.M., Ribier, A., Rondot, B. and Vanlerberghe, G. (1979) Int. J. Cosmetic Sci. 1:306–314.

- Kiwada H.,Nimura H. and Kato Y (1985,b) Chem.. Pharm. Bull. 33: 2465.

- Kiwada, H., Nakajima, I., Matsuura, H., Tsuji, M. and Kato, Y. (1988) Chem. Pharm. Bull. 36:1841.

- Kiwada, H., Nimura, H., Fujisaki, Y., Yamada, S. and Kato, Y. (1985a) Chem. Pharm. Bull. 33: 753.

- Manconi, M., Sinico, C., Valenti, D., Loy G., and Fadda, A. M., (2002) Int J Pharm, 234:237–248.

- Manosroi, A., Wongtrakul, P., Manosroi, J., Sakai, H., Sugawara, F., and Yuasa, M., (2003) Colloids and Surfaces B: Biointerfaces 30: 129-138.

- Niemiec, S.M., Hu, Z., Ramachandran, C., Wallach, D.F.H. and Weiner, N. (1994) S.T.A. Pharm. Sci. 4: 145.

- Sazoka F C & Papahadjopoulos D, (1978) Proc Natl Acad Sci U S A, 75 4194.

- Stafford, S., Baillie, A.J. and Florence A.T. (1988) J. Pharm. Pharmacol 40: 26P.

- Uchegbu I.F., Turton, J.A., Double J.A. and Florance A. T. (1994) Biopharm. Drug Dispos. 15:691.

- Uchegbu, Vyas S. P. and Suresh P. Vyas (1988) Int J Pharm, 172: 33–70.

- Uchegbu, I.F., Double, J.A., Turton, J.A. and Florence, A.T. (1995) Pharm. Res. 12: 1019–1024.

- Yoshida, A., Manosroi A., Manosroi, J., and Yamauchi, M.A., (1995) Colloids Surf. B: Biointerfaces. 4:423.

- Yoshioko, T. and Florence, A.T. (1994) Int. J. Pharm. 108:117– 123.

19

Solid Lipid Nanoparticles

Solid lipid nanoparticles (SLNs) have attracted increasing scientific and commercial attention as novel colloidal drug carrier for intravenous applications as they have been proposed as an alternative particulate carrier system (Muller and Lucks, 1996; Almeida *et al.*, 1997; zur Muhlen *et al.*, 1998). The solid lipid nanoparticles (SLN) are sub-micron size range colloidal carriers (50–1000 nm), which are composed of physiological lipid, dispersed in water or in an aqueous surfactant solution. SLNs as colloidal drug carrier combine advantages of polymeric nanoparticles, fat emulsions and liposomes simultaneously, avoiding some of their disadvantages. The main features of SLNs are the excellent physical stability, protection of incorporated labile drugs from degradation, controlled drug release (fast or sustained) depending on the incorporation model, good tolerability and site-specific targeting. Potential disadvantages such as insufficient loading capacity, drug expulsion after polymorphic transition during storage and relatively high water content of the dispersions (70–99.9%) have been observed. SLN formulations for various application routes (parenteral, oral, dermal, ocular, pulmonary, rectal) have been developed and thoroughly characterised *in vitro* and *in vivo*. A first product has recently been introduced to the Polish market (Nanobase, Yamanouchi) as a topically applied moisturiser.

This chapter highlights the main features of SLNs, including the concept of SLNs, different methods of production, and their applications. Special attention is paid to the relation among drug incorporation, the heterogeneity of the lipid particle, and the presence of other colloidal species.

Advantages of SLNs as Alternative Particulate Carrier

Some of the advantages cited in the literature are mentioned (Muller *et al.,* 1995; zur Muhlen *et al.,* 1998):

- Small size and relatively narrow size distribution, which provide biological opportunities for site-specific drug delivery by SLNs.
- Controlled release of active drug over a long period can be achieved.
- Protection of incorporated drug against chemical degradation.
- Possible sterilisation by autoclaving or gamma irradiation.

- SLNs can be lyophilised as well as spray dried.
- No toxic metabolites are produced.
- Avoidance of organic solvents.
- Relatively cheaper and stable.
- Ease of industrial scale production by hot dispersion technique.
- Incorporation of drug can reduce distinct side effects of drug, e.g. Thrombophlebitis that are associated with IV injection of diazepam or etomidate.
- Surface modification can easily be accomplished and hence can be used for site - specific drug delivery system.

SLNs Versus Other Colloidal Drug Carriers

SLN have been proven to be a better alternative carrier system in comparison with conventional O/W emulsion if a prolonged release or a protection of drug against chemical degradation is required (zur Muhlen *et al.*, 1998). Incorporation of the drug into the solid lipid matrix might surely be a better protection than that can be achieved in the oily internal face of emulsion and liposomes. Prolonged release from emulsions does not appear to be feasible which can be achieved to a certain extent from SLN.

Compared to polymeric nanoparticles, the SLNs possesses some genuine advantages. Apart from the lower cytotoxicity, due to the absence of solvents in the production process, and a relatively low cost for the excipients the major advantage is that its large-scale production is possible by the simple process of high-pressure homogenisation. Such equipment already exists in pharmaceutical industry for the production of emulsions for parenteral nutrition and emulsions as drug carriers. While compared to liposomes the SLNs possesses the advantage of offering better protection to drug against chemical degradation there is no or little access of water in the inner core of lipid particles. Depending on the nature of drug, a higher payload might be achieved. In addition, the SLNs provide more possibilities to modify the drug release profile.

INGREDIENTS AND FORMULATION PROCESSES

Ingredients

General ingredients include the drug, solid lipids, emulsifiers, and water. Depending on the application, other ingredients might be present (osmotic agents, matrices for lyophilisation, buffers, etc.) (Table 19.1).

The danger of acute and chronic toxicity resulting from the SLN lipids is rather low because, in general, physiological lipids are used (there are few exceptions, such as amphiphilic calixarenes. The term "lipid" is generally used in a very broad sense and includes triglycerides (e.g., tristearin), partial glycerides (e.g., monostearate), fatty acids (e.g., stearic acid), steroids (e.g., cholesterol), and waxes (e.g., cetyl palmitate). More attention should be given to the physicochemical properties of the lipid and to classifying them in relation to their interactions with water. The choice of emulsifier depends on the administration route and is more limited for parenteral administrations. A large variety of ionic and nonionic emulsifiers of different molecular weight have been used to stabilise the lipid dispersion. The most frequently used compounds include different kinds of poloxamers, polysorbates, lecithin, and bile acids. In many cases, the combination of emulsifiers was more efficient at preventing particle agglomeration than was the use of a single surfactant.

Table 19.1: List of lipids used for the preparation of solid lipid nanoparticles

Triglycerides	*Hard fat types*	*Emulsifiers / Coemulsifiers*
Trilaurin Tristearin Trimyristin Tripalmitin Tribehenin Hydrogenated coco-glycerides (Softisan® 142)	Witepsol® (available in different grades W35, H35, H42 and E85) Glyceryl monostearate Glyceryl palmitostearate Cetyl palmitate Stearic acid Palmitic acid Decanoic acid Behenic acid Acidan N12	Soybean lecithin Egg lecithin Phosphatidylcholine Poloxamer 188 Poloxamer 407 Poloxamer 908 Tyloxapole Polysorbate 20 Polysorbate 60 Polysorbate 80 Sodium cholate Sodium glycocholate Taurocholic acid Taurodeoxycholic acid Butanol

Processes/Production Techniques of SLN

Different approaches exist for the production of finely dispersed SLN dispersions. In this section, the various methods are described briefly, also with regard to scaling up possibility, a prerequisite for the introduction of a product to the market. To manufacture SLNs, the hot high-pressure homogenisation above the melting point of the lipid and subsequent re-crystallisation is recommended (melt emulsification), but the cold high-pressure homogenisation (high pressure milling of lipid suspensions) for thermo labile drugs exists, too. Other production methods for SLNs as the production from microemulsions, the precipitation and dispersing by ultrasound are published and differ normally in obtained particle size distribution.

High Pressure Homogenisation

HPH has emerged as a reliable and powerful technique for the preparation of SLNs. HPH has been used for years for the production of nanoemulsions for parenteral nutrition. In contrast to other techniques, scaling up represents no or minor problems in most cases. High pressure homogenisers push a liquid with high pressure (10 to 200 MPa) through a narrow gap (in the range of few microns). The fluid accelerates on a very short distance to very high velocity (over 1000 km/h). Very high-shear forces disrupt the particles down to the submicron range. Typical lipid contents range between 5 to 10% of the fluid and represent no problem to the homogeniser. Even lipid concentrations up to 40% have been homogenised to lipid nanodispersions. Two general approaches of the homogenisation step, the hot and the cold homogenisation techniques, can be used for the production of SLN. In both cases, a preparatory step involves incorporating the drug into the bulk lipid by dissolving or dispersing the drug in the lipid melt.

Hot Homogenisation Technique

The hot homogenisation technique (Scheme 19.1) can be applied to lipophilic and insoluble drugs. Even many heat sensitive drugs can be processed because the exposure time to high temperatures is relatively short. Hot homogenisation is carried out at temperatures above the melting point of the lipid and can therefore be regarded as the homogenisation of an emulsion. A pre-emulsion of the drug-loaded lipid melt and the aqueous emulsifier phase (same temperature) is obtained by a high-shear mixing device (Ultra-Turrax). The quality of the pre-emulsion affects the quality of the final product to a large extent, and obtaining droplets in the size range of a few micrometers is desirable. The primary product of the hot homogenisation is a nanoemulsion resulting from the liquid state of the lipid. Solid particles are expected to be formed by the cooling of the sample to room temperature or below. Because of the small particle size and the presence of the emulsifiers, lipid crystallisation may be highly retarded, and the sample may remain as a supercooled melt (nanoemulsion) for several months. The technique is found unsuitable for incorporating hydrophilic drugs into SLNs because of higher partition of drug in water during homogenisation resulting in low entrapment efficiency.

Melting of the lipid
↓
Dissolution of the drug in the melted lipid
↓
Mixing of the preheated dispersion medium and the drug lipid melt
↓
Premix using a stirrer to form a coarse pre-emulsion
↓
High-pressure homogenisation at a temperature above the lipids melting point
↓
O/W - nanoemulsion
↓
Solidification of the nanoemulsion by cooling down to room temperature to form SLN

Scheme 19.1: SLN preparation using hot homogenisation technique

Cold Homogenisation Technique

For hydrophilic drugs the cold homogenisation technique is the method of first choice (Scheme 19.2). The first preparatory step is the same as in the hot homogenisation procedure and includes the solubilisation or dispersion of the drug in the melt of bulk lipid. However, different steps follow. The drug-containing melt is cooled very rapidly (e.g., by means of dry ice or liquid nitrogen). The high cooling rate favours a homogenous distribution of the drug within the lipid matrix. The solid, drug-containing lipid is milled by means of ball or mortar milling in the range of 50 to 100 µm. Low temperatures increase the fragility of the lipid and, therefore, favour particle disruption. The solid lipid microparticles are dispersed in a chilled emulsifier solution. A pre-suspension is formed by high speed stirring of the particles in a cold aqueous surfactant solution. This pre-suspension is then homogenised at or below room temperature forming SLNs, the homogenising conditions are generally five cycles at 500 bar. In case of a too low solubility of the hydrophilic drug in the melted lipid, surfactants can be used for solubilisation of the drug. This homogenisation technique avoids and minimises melting process of lipid and is suitable for thermo-sensitive and thermo-labile drugs. (Muller *et al.*,1995).

Melting of the lipid
↓
Dissolution / solubilisation of the drug in the melted lipid
↓
Solidification of the drug loaded lipid in liquid nitrogen or dry ice
↓
Grinding in a powder mill (50–100µm particles)
↓
Dispersion of the lipid in the cold aqueous dispersion medium
↓
Homogenisation at room temperature or below
↓
Solid lipid nanoparticles

Scheme 19.2: *SLN preparation using cold Homogenisation Technique*

Solvent Injection Method

The production of polymeric nanoparticles by dilution of polymer solutions in water has been described by De Labouret *et al*. The particle size was critically determined by the velocity of the distribution processes. Nanoparticles were produced only with polar solvents, which distribute very rapidly into the aqueous phase (e.g., acetone, ethanol, isopropanol, methanol), whereas larger particle sizes were obtained with more lipophilic solvents. The process can also be easily used for the production of lipid nanodispersions. A requirement is the solubility of the lipid in the polar organic solvent, which limits the application range of this procedure. A further disadvantage is the low concentration of the lipid nanoparticles (typically 1% or less). Higher amounts of the organic solvent increase the solubility of the lipid in the aqueous phase and lead to an increase in particle size resulting from Ostwald ripening. The main advantage of the method is the avoidance of thermal stress.

Microemulsion-Based SLNs Preparation

SLNs preparation techniques that are based on the dilution of microemulsions have been developed by Gasco. It should be mentioned that there are different definitions and opinions about the structure and dynamics of microemulsion in the scientific community.

Firstly, a warm microemulsion is prepared by stirring, containing typically 10% molten solid lipid, 15% surfactant and up to 10% cosurfactant. This warm microemulsion is then dispersed under stirring in excess cold water (typical ratio 1:50) using an especially developed thermostated syringe. The excess water is removed either by ultra-filtration or by lyophilisation in order to increase the particle concentration.

Experimental factors such as microemulsion composition, dispersing device, temperature and lyophilisation on size and structure of the obtained SLNs have been studied intensively. It has to be remarked critically, that the removal of excess water from the prepared SLNs dispersion is a difficult task with regard to the particle size. Also, high concentrations of surfactants and cosurfactants (e.g. butanol) are necessary for formulating purposes, however less desirable with respect to regulatory purposes and application.

Preparation by w/o/w Double Emulsion Method

Recently, a novel method based on solvent emulsification evaporation for the preparation of SLNs loaded with hydrophilic drugs has been introduced to the scientific community. Here, the hydrophilic drug is encapsulated-along with a stabiliser to prevent drug partitioning to the external water phase during solvent evaporation in the internal water phase of a W/O/W double emulsion. This technique has been used for the preparation of sodium cromoglycate-containing SLNs, however, the average size was in the micrometer range so that the term "lipospheres" in the sense as a term for nanoparticles is not used correctly for these particles.

Preparation by Solvent Emulsification-Evaporation or -Diffusion

Different academic groups have attempted the production of SLN via precipitation. In the solvent emulsification-evaporation, lipophilic material is dissolved in a water immiscible organic solvent (e.g., cyclohexane) that is emulsified in an aqueous phase to give an oil/water (O/W) emulsion. On evaporation of the solvent by reduced pressure, solid lipid nanoparticles dispersion is formed. The mean diameter of the obtained particles was 25 nm, with cholesterol acetate as the model drug and using a lecithin/sodium glycocholate blend as the emulsifier. Mean particle size of the final particles ranged from 30 to 100 nm, depending on the lecithin/cosurfactant blend. The smallest particle diameters were obtained by using bile salts as cosurfactants. Comparable small-particle-size distributions are not achievable by melt emulsification of a similar composition. The mean particle size depends on the concentration of the lipid in the organic phase. Very small particles could only be obtained with low fat loads (5 wt%) related to the organic solvent. With increasing lipid content, the efficiency of the homogenisation declines because of the higher viscosity of the dispersed phase. The advantage of this procedure over the cold homogenisation process described before is the avoidance of any thermal stress. A clear disadvantage is the use of organic solvents. Problems might arise due to solvent residues in the final dispersion. Typically, lipid concentrations in the final SLN dispersion range around 0.1 g/l, therefore, the particle concentration has to be increased by means of, e.g. ultra-filtration or evaporation (Trotta et al., 2003; Sjostrom et al., 1995).

CHARACTERISATION OF SLN

Appropriate characterisation of the solid lipid nanodispersion is a necessary and very difficult task because of the submicron size of the particles and the complexity of the system, which also includes dynamic phenomena. Any particle separation from the aqueous environment or only dissolution with water could easily lead to misleading results due to particle aggregation and changed samples if stabilisers are removed from the particle surface. Therefore, non-invasive investigation techniques without the need of dilution have been applied whenever possible. Nuclear magnetic resonance (1H-NMR) and electron spin resonance spectroscopy (ESR), fluorescence spectroscopy, X-ray diffraction, measurements of refractive index and density, Raman spectroscopy were used beside invasive methods (transmission electron microscopy (TEM), field- flow fractionation (FFF), photon correlation spectroscopy (PCS) and laser diffraction (LD)). The SLNs are generally characterised for size, density, electrophoretic mobility, angle of contact and specific surface area.

Parameter	Characterisation method
Particle size and size distribution	Photon correlation spectroscopy (PCS) Laser defractometry Transmission electron microscopy Scanning electron microscopy Atomic force microscopy Mercury porositometry
Charge determination	Laser doppler anemometry Zeta potential meter
Surface hydrophobicity	Water contact angle measurements Rose Bengal (dye) binding Hydrophobic interaction chromatography X-ray photoelectron spectroscopy
Chemical analysis of surface	Static secondary ion mass spectrometry Sorptometer
Carrier-drug interaction	Differential scanning calorimetry
SLNs dispersion stability	Critical flocculation temperature (CFT)
Release profile	*In vitro* release characteristics under physiologic and sink conditions
Drug stability	Bioassay of drug extracted from nanoparticles Chemical analysis of drug

Size and Morphology

The particle size is one of the most important parameters of SLNs. Particle size and sizing of sub-optical particulates is a different procedure, as it involves not only procedural variability, but some of the surface associated properties may even change during sizing procedure. Two main techniques are being used to determine the particle size distribution of nanoparticles and include photon correlation spectroscopy (PCS) and electron microscopy (EM) (Reviewed in Kreuter, J. 1983; Kreuter, J. 1991; Fusai *et al.*, 1997). The latter include scanning electron microscopy (SEM), transmission electron microscopy (TEM) and freeze-fracture techniques.

A given preparation when determined for size using different procedures, it was deduced that results co-ordinate well with better agreement when freeze-fracturing and photon correlation spectroscopy are quantitatively compared. The electron microscopy however could be adopted as an alternative option, which measures individual particles for size and its distribution. It is much less time consuming. Additionally, freeze fracturing of particles allows for morphological determination of inner structure of particles. In combination with freeze fracture procedures, TEM permits differentiation among nanocapsules, nanoparticles and emulsion droplets. Scanning electron microscopy is much less time consuming. However, particles being based on organic material and non-conductive hence require gold coating. The thickness of gold coat may vary from 30–50 nm. Thus determined size should be denoted as gold-coated particle size rather than as particle size (Fig.19.1).

The most widely used method to characterise the size of solid lipid nanoparticles is photon correlation spectroscopy (PCS) and laser diffraction (LD). PCS (also known as dynamic light scattering) measures the fluctuation of the intensity of the scattered light caused by particle movement and covers a size range from a few nanometers to about 3 μm. This method is based on the dependence of the diffraction angle on the particle radius. Smaller particles cause more intense scattering at high angles than do larger ones.

This method requires only very small amounts of sample and is rapid and easy to perform, and its range of operation (nominally between a few nanometers and a few micrometers) covers the relevant range for lipid nanoparticle suspensions. PCS analyses the Brownian motion of the particles in the dispersion medium. Light microscopy is not sensitive to the nanometer size range but gives a fast indication of the presence of microparticles. Electron microscopy provides, in contrast to PCS and LD, direct information on the particle shape. However, the investigator should pay special attention to possible artifacts that may be caused by the sample preparation.

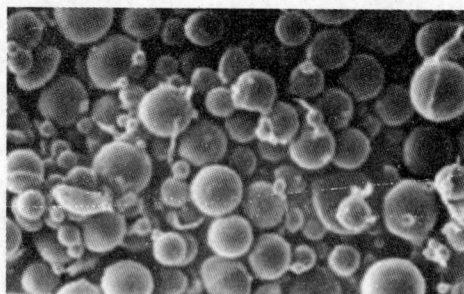

Fig. 19.1: Scanning electron microscope photograph of solid lipid nanoparticles

Atomic force microscopy (AFM) is an advanced nanoscopic technique that has been applied for the characterisation of solid lipid nanoparticles (zur Muhlen *et al.*, 1996). The AFM images can be obtained in an aqueous medium and for this reason it is an effective means for the investigation of nanoparticle behaviour in biological environment. Mercury porositometry is equally suitable technique for the sizing of nano-particulates (Kreuter,

J. 1983). The freeze-dried nanoparticles are filled in a dilatometer under vacuum then measured with the help of a mercury pressure porositometer. The method largely measures particulate agglomerates as mercury fails to penetrate to a greater extent within the primary particles.

Specific Surface Area

The specific surface area of freeze-dried SLNs is generally determined with the help of Sorptometer (Kreuter, J. 1983). The calculation method using the equation can be used in the calculation of specific surface area.

$$A = 6 \, / \, \partial. \, d$$

Where A is the specific surface area, ∂ is the density and d is the diameter of the particle.

In most of the cases, the measured and calculated specific surface areas fairly compare while in some cases the residual surfactant could affect deviation in measured values. The surfactant coating apparently reduces the specific surface area.

Surface Charge and Electrophoretic Mobility

The nature and intensity of the surface charge of SLNs is very important as it determines their interaction with the biological environment as well as their electrostatic interaction with bioactive compounds. For measurement, a dilute suspension of the nanoparticles is subjected to a weak electric field, and the mobility of the particles is determined by Laser Doppler Anemometry. This technique is based on the evaluation of a frequency (Doppler) shift that is observed for the light scattered from the particles' motion in the electric field. As a result, the electrophoretic mobility (velocity of the particles/electric field strength) of the nanoparticles is obtained. The zeta potential can be obtained by measuring the electrophoretic mobility applying the Helmholtz-Smoluchowski equation. Generally, the electrophoretic mobility of SLNs is determined in phosphate saline buffer (PBS, pH 7.4) and human serum. The aggregated bands of SLNs are visualised distinctively. It is important that free drug adherent or solubilised in aqueous phase and residual surfactant should be removed before electrophoretic mobility is determined. Phosphate saline buffer (PBS) relatively reduces the absolute charge value due to ionic interaction of buffer components with the charged surface of nanoparticles. In the study of solid lipid nanoparticles, zeta potential determinations have mainly been employed with respect to conclusions about the physical stability or instability, respectively, of the formulations during storage or on interaction with electrolytes or (simulated) biological fluids.

Surface Hydrophobicity

The surface hydrophobicity of nanoparticles has an important influence on the interaction of colloidal particles with the biological environment (e.g. protein adsorption and cell adhesion). The hydrophobicity and hydrophilicity collectively determine the bio-fate of nanoparticles and their contents. Hydrophobicity regulates the extent and type of hydrophobic interactions of nanoparticulates with blood components.

Several methods, including hydrophobic interaction chromatography, two-phase partition, adsorption of hydrophobic fluorescent or radiolabelled probes, and contact angle measurements have been adopted to evaluate surface hydrophobicity (Carstensen *et al.*, 1991). The measurement of angle of contact suggests about the hydrophobicity or hydrophilicity of the nanoparticles. The water contact angle is measured only on plain surface hence nanoparticles are compressed as tablet/pellet. To study the effect of blood components on resultant *in vivo* hydrophilicity or hydrophobicity, the particles are first incubated with blood serum, then centrifuged and lyophilised. The dried nanoparticles are then compressed and angle of contact with water (water contact angle) is determined. The serum components decrease the contact angle by 20°. This suggests that blood components are adsorbed strongly and affect subsequent wettability characteristics of the nanoparticles. Recently, several sophisticated methods of surface chemistry analysis are used. For example, X-ray Photoelectron Spectroscopy (XPS) permits the identification of specific chemical groups on the surface of nanoparticles.

Density

In addition to surface scanning electron microscopy, transmission electron microscopy following freeze fracturing could successfully be used in morphological investigation of the nanoparticles. Within the interior, continuous or some structural imperfections exist that also provide an indication in regard to density distribution across the matrix. Some polymeric nanoparticles specially polycyanoacrylate and poly(methyl methacrylate) seem to have porous interior, also exhibit more irregular and rough surface.

The density of nanoparticles is determined with helium or air using a gas Pycnometer (Kreuter, J. 1983). The value obtained with air and with helium may differ noticeably from each other. The difference is much more pronounced due to specific surface area and porosity of the structure.

Crystallinity and Polymorphism

When preparing lipid nano- and microparticles from solid, crystalline raw materials, it is usually expected that the lipid matrix of the particles is or will become solid after the dispersion step. It has, however, turned out that some matrix materials do not crystallize easily in the colloidally dispersed state after processing in the heat for example, in melt-homogenisation. Shorter chain triglycerides like tricaprin, trilaurin, or trimyristin are particularly problematic in this respect, but retarded crystallisation has also been observed for dispersions of more complex glycerides. Differential scanning calorimetry (DSC) and X-ray diffraction (XRD) are the techniques most widely used for the characterisation of crystallinity and polymorphism of solid lipid particles. Although DSC is usually more sensitive in detecting crystalline material, XRD is much more reliable in determining the type of polymorph present in the dispersions because it provides structural data. In contrast, DSC can detect the type of polymorph only indirectly via the transition temperatures and enthalpies. Because these parameters may be different from those observed in the bulk material, particularly for small colloidal particles, assignment of polymorphic forms in DSC curves should be supported by X-ray data. In DSC the sample is subjected to a controlled temperature program, usually a temperature scan, and the heat flow to or from the sample is monitored in comparison to an inert reference. The resulting curves, which show the phase transitions in the monitored temperature range, such as crystallisation, melting, or polymorphic transitions can be evaluated with regard to phase transition temperatures and transition enthalpy. DSC is thus a convenient method to confirm the presence of solid lipid particles via the detection of a melting transition.

In the characterisation of solid lipid nanoparticles, the major points of interest are usually the confirmation of the solid, crystalline state of the particles and the identification of the polymorphic form of the lipid matrix. This can be done by comparison to literature data or to measurements of the corresponding bulk materials. The X-ray diffractograms of the lipid matrix materials usually display only few major reflections characteristic of the packing of the alkyl chains. The lipids crystallise in lamellar organisations; with the alkyl chains packed side by side in different arrangements and oriented either perpendicular to or tilted toward the plane of the single layers. Typically, these arrangements display a strong small-angle reflection, indicating the repeating distance of the single layers.

With the help of XRD, the differences in polymorphism between glyceride nanoparticles and the corresponding bulk material were clearly demonstrated. Moreover, this method has been applied to evaluate the factors that affect the rate of polymorphic transitions in glyceride nanoparticles such as the type and chain length of the lipid, the presence of drug or liquid oil, the type of surfactant, or the particle size.

The X-ray reflections of solid lipid nanoparticles are usually much broader than those of the bulk material as a result of the small particle size and, potentially, also of a decrease in crystalline order. Fine details may thus not be recognisable in the resulting, more diffuse diffractograms. Assignment of polymorphs may become increasingly difficult with the complexity of the material under investigation (e.g., complex glyceride mixtures), particularly in cases in which there is also very limited knowledge about the structure and behaviour of the bulk material. NMR is a very useful tool for investigating colloidal systems. NMR active nuclei of interest are ^{1}H, ^{13}C, ^{19}F, and ^{31}P. Because of the different chemical shifts, it is possible to attribute the NMR signals to particular molecules or their segments. Simple 1H-NMR spectroscopy permits an easy and very rapid detection of supercooled melts caused by the low line widths of the lipid protons. This method is based on the different proton relaxation times in the liquid and semisolid/solid states.

Molecular Weight Measurements of Nanoparticles

Molecular weight of the polymer and its distribution in the matrix can be evaluated by gel permeation chromatography (GPC) using a refractive index detector. Sukuma and co-workers (1997) determined the number average and weight average molecular weight of macromolecules on the polystyrene nanoparticles having surface grafted hydrophilic polymeric chains and correlated these parameters with a good water dispersibility of the system. Using gel permeation chromatography, it was shown that PACA nanoparticles are built by an entanglement of numerous small oligomeric subunits rather than by the rolling up of one or few long polymer chains.

Nanoparticle Recovery and Drug Incorporation Efficiency

The nanoparticle recovery which is also referred to as nanoparticle yield in the literature (Go vender *et al,* 1999) can be calculated using the following equation.

Drug incorporation efficiency has been expressed both as drug content (% w/w), which is also referred as drug loading in the literature (Govender *et al.*, 1999) and Drug entrapment (%), represented by following equations:

$$\text{SLNs Recovery(\%)} = \frac{\text{Analysed weight of SLNs}}{\text{Theoretical weight of SLNs}} \times 100$$

$$\text{Drug content (\%w/w)} = \frac{\text{Mass of drug in SLNs}}{\text{Mass of SLNs recovered}} \times 100$$

$$\text{Drug entrapment (\%)} = \frac{\text{Mass of drug in nanoparticles}}{\text{Mass of drug used in the formulation}}$$

In vitro Release

In vitro release profile can be determined using standard dialysis, diffusion cell or recently introduced modified ultrafiltration technique (Kreuter, J. 1983; Kruter, J. 1991; Magenheim et al, 1993). *In vitro* drug release from the SLNs can be evaluated in phosphate buffer utilising double chamber diffusion cells on a shaker stand. A millipore hydrophilic low-protein binding membrane is placed between the two chambers. The donor chamber is filled with SLNs suspension and the receptor chamber with plain buffer. The receptor compartment is assayed at different time intervals for the released drug using standard procedures. Magenheim and co-workers (1993) used a modified ultrafiltration technique to determine the *in vitro* release behaviour of the nanoparticles. The nanoparticle suspension is added directly into a stirred ultrafiltration cell-containing buffer. At different time intervals aliquots of the dissolution medium are filtered through the ultrafiltration membrane using less than 2 bar positive nitrogen pressure and assayed for the released drug using standard procedures.

In vivo Fate and Biodistribution of Nanoparticles

Following intravenous administration, the colloidal carriers first come into contact with plasma/serum proteins before they reach target cells. Most notably, the interaction of the colloidal carriers with the phagocytes often requires some serum components and then subsequently interaction with complement receptors, Fc receptors and sugar/lectin receptors on the macrophage, lymphocytes or other cells. Soluble carriers can be pinocytosed via Fc or lectin receptors. A number of other receptors are expressed on different cell types, which negotiate the transportation of various endogenous ligands or colloidal carriers appended with their synthetic mimics (reviewed in Vyas and Sihorkar, 2000; Vyas *et al.*, 2001). Normally, intravenously injected colloidal carriers follow their interactions with at least two distinct groups of plasma proteins. It is now recognised that phagocytosis of particulates by elements of RES (liver, spleen, bone marrow) and specially with reference to liver (Kupffer cells) is regulated by the presence and balance between two groups of serum components:

opsonins that promote phagocytosis, and dysopsonins, that suppress the process (Absolom, 1986; Moghimi & Patel, 1989; Moghimi & Patel, 1998). The so-called opsonins adsorb on to the surface of the colloidal carriers and render particles recognisable and more "palatable" to the RES (Fig. 19.2). Thus they mediate their endocytosis by the fixed macrophages of the reticuloendothelial system and circulating monocytes. Immunoglobulins and components of complement systems (particularly C3 and C5) are known as classical opsonin molecules, while fibronectin, C-reactive protein and tuftsin are also known to enhance recognition of various particulates by different macrophages. Immunoglobulin IgG and secretory IgA are the best-known dysopsonins (Absolom, 1986). The mode of dysopsonins is not well documented, however, their hydrophilicity could be assumed as a responsible mechanism of action. Recently, efforts are being waged to "disguise" the recognition of particulates by RES thus make the nanoparticles escape RES capture. The central dogma in the opsonin driven phagocytosis (opsono-phagocytosis) is the higher protein adsorbability of hydrophobic relative to hydrophilic surfaces. The same has been related to the enhanced uptake of more hydrophobic particles by phagocytosis *in vitro* and rapid removal of hydrophobic particles *in vivo*.

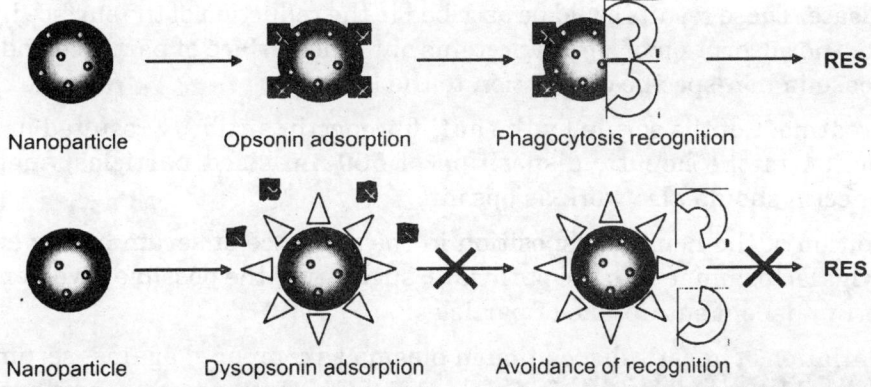

Fig. 19.2: *In vivo fate of nanoparticles after adsorption of serum components*

Essentially, the macrophages located in the reticuloendothelial systems play a crucial role in opsonin mediated phagocytosis of the injected particulate systems. Polystyrene particles as small as 60 nm showed higher clearance rates from circulation (Illum et al., 1987). Similarly, short circulation half lives were observed irrespective of the compositions of the injected microparticulate systems of albumin, poly(lactic acid), poly(lactide-co-glycolide), poly(cyanoacrylate) or polyacryl starch (reviewed in Stolnik *et al.*, 1995). Therefore, using these systems, it is only possible to target drugs to RES-rich organs. Wide ranges of serum components, which are expressed on either at the metastatic states or as a result of changes in circadian rhythm of the different target sites, are thought to play key roles in determining the *in vivo* fate of the particulate systems. Polystyrene particles (PS) (60 nm in diameter) and colloidal gold particles (17 nm in diameter) were found to be opsonised by fibronectins but the adsorption was allegedly prevented after the coating of the particles with polaxamine-908 (Moghimi *et al., 1993*). In another study, Ogawara and co-workers (1999) demonstrated that serum components play an important role in the hepatic disposition of polystyrene particles and the complement C3b and fibronectins are involved as serum opsonins. In a very unique set of studies they tried to identify the entity of several serum opsonins and dysopsonins responsible for the hepatic uptake of polystyrene particles of 50 nm and 500 nm. The results of their studies are summarised:

i. Pretreatment of liver by trypsin significantly suppressed the serum dependent hepatic uptake of both types of particles (50 nm and 500 nm), suggesting that serum components involved in opsonisation are proteinaceous in nature.

ii. Pretreatment of serum with anti-CD3 antibody reduced the promotive effect of serum on the hepatic uptake of 500-nm particles (whereas it was already established that serum in the perfusate inhibited and promoted the hepatic disposition of 50-nm and 500-nm particles at 37°C, respectively). This suggested that complement factor C3b is involved.

iii. Hepatic disposition of both particles at 4°C was reduced by addition of serum in the perfusate. These results could be ascribed to the reduction of the surface hydrophilicity due to the adsorption of serum proteins onto the surface of particles and to resultant decrease in non-specific disposition to the liver.

iv. Pretreatment of the serum by the anti-fibronectin antibody resulted in a significant reduction in the hepatic disposition of 500-nm sised particles, suggesting that fibronectin should also work as opsonin.

v. Inhibition of the hepatic disposition in the presence of serum by the addition of N-acetylgalactosamine into the perfusate, suggesting the possible involvement of lectin in serum-dependent uptake of particles.

vi. Potentiation of hepatic disposition in plasma as compared against serum, suggesting the possible involvement of blood-coagulation factors, such as fibronigen as an opsonin.

From these results, serum is inferred to function both as the opsonin to enhance the hepatic uptake of particles and as an inhibitor by reducing non-specific interaction between particles & serum components (a possible dysopsonic effect). In a very interesting study, Luck and co-workers (1999) analysed the mechanisms for C3 binding to the particle surface and subsequent inactivation by cleavage using two-dimensional electrophoresis (2-DE). It could be demonstrated that 2-DE analysis provides the possibility to distinguish between adsorption and covalent attachment of C3 to particulate surfaces. The findings suggest that covalent binding of the C3 component C3b to the particles' surface caused complement activation. The authors stated that the influence of the incubation medium on the *in vitro* protein adsorption of particulate drug carriers has to be considered when a correlation between the protein adsorption pattern and the *in vivo* behaviour of the particles is to be correlated.

PROTOCOL 19.1

Preparation of Solid Lipid Nanoparticles by Hot Homogenisation

Hot Homogenisation Techniques

Materials

Cetyl palmitate

Poloxamer

(Polyoxyethylene-polyoxypropylene-block copolymer)

Water for injection q.s.

Drug (any lipophilic drug)

Procedure

1. Heat the lipid to 70 °C or above the 5–10 °C of melting point and mix the drug to be encapsulated.

2. Prepare a solution of poloxamer 188 in water for injection and heat it to 70 °C.

3. Disperse the mixture at 70°C with the help of an ultraturrex.

4. Subject the obtained premix for high-pressure homogenisation, adjust temperature to 70 °C.

5. Repeat the cycles at 700 bar.

6. A SLN dispersion will be obtained (Scheme 19.3)

Characterisation of Solid Lipid Nanoparticles

- Particle size and shape
- Surface charge
- Polymorphism and crysallinity
- Drug entrapment and release kinetics
- *In-vivo* behaviour

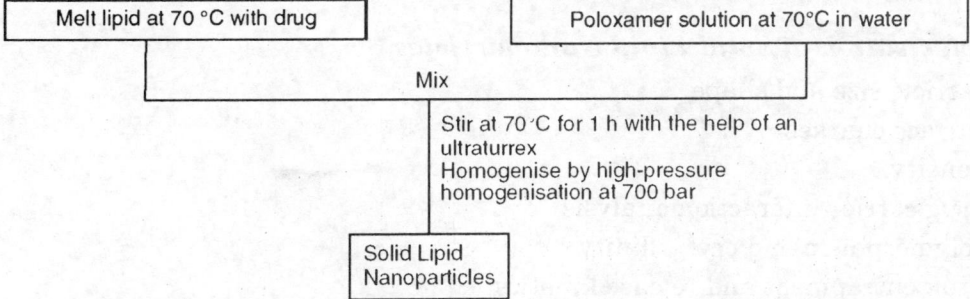

Scheme 19.3: *Preparation of solid lipid nanoparticles by hot homogenisation*

PROTOCOL 19.2

Preparation of Solid Lipid Nanoparticles by Cold Homogenisation

Cold Homogenisation Techniques

Material

Cetyl palmitate
Poloxamer (Polyoxyethylene-polyoxypropylene-block copolymer)
Lipoid S 75
Water for injection q.s.
Drug (any lipophilic drug)

Procedure

1. Dissolve the drug in the melted lipid.

2. Solidify the obtained matrix in liquid nitrogen or dry ice and with a mortar mill grind the matrix up to a fine powder of particle size between 50 μm and 100 μm.

3. Disperse the obtained powder in an aqueous surfactant solution and homogenize at temperatures of approx. 5 to 10°C below the melting point (1500 bar, 10 cycles) (Scheme 19.4).

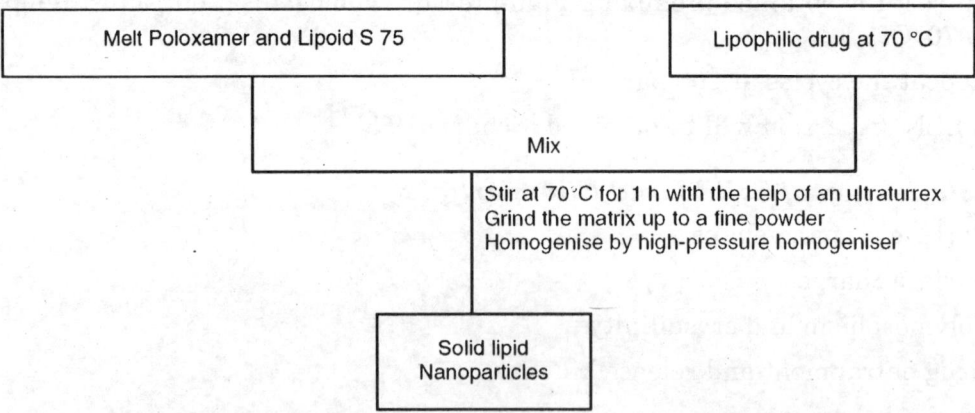

Scheme 19.4.: *Preparation of SLN by cold homogenisation method*

Characterisation of Solid Lipid Nanoparticles

- Particle size and shape
- Surface charges
- Density
- Drug carrier interaction analysis
- Polymorphism and crystallinity
- Drug entrapment and release kinetics
- *In-vivo* behaviour

PROTOCOL 19.3

Preparation of Solid Lipid Nanoparticles by Microemulsion (O/W) Technique

Materials

Stearic acid

Epikuron 200

Sodium taurocholate

Cremophor® EL (polyethoxylated castor oil, average MW 2513)

Sodium hexadecyl phosphate

Drugs (tobramycin; TOB)

Procedure

- Weigh stearic acid (internal phase, 0.7 mmol), Epikuron 200 (surfactant, 0.14 mmol), sodium taurocholate (cosurfactant, 0.69 mmol) water (111.1 mmol) and TOB (0.026 mmol) as ion-pair complex.
- Dissolve mixture completely in hexadecyl phosphate at (1:2 ratio of mixture: hexadecyl phosphate) in water bath at 50 °C.
- Pour the resultant organic solution into double filtered cold water (2–3 °C) at a 1:5 microemulsion: water (v/v) ratio under mechanical stirring.
- Adjust the pH value of the acidic aqueous phase to 1.10 by addition of 0.1 M hydrochloric acid.
- Wash three times by diaultrafiltration (Diaflo YM 100 membrane, cut off MW 100000 Da)
- Centrifuge the entire dispersed system (4000 rpm for 10 min,) and re-suspend in distilled water. Lyophilise the resultant dispersion to get dried powder (Scheme 19.5).

PROTOCOL 19.4

Preparation of Solid Lipid Nanoparticles with Clobetasol Propionate by Solvent Diffusion Method

Materials

Monostearin as lipid material of SLN

Polyvinyl alcohol (PVA) as a dispersing agent in water phase.

Procedure

- Weigh monostearin (396 mg) and drug (clobetasol propionate, 4 mg)
- Dissolve completely in a mixture of acetone (12 ml) and ethanol (12 ml) in water bath at 50 °C.
- Pour the resultant organic solution into 240 ml of an acidic aqueous phase containing 1% PVA (w/v) under mechanical agitation with 400 rpm at room temperature for 5 min.

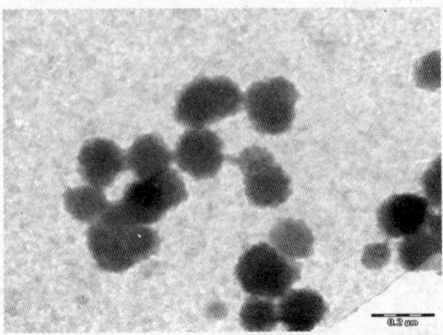

Fig 19.3: *TEM photograph of different MTX-loaded SLNs formulations (stabilised by 1% w/w soya lecithin)*

- Adjust the pH value of the acidic aqueous phase to 1.10 by addition of 0.1 M hydrochloric acid.
- The SLN suspension will be quickly produced.
- Centrifuge the entire dispersed system (4000 rpm for 10 min,) and re-suspend in distilled water. Lyophilise the resultant dispersion to get dried powder.

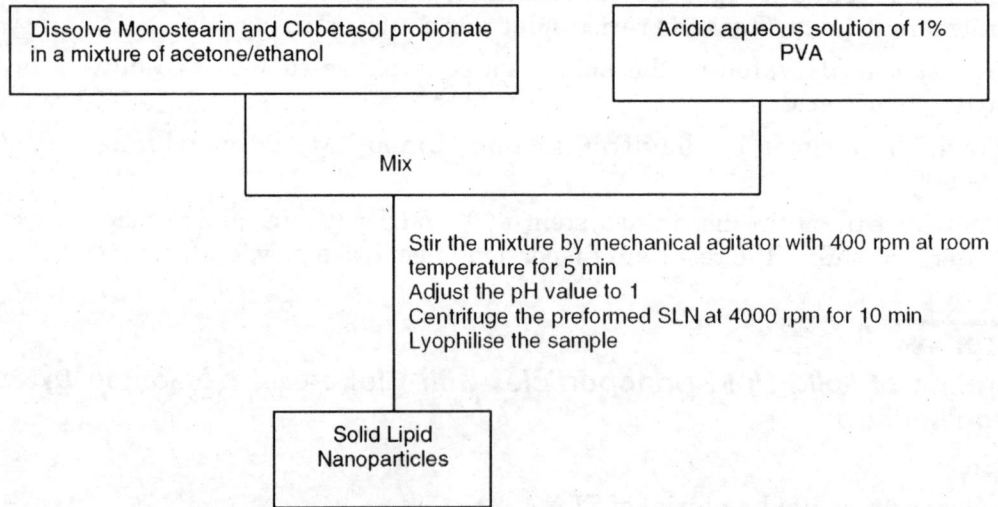

Scheme 19.5.: *Preparation of SLN by solvent diffusion method*

Lyophilisation of SLN Dispersion

Keep SLN dispersion (1.0% of lipid content, w/v) under −75 °C in a deep-freeze for 5 h and then move the samples to the freeze-drier. Lyophilise for 72 h to get the SLN powder.

Recovery of SLN

The recovery of SLN is defined as the weight ratio of the freeze-dried SLN to the initial loading of monostearin and drug and can be calculated from.

Recovery=analysed weight of SLN ×100/theoretical weight of SLN

Morphological Examination

For morphological examination of the SLNs, transmission electron microscopy (TEM) is usually perform. Stain the samples with 2% (w/v) phosphotungstic acid and place on copper grids with films for viewing by TEM (Fig. 19.3).

Mean Diameter and Zeta Potential

It is determined with Zetasiser (Malvern, UK). Dilute the suspension 20 times with the original dispersion medium of preparation for size determination while use undiluted sample for the determination of zeta potential.

Drug Content

Dissolve the freeze dried SLNs in ethanol under water bath at 65 °C for 30 min and then cool to room temperature, to preferentially precipitate the lipid. Measure the drug content in the supernatant after centrifugation (4000 rpm for 15 min) using suitable method, spectrophotometrically or by means of a HPLC method.

Drug recovery =analysed weight of drug in SLNs×100/theoretical weight of drug loaded in system

Drug content=analysed weight of drug in SLNs×100/analysed weight of SLN.

PROTOCOL 19.5

Production of Lipospheres (LS) by Melt Dispersion Technique, Solvent Evaporation or w/o/w Double Emulsion Method

Melt Dispersion Technique

- Weigh five grams of a lipidic mixture, with/without 200 mg of lipophilic model drug and melt at 70°C then emulsify into 150 ml of an external aqueous phase containing a suitable surfactant.
- Eight natural or synthetic emulsifiers were employed, namely gelatin (200 bloom), pectin, carrageenan, PVA, polyoxyethylene 20 sorbitan trioleate (polysorbate 85, tween 85) and lauryl sarcosine.
- Stir the emulsion using a mechanical stirrer equipped with a three-blade rotor with a diameter of 55mm.
- Then heat the emulsion to the same temperature as the melted lipidic phase. Cool the milky formulation rapidly to about 20°C by immersing the formulation flask in a cool water bath without stopping the agitation to yield a uniform dispersion of LS. Wash the obtained LS with water and isolate by filtration through a paper filter.

Solvent Evaporation Technique

- Dissolve five grams of the lipid matrix in 10 ml of ethyl acetate at 50°C.

- Emulsify in 150 ml of an external aqueous phase containing the surfactant agent using a mechanical stirrer.
- Stir the resulting oil-in-water emulsion for 6–8 h under ambient conditions to allow the solvent evaporation.
- Collect the liposheres by filtration through a paper filter.

PROTOCOL 19.6

Preparation of MTO-SLN by Film Dispersion–Ultrasonication Method

Materials

Mitoxantrone (MTO)

Compritol®888 ATO,

Lecithin

Polyoxyl (40) stearate (S-40i),

Pluronic F68,

Tween 80 and 60

Procedure

- Dissolve lecithin and Compritol®888 in 5mL chloroform
- Evaporate the above solution under reduced pressure to form a thin layer of uniform film at the bottom of the bottle
- Add 10 ml of aqueous phase containing surfactant S-40 and MTO
- Sonicate the resultant lipid dispersion for several minutes to get MTO-SLN.

Use the amounts of Compritol®888, lecithin, S-40 and MTO as the tested variables or independent variables, and encapsulation yield (EY), drug content (DC) and *in vitro* cumulative release rate (Q_t at time t) as the evaluation indexes.

PROTOCOL: 19.7

Preparation of Semisolid SLN Dispersion by One Step Production Process

Materials

Compritol 888 ATO

Miglylol 812 (caprylic:capric triglycerides)

Retinol

Procedure

- Weigh compritol, miglylol lipidic mixture with/without retinol and melt at 85°C then disperse into external aqueous phase containing a suitable surfactant
- Stir the emulsion using a mechanical stirrer and pass through a Lab 40 high-pressure homogeniser (500 bar, 3 cycles)
- Then heat the emulsion to the same temperature as the melted lipidic phase. Cool the milky formulation rapidly to about 20°C by immersing the formulation flask in a

cool water bath without stopping the agitation to yield a uniform dispersion of SLN as nanoemulsion

- Wash the obtained SLNs with water and isolate by filtration through a paper filter.

PROTOCOL 19.8

Preparation of Cationic SLN by a Solvent Emulsification/Evaporation Technique

Materials

Precirol® ATO
DOTAP
Tween 80

Procedure

- Dissolve Precirol® ATO in dichloromethane (5%, w/v) then emulsify into an external aqueous phase containing cationic lipid DOTAP (0.1–0.4%) and the surfactant Tween 80 (0.4–0.1%).
- Sonicate the resultant emulsion for 0.5–1.0 min at 50W
- Evaporate the organic solvent from above mixture under reduced pressure with agitation to get SLN particles
- Wash SLNs by centrifugation (3000 rpm, 20 min, three times)

SUGGESTED READINGS

- Almeida, A.J. Runge, S. Muller, R.H. (1997) Int. J. Pharm. 149, 255–265.
- Absolom, D. R. (1986) Methods Enzymol., 132, 281–318.
- Bunjes, H., Koch, M.H.J., and Westesen, K., (2000) Langmuir, 16, 5234.
- Bunjes, H., Westesen, K., and Koch, M.H.J. (1996) Int. J. Pharm., 129, 159.
- Hu, F.Q. Yuan, H. Zhang, H.H. Fang, M. (2002) Int. J. Pharm. 239, 121–128.
- Finsey, R., (1994) Adv. Colloid Interface Sci. 52, 79.
- Freitas, C. and Müller, R.H., (1999) Eur. J. Pharm. Biopharm. 47, 125.
- Garti, N. and Sato, K., Crystallisation and Polymorphism of Fats and Fatty Acids, Marcel Dekker, New York, 1988.
- Illum, L. and Davis, S.S. (1983) J. Pharm. Sci., 72, 1086–1090.
- Illum, L. and Davis, S.S. (1984) FEBS Lett. 167, 79–82.
- Illum, L. and Davis, S.S. (1986) Int. J. Pharm., 29, 53.
- Illum, L., Davis, S.S., Muller, R.H., Mak, E. and West, P. (1987) Life Sci., 40, 367–374.
- Illum, L., Jones, P.D.E., Baldwin, R.W. and Davis, S.S. (1984) Microspheres and drug therapy: pharmaceutical, immunological and medical aspects (Davis, S.S., Illum, L., Mcvie, J.G. and Tomlinson, E., Eds.), Elsevier, Amsterdam, 353–363.
- Jores, K., Mehnert, W., and Mäder, K., (2003) Pharm. Res., 20, 1274.
- Kreuter, J. (1983) Int. J. Pharm., 14, 43–58.

- Kreuter, J. (1994) Eur. J. Drug Metab. Pharmacokinet., 19, 253–256.
- Kreuter, J. and Haenzel, I. (1978) Infect. Immun., 19, 667–675.
- Kreuter, J. and Speiser, P. (1976) J. Pharm. Sci., 65, 1624–1627.
- Kreuter, J., Alyautdin, R.N., Kharkevich, D.A. and Ivanov, A.A. (1995) Brain Res., 674, 171–174.
- Kreuter, J., Berg, U., Liehl, E., Soiva, M. and Speiser, P.P. (1986) Vaccine, 4, 125–129.
- Kreuter, J., in: Kreuter, J. (Ed.) Colloidal drug delivery systems, Marcel Dekker, New York, 1994, 219–343.
- Kreuter, J., Liehl, E., Berg, U., Soiva, M. and Speiser, P.P. (1988) Vaccine, 6, 253–256.
- Kreuter, J., Nanoparticle-Based Drug Delivery Systems, (1991) J Control Rel. 16, 169.
- Kreuter, J., Stieneker, F. and Lower, J. (1991) Proc. Int. Symp. Controlled Release Bioact. Mater., 18, 277–278.
- Lippacher, Muller, R.H. Mader, K. (2001) Int. J. Pharm., 214, 9–12.
- Lu, B, Xiong, S.B., Yang, H., Yin, X.D., Chao, R.B. (2006) Eur. J. Pharma Sci., 28, 86–95.
- Luck, M., Schroder, W., Paulke, B.R., Blunk, T. and Muller, R.H. (1999) Biomaterials, 20, 2063–2068.
- Trotta, M., Debernardi, F., Caputo, O., (2003) Int. J. Pharm. 257, 153–160.
- Gasco, M.R., (1993) US Patent No. 5250236.
- Gasco, M.R (1997) Pharm. Technol. Eur. 9, 52–58.
- Magenheim, M.Y. Levy, S. Benita, (1993) Int. J. Pharm. 94, 115–123.
- Mehnert, W., Mader, K., (2001) Adv. Drug Deliv. Rev. 47, 165–196.
- Meyer, O., Kirpotin, D., Hong, K.L., Sternberg, B., Park, J.W., Woodle, M.C., Papahadjopoulos, D., (1998) J. Biol. Chem. 273, 15621–15627.
- Middaugh, C.R., Evans, R.K., Montgomery, D.L., Casimiro, D.R., (1998) J. Pharm. Sci. 87, 130–146.
- Moghimi, S.M. and Patel, H.M. (1989) Biochim. Biophys. Acta, 984, 379–383.
- Moghimi, S.M. and Patel, H.M., (1998) Adv. Drug Deliv. Rev. 32, 45–60.
- Moghimi, S.M., Muir, I.S., Illum, L., Davis, S.S., Kolb-Bachofen, V. (1993) Biochim. Biophys. Acta, 1179, 157–165.
- Ogawara, K., Yoshida, M., Kubo, J., Mnishikawa, M., Takakura, Y., Hashida, M., Higaki, K. And Kimura, T. (1999) J. Control. Rel., 61, 241–250.
- Cavalli, R., Marengo, E. Rodriguez L., Gasco M.R. (1996) Eur. J. Pharm. Biopharm. 43, 110–115.
- Miiller, R.H. Lucks J.S., (1996) European Patent No. 0605497,
- Miiller, R.H. Maaben S., Weyhers, H. Specht, F. Lucks J.S, (1995) Pharm. Res. 12, 39–48.
- Miiller R.H., Mehnert W., Lucks, J.S. Schwarz, C. zur Miihlen, A. Weyhers, H Freitas, C. Riihl, D. (1995) Eur. J. Pharm. Bio-pharm. 41, 62–69.
- Cortesi, R, Esposito, E Luca, G, Nastruzz, C. (2002) Biomaterials 23, 2283–2294.
- Santos Maia, C., Mehnert, W., and Schäfer-Korting, M., (2000) Int. J. Pharm., 196, 165.
- Siekmann, B. and Westesen, K., (1996) Eur. J. Pharm. Biopharm. 43, 104.
- Siekmann, B. and Westesen, K., (1994) Pharm. Pharmacol. Lett. 3, 225.
- Storhoff, J.J. and Mirkin, C.A. (1999) Chem. Rev., 99, 1849-1862.
- Jenning , V., Thunemann A. F., Gohla S. H. (2000) Int J Pharm 199, 167–177.

- Vyas, S.P. and Malaiya, A. (1989) J. Microencaps., 6, 493–499.
- Vyas, S.P. and Sihorkar, V. (2000) Adv. Drug Deliv. Rev., 43, 101–164.
- Washington, C., Photon correlation spectroscopy, in Particle Size Analysis in Pharmaceutics and Other Industries, Ellis Horwood, New York, 1992, 135.
- Westesen, K., Bunjes H., and Koch, M.H.J., (1997) J. Controlled Rel. 48, 223.
- Mei, Z. Chen, H. Weng, T. Yang, Y. Yang X. (2003) Eur J Pharm Biopharm 56, 189–196.
- Zur Muhlen, E. zur Muhlen, H. Niehus, W. Mehnert, (1996) Pharm. Res. 13, 1411–1416.
- Zur Muhlen, C. Schwarz, W. Mehnert, (1998) Eur. J. Pharm. Biopharm. 45, 149–155.
- Zur Muhlen, W. Mehnert, (1998) Pharmazie 53, 552.

20
Drug Conjugates

The technology of bioconjugation has affected nearly every discipline in the life sciences. It includes the linking of two or more molecules to form a novel complex having the combined properties of its individual components. Natural or synthetic compounds with their individual activities can be chemically combined to create unique substances possessing carefully engineered characteristics. The application of the available crosslinking reactions and reagent systems for creating novel conjugates with peculiar activities has made possible the assay of minute quantities of substances, the *in vivo* targeting of molecules, and the modulation of specific biological processes. Modified or conjugated molecules have been used for purification, detection or localisation of specific cellular components, and in the treatment of diseases.

Crosslinking and modifying agents produced with the help of conjugation techniques can be applied to alter the native state and function of peptides and proteins, sugars and polysaccharides, nucleic acids and oligonucleotides, lipids and almost any other imaginable molecule that can be chemically derivatised. The structure and function of natural and synthetic molecules can be investigated and receptor-ligand interactions can be revealed with the help of modification or conjugation strategies.

BIOCONJUGATE CHEMISTRY

Modification and conjugation techniques are based on two interrelated chemical reactions; the reactive functional groups present on the various crosslinking or derivatising reagents and functional groups present on the target macromolecules to be modified. Without both types of functional groups being available and chemically compatible, the process of derivatisation would be impossible. Reactive functional groups on crosslinking reagents, tags and probes provide the means to label specifically certain target groups on ligands, peptides, proteins, carbohydrates, lipids, synthetic polymers, nucleic acids, and oligonucleotides. Knowledge of the basic mechanisms by which the reactive groups couple to target functional groups provide the means to design intelligently a modification or conjugation strategy. Choosing the correct reagent systems that can react with the chemical groups available on target molecules constitute the basis for successful chemical modification (Hermanson, 1996).

BIOCONJUGATE REAGENTS

The principal reactive functional groups commonly present on bioconjugate reagents are now commercially available. These reagents are used to solve almost any conceivable modification or conjugation problem.

Zero-length crosslinkers are smallest available reagent systems for bioconjugation. These compounds mediate the conjugation of two molecules by forming a bond containing no additional atoms. Thus, one atom of a molecule is covalently attached to an atom of a second molecule with no intervening linker or spacer. In many conjugation schemes, the final complex is bound together by virtue of chemical components that add foreign structures to the substances being crosslinked, i.e. EDC [1-Ethyl-3-(3-dimethylaminopropyl)carbod iimide hydrochloride], EDC plus N-Hydroxysulphosuccinimide, CMC[1-Cyclohexyl-3-(2-morpho-linoethyl) carbodiimide], N,N' -Carbonyldiimidazole(Chu *et al., 1986;* Ghose *et al., 1990).*

Homobifunctional crosslinkers are used for modification and conjugation of macromolecules consisted of bioreactive compounds containing the same functional group at both ends. Most of these homobifunctional reagents are symmetrical in design with a carbon chain spacer connecting the two identical reactive ends, i.e. formaldehyde, glutaraldehyde, carbohydrazide, DST (disuccinimidyl tartarate), etc.

Heterobifunctional crosslinkers contain two different reactive groups that can couple to two different functional targets on macromolecules, the result is the ability to direct the crosslinking reaction to selected parts of target molecules, thus guiding better control over the conjugation process, i.e. SPDP [(N-Succinimidyl 3 - (2-pyridyldithio) propionate], ABH [p-Azidobenzoyl hydrazide], APG [p-Azidophenyl glyoxal], etc.

Trifunctional crosslinkers are relatively new form of conjugation reagents, possessing three different reactive or complexing groups per molecule, i.e. 4-Azido-2-nitrophenyl-biocytin-4-nitrophenyl ester.

Tags and probes are relatively small modifying agents and are used to label proteins, nucleic acids, and other molecules. These compounds often contain groups that provide sensitive detectability by virtue of some intrinsic chemical or atomic property such as fluorescence, visible chromogenic character, radioactivity, or bioaffinity towards another protein. Most probes can be designed to contain a reactive portion capable of coupling to the functional groups of biomolecules. After modification of a protein via this reactive part, the probe becomes permanently attached, thus intact tagging it with a unique detectable property. Subsequent interactions that the protein is allowed to undergo can be followed through tags visibility, i.e. fluorescent labels such as fluorescein derivatives, rhodamin derivatives; biotinylation reagents such as D-biotin, biotin-hydrazide, photobiotin; iodination reagents such as chloramine-T, Iodo-beads, Iodo-Gen.

BIOCONJUGATE APPLICATIONS

Bioconjugation techniques are used in the preparation of unique conjugates and labelled molecules for use in particular application areas. These include hapten-carrier immunogen conjugates and antibody-enzyme conjugates.

Hapten-carrier immunogen conjugates, i.e. carbodiimides mediated hapten carrier conjugates and glutaraldehyde mediated hapten carrier conjugates, are used in antibody production, in immune response research and in the creation of vaccines.

Antibody-enzyme conjugates, i.e. NHS ester-maleimide-mediated conjugates, glutaraldehyde mediated conjugates are used in immunoassays, targeting and detection techniques. The development of enzyme-linked immunosorbent assay (ELISA) systems and the ability to make conjugates of specific antibodies with enzymes has provided the means to quantify or detect hundreds of important analytes. The use of enzymes as labels in immunoassay procedures surpassed radioactive tags as the means of detection, primarily due to the long-term stability potential of an enzyme system and the hazards and waste problems associated with radioisotopes.

In addition to labelling immunoglobulins with enzymes to provide detectability through their catalytic action on a substrate, antibody molecules also can be labelled or tagged with small compounds that can provide indigenous traceable properties. Labelled antibodies, i.e. fluorescently labelled antibodies, radiolabelled antibodies and biotinylated antibodies are also having immense uses in immunoassays, targeting and detection techniques. Antibody-liposomes conjugates may possess encapsulated components that can be used for detection of therapy. Liposomes possessing antibodies directed against tumour cell antigens can deliver encapsulated toxins or drugs to the associated cancer cells, affecting toxicity and cell death (Fig. 20.1). Biotin, avidin and proteins can also be appended onto the surface of liposomes with the help of various conjugation techniques for different, however specific therapeutic applications.

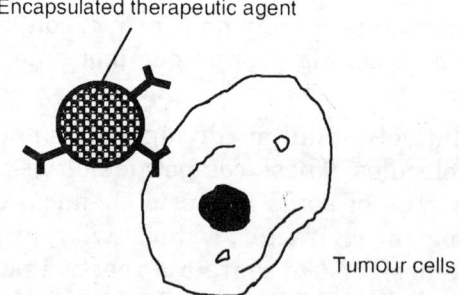

Encapsulated therapeutic agent

Tumour cells

Fig. 20.1. *Antibody-liposomes immunotherapeutic system*

Avidin or streptavidin conjugates are used in immunoassays. The specificity of antibody molecules provides the targeting capability to recognise and bind particular antigen molecules. If there are biotin labels on the antibody molecule, it creates multiple sites for binding of avidin and streptavidin. If avidin or streptavidin in turn labelled with an enzyme, fluorophore, etc., then a very sensitive antigen-detection system is created. The potential for more than one labelled avidin to become attached to each antibody through its multiple biotinylation sites is the key to dramatic increase in assay sensitivity over that obtained through the use of antibodies directly labelled with a detectable tag (Fig. 20.2).

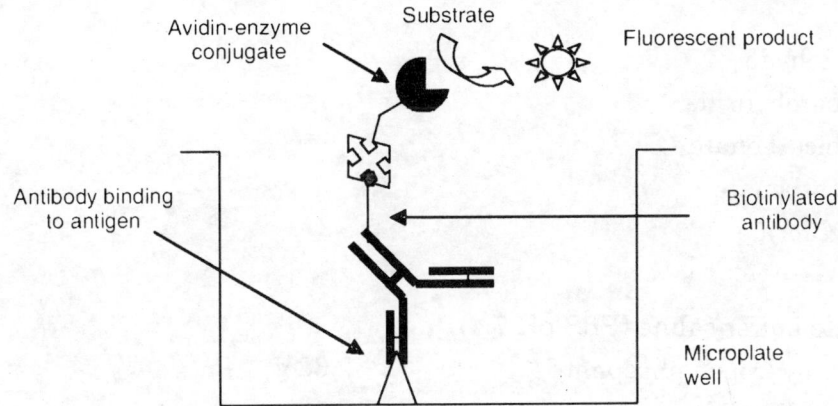

Fig. 20.2. *The basic design of the labelled avidin-biotin (LAB) assay system*

Enzymatic labelling of DNA and chemical modification of nucleic acids and oligo-nucleotides can be done effectively with the help of bioconjugation techniques. To modify the unique chemical groups on nucleic acids, novel methods have been developed which allow derivatisation through discrete sites on the available bases, sugars, or phosphate groups. These conjugation methods can be used to add a functional group or a label to an individual nucleotide or to one or more sites in oligonucleotide probes or full-sized DNA or RNA polymers.

PROTOCOL 20.1

Glutaraldehyde Based Hapten-Carrier Conjugation

In bioconjugation techniques, glutaraldehyde is used as homobifunctional crosslinking reagent in one or two step conjugation procedure to prepare hapten-carrier conjugates. Glutaraldehyde reacts with primary amino groups to create Schiff bases or double-bond addition product. The conjugates formed in the reaction of glutaraldehyde with protein carriers and peptide haptens are usually of high molecular weight and may cause precipitation products. Various types of procedures are discussed in the literature to form glutaraldehyde conjugates. In some methods neutral pH environment in phosphate buffer (pH 6.8–7.4) is used while in others alkaline conditions in carbonate buffer (pH 8–9) are used. In general, the higher pH conditions will be more effective to form Schiff base intermediates and result in greater conjugation yields with higher molecular weight conjugates. One step glutaraldehyde method is utilised in the following procedure in which by varying the pH and the amount of glutaraldehyde added to the reaction, the yield and molecular weight of the conjugate formed could be controlled.

Materials, Chemicals and Buffers

Materials

For column separations, following pre-poured column can be used:

For 1.25 ml to 2.5 ml sample volumes: Sephadex G-50.

Chemicals

Glutaraldehyde

Sodium borohydride

Sodium bicarbonate

Sodium carbonate

Sodium chloride

Buffers

Phosphate buffer saline (PBS pH 7.4)

Disodium hydrogen phosphate	2.38 g
Potassium dihydrogen phosphate	0.19 g
Sodium chloride	8.0 g
Distilled water	to 1000 ml

Procedure

- Dissolve carrier protein (or another carrier that contains amino groups) in 0.1 M sodium carbonate, 0.15 M NaCl, pH 8.5, at a concentration of 2 mg/ml.

- Add peptide hapten to the carrier solution to obtain a concentration of about 2 mg/ml. Determine, the molar ratio of peptide to carrier. 20:1 to 40:1 (peptide: carrier) ratio result in good immunogens.

- Add fresh glutaraldehyde and thoroughly mixed with the peptide/carrier solution to obtain a 1% final concentration. Allow to react for 2–4 hours at 4°C.

- Mix the solution periodically on a rotary flask shaker. (Caution: Use of fume hood is recommended when working with glutaraldehyde. Avoid contact with skin and clothing.)

- The conjugation may be stabilised by the addition of a reductant, e.g. sodium borohydride or sodium cynoborohydride which is usually recommended for specific reduction of Schiff bases, but since the conjugate has already been formed at this point, sodium borohydride reduces the Schiff bases and eliminates any remaining aldehyde group as well. Add sodium borohydride to the final concentration of 10 mg/ml and allow to react for 1 hour at 4°C.

- Finally, purify conjugate by gel electrophoresis using Sephadex G-25 or dialysis to remove excess reagent. Some precipitation may occur in the final product due to the presence of high molecular weight conjugates. If turbidity is evident, dialyse against PBS at pH 7.4 instead of gel filtering.

Conjugation of Proteins to Liposomes

Conjugation of liposomes with proteins may be done through reactive functional groups on the head groups of phospholipids with homobifunctional or heterobifunctional crosslinking reagents, with carbodiimides, by reductive amination, by NHS ester activation of carboxylates, or through the noncovalent use of avidin-biotin interaction. The resultant protein-liposomes composition is highly dependent on the size of each liposome, the amount of protein charged to the reaction, and the **molar** quantity of reactive lipid present in the bilayer construction. Liposome protein coupling occasionally induces vesicle aggregation due to unique properties or concentration of the protein used, or it may be a result of liposome to liposome crosslinking during the conjugation process hence amount of protein charged to the reaction has to be adjusted to solve an aggregation problem (Scheme 20.1).

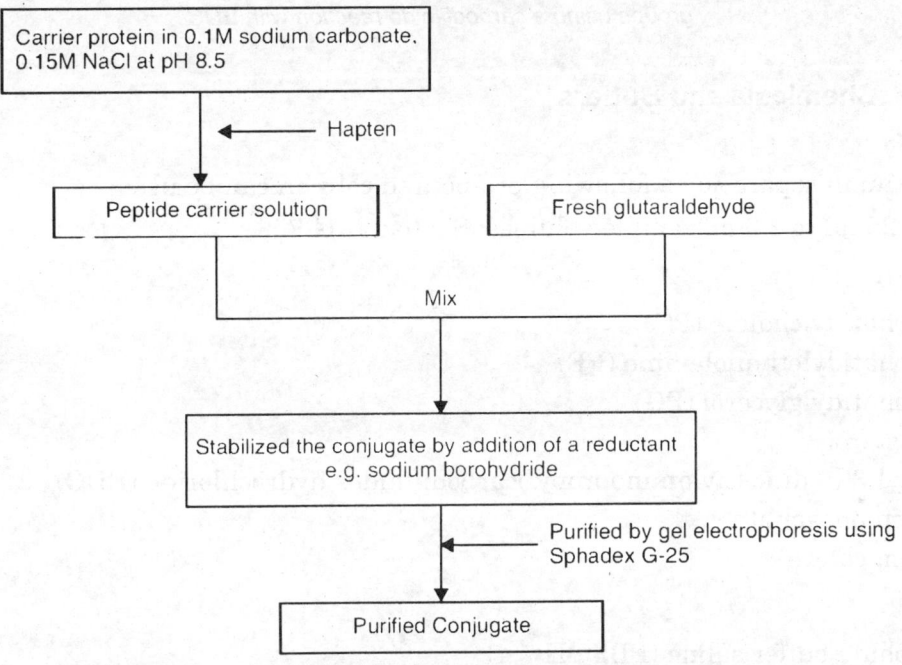

Scheme 20.1: *Glutaraldehyde based hapten-carrier conjugation*

PROTOCOL 20.2

Carbodiimide Based Conjugation to Phosphatidylethanolamine Lipid Derivatives

Liposomal membrane is composed of underivatised PE that contains an amino group that participates in the carbodiimide reaction with carboxylate groups of proteins. Carboxylate groups are activated by water-soluble carbodiimide EDC to form active ester intermediate that can react with PE to form an amide linkage (Fig. 20.3). (Hoare and Koshland, 1966, Chu *et al*, 1986, Ghose *et al,* 1990) Unfortunately, since abundance of both amide and carboxylates present on proteins, EDC coupling of proteins to the surface of liposomes often results in considerable protein to protein crosslinking. Sometimes vesicle aggregation also occurs due to protein coupling to more than one liposomes. This polymerisation problem can be avoided by first blocking the amino groups of the protein with citraconic acid, which has been used successfully with antibodies.

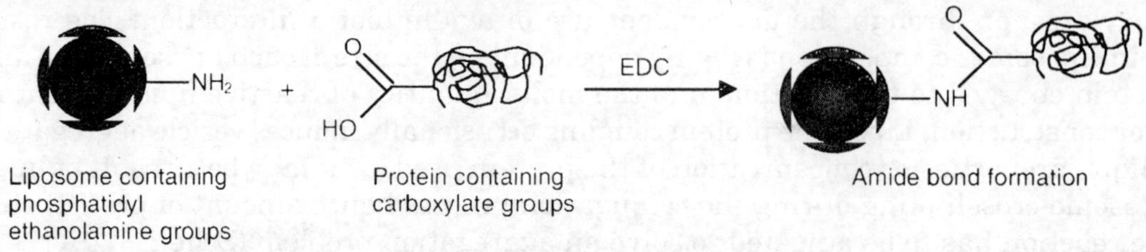

Liposome containing
phosphatidyl
ethanolamine groups

Protein containing
carboxylate groups

Amide bond formation

Fig. 20.3. Reaction showing the conjugation of protein with a liposome containing PE groups using a carbodiimide reaction with EDC

Materials, Chemicals and Buffers

Materials

For column separations, following pre-poured column can be used:

For 1.25 ml to 2.5 ml sample volumes: Sephadex G-75.

Chemicals

Phosphatidylcholine (PC)

Phosphatidylethanolamine (PE)

Phosphatidylglycerol (PG)

Cholesterol

1-Ethyl-3-(3-dimethylaminopropyl)carbodiimides hydrochloride (EDC)

Sodium phosphate

Sodium chloride

Buffers

Phosphate buffer saline (PBS pH 7.4)	
Disodium hydrogen phosphate	2.38 g
Potassium dihydrogen phosphate	0.19 g
Sodium chloride	8.0 g
Distilled water	to 1000 ml

Procedure

- Prepare liposomal suspension containing PE by mixing PC: cholesterol: PG: PE in a molar ratio of 8:10:1:1 by any suitable method.

- Adjust the concentration to about 5 mg lipid/ml buffers. The final liposomal suspension should be in 10 mM sodium phosphate, 0.15 M NaCl, pH 7.4.

- Dissolve the protein in PBS, pH 7.4, and add an aliquot to the liposomal suspension. The amount of protein to be added can vary considerably, depending on the abundance of protein and the desired final density required. From 1mg protein/ml to 20 mg protein/ml liposome suspension can be reacted.

- Add 10 mg EDC/ml of lipid/protein mixture and solubilised using a vortex mixer. Allow to react for 2 hours at room temperature. Scale back the amount of EDC added to the reaction if liposomes aggregation or protein precipitation occurs during the crosslinking process.
- Purify the conjugate by gel filtration using a column of Sephadex G-75.

PROTOCOL 20.3

Glutaraldehyde Based Conjugation to Phosphatidylethanolamine Lipid Derivatives

Glutaraldehyde, a homobifunctional crosslinker reacts with PE residues present on the liposome surface to form an activated surface reactive aldehyde group. A two-step conjugation reaction via glutaraldehyde is a suitable method when working with liposomes, since precipitated protein would be difficult to remove from vesicle suspension (Fig. 20.4).

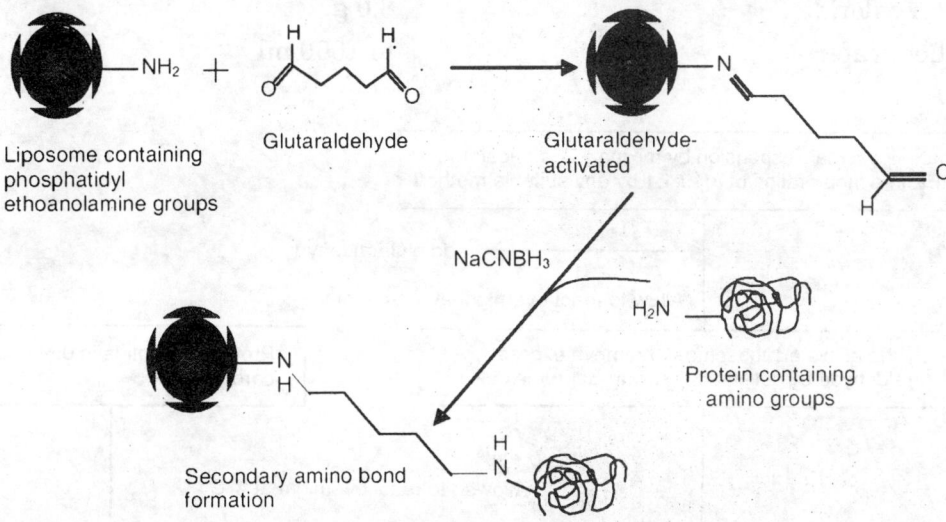

Fig. 20.4. *Reaction showing glutaraldehyde activation of PE-containing liposomes used to couple protein molecules*

Materials, Chemicals and Buffers
Materials

For column separations, following column can be used:

For 1.25 ml to 2.5 ml sample volumes: PD-10 (Sephadex G-50).

Chemicals

Phosphatidylcholine

Phosphatidylethanolamine

Phosphatidylglycerol

Cholesterol

Glutaraldehyde

Sodium borohydride

Sodium bicarbonate

Sodium carbonate

Sodium chloride

Buffer

Phosphate buffer saline (PBS pH 6.8)

Disodium hydrogen phosphate	2.80 g
Potassium dihydrogen phosphate	0.19 g
Sodium chloride	8.0 g
Distilled water	to 1000 ml

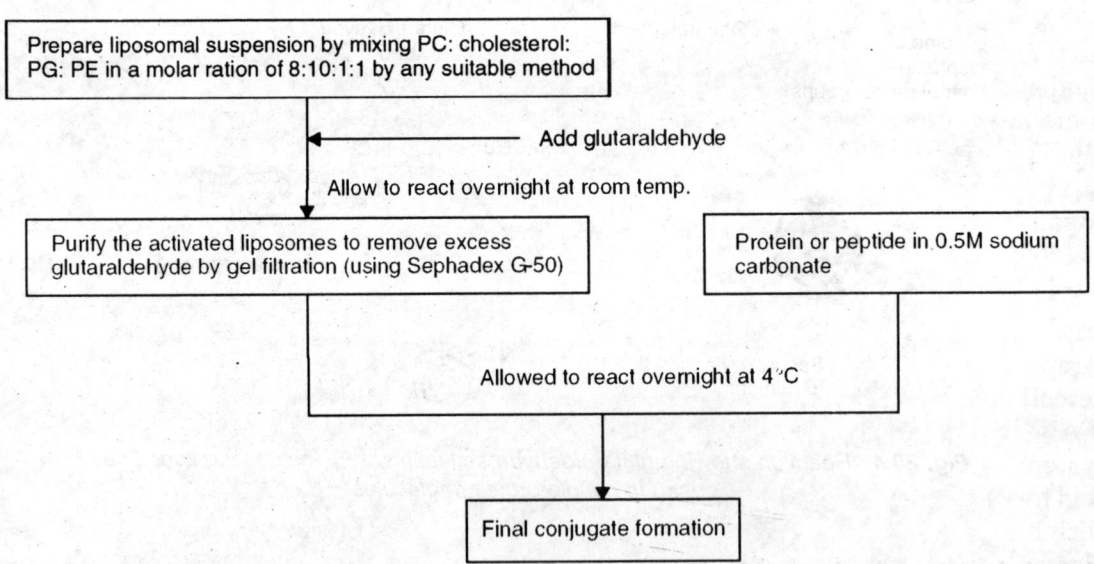

Scheme 20.2: *Formation of glutaraldehyde based conjugation to phosphatidylethanolamide lipid derivatives*

Procedure

- Prepare liposomal suspension containing PE by mixing PC: cholesterol: PG: PE in a molar ratio of 8:10:1:1 by any suitable method.

- Adjust the concentration to about 5 mg lipid/ml buffer. The final liposomal suspension should be in 10 mM sodium phosphate, 0.15 M NaCl, pH 7.2.

- Add glutaraldehyde to the liposomal suspension to obtain final concentration of 1.25% v/v and allow to react overnight at room temperature under a nitrogen blanket.

- Purify the activated liposomes to remove excess glutaraldehyde by gel filtration (using Sephadex G-50) or by dialysis against PBS, pH 6.8.
- Prepare protein or peptide solution in 0.5 M sodium carbonate (pH 9.5) at a concentration of 10 mg/ml.
- Mix this protein or peptide solution with activated liposomal suspension for conjugation reaction to be accomplished.
- Usually 4 mg of protein per milligram of total lipid is required for acceptable conjugation.
- Allow to react overnight at 4°C under an atmosphere of nitrogen.
- Add sodium borohydride to the final concentration of 10 mg/ml for reduction of resultant Schiff bases and any excess of aldehyde (Scheme 20.2).

Avidin-Biotin System

Avidin-biotin system is one of the most popular conjugation techniques of noncovalent conjugation, which is used, in specific targeting applications and assay designs. Avidin is a glycoprotein that contains four identical subunits and each subunit contains one binding site for biotin and one for oligosaccharide modification. This interaction may be used to enhance the signal strength of immunoassay systems. The only disadvantage is the tendency of avidin molecule to bind non-specifically to the components other than biotin due to its high pI (isoelectric point) and carbohydrate content. Streptavidin is another biotin binding protein isolated from *Streptomyces avidinii* having less nonspecificities of avidin. Streptavidin, similar to avidin, contains four subunits, each with a single biotin-binding site. Avidin and streptavidin are used in bioconjugation techniques to conjugate other proteins or label with various detection reagents without loss of biotin binding activity.

There are various basic immunoassays based on avidin-biotin interaction. Biotinylated antibody creates multiple sites for the binding of avidin or streptavidin. If avidin or streptavidin is labelled with enzyme or fluorophore, etc. then a very sensitive antigen detection system can be created. Some of the assay systems are, labelled avidin-biotin (LAB) assay system, bridged avidin-biotin system (BRAB), and avidin-biotin complex (ABC) system. Similar techniques are used to develop avidin-biotin system for detection of nucleic acid hybridisation in which avidin labelled complexes are used to detect DNA probes labelled with biotin after binding with their complementary DNA target. Avidin-biotin system can also be used in the nonenzyme assay systems in which labelled avidin molecules can be utilised for detection of biotinylated molecule after it has bound to its target. Similarly, in radioimmunoassay designs, radiolabelled avidin can be employed as a universal detection reagent. In the tumour imaging techniques, avidin labelled ^{125}I can be used to localise biotinylated monoclonal antibodies directed against tumour cells *in vivo*.

PROTOCOL 20.4

Preparation of Avidin-HRP or Streptavidin-HRP Conjugates

Horseradish peroxidase can be conjugated with avidin or streptavidin by periodate oxidation and reductive amination. Periodate oxidation of polysaccharide components of the glycoprotein molecule (HRP and avidin) produces reactive aldehyde groups. Another protein (biotin) can be conjugated with these reactive aldehyde groups by reacting the aldehyde with amines to form Schiff bases with subsequent reduction using sodium cynoborohydride to create stable secondary amino bonds (Fig. 20.5).

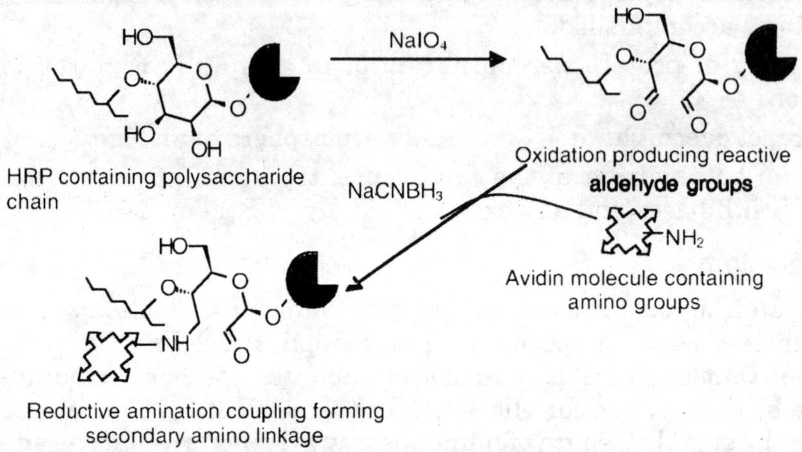

Fig. 20.5. *Schematic diagram showing the conjugation of HRP with avidine by the process of reductive amination and periodate oxidation*

Materials and Chemicals

Materials

For column separations, following pre-poured column can be used:

For 1.25 ml to 2.5 ml sample volumes: Sephadex G-25.

Chemicals

Horseradish peroxidase (HRP)

Sodium periodate

Ethanolamine

Sodium cynoborohydride

Sodium bicarbonate

Sodium phosphate

Sodium carbonate

Sodium chloride

Procedure

- Dissolve HRP in water or 0.01 M NaCl, pH 7.2, at a concentration of 10–20 mg/ml. Prepare sodium periodate solution in water at a concentration of 0.088 M. It must be protected from light.

- Immediately, add 100 µl of sodium periodate solution and mix to each ml of the HRP solution.
- Allow to react in the dark for 20 minutes at room temperature. As the reaction proceeds, the colour changes will be apparent from brownish/gold to green (Scheme 20.3).

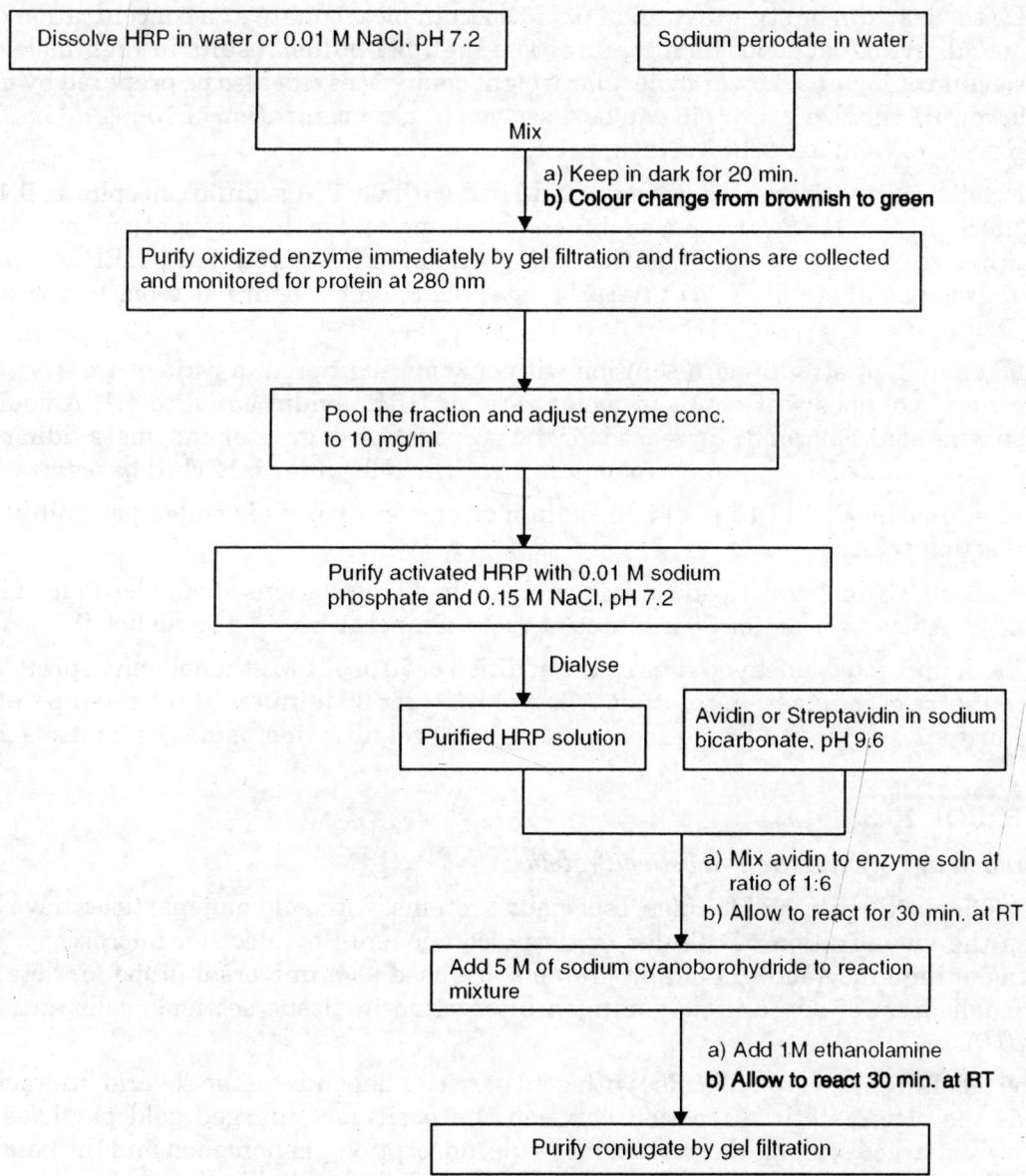

Scheme 20.3: *Preparation of Avidn- HRP or Streptavidin –HRP Conjugate*

- Purify oxidised enzyme immediately by gel filtration using column of Sephadex G-25. Fractions (0.5 ml) are collected and monitored for protein at 280 nm. HRP may also be detected at 403 nm.

- Pool the fractions and adjust enzyme concentration to 10mg/ml for the conjugation step. HRP can be stored freeze-dried for a long period without loss of activity. It should not be stored at room temperature due to the risk of polymerisation.

- Dissolve avidin or streptavidin in 0.2 M sodium bicarbonate at a concentration of 10 mg/ml, pH 9.6 at room temperature. The high pH buffer results in high molecular weight conjugates. Lower molecular weight conjugates can also be prepared by using lower pH value, e.g. protein can be dissolved at a concentration of 10 mg/ml in 0.1 M sodium phosphate, 0.15 M NaCl, pH 7.2.

- Finally, purify the periodate activated HRP with 0.01 M sodium phosphate, 0.15 M NaCl, pH 7.2. HRP can be used directly at 10 mg/ml for the conjugation using lower pH environment. For conjugation using higher pH environment, HRP should be dialysed against 0.2 M sodium carbonate, pH 9.6 for 2 hours at room temperature prior to use.

- Mix avidin or streptavidin solution with enzyme solution at a ratio of 1:6 (v/v). This ratio of volumes will result in molar ratio of HRP: avidin equal to 4:1. Amount of enzyme solution can be increased for the preparation of greater enzyme: avidin ratio. Allow to react for 2 hours at room temperature to form initial Schiff bases.

- In a fume hood, add 10 µl of 5 M sodium cyanoborohydride is added per milliliter of reaction solution.

  Caution: Cyanoborohydride is extremely toxic. All operations should be done in fume hood. Allow to react for 30 minutes at room temperature (in a fume hood).

- Block unreacted aldehyde sites by the addition of 50 µl of 1 M ethanolamine, pH 9.6, per millilitre of conjugation solution. Allow to react for 30 minutes at room temperature. Purify the conjugate from excess reactants by gel filtration using Sephadex G-25.

PROTOCOL 20.5

Preparation of Colloidal Gold-labelled Proteins

The labelling of targeting molecules, especially proteins, with gold nanoparticles have been used in the visualisation of cellular or tissue components by electron microscopy. Gold labelling of immunoglobulin binding proteins are used as a universal probe for detection and visualisation of any antibody-antigen interaction in tissue sections, cells and blots (Fig. 20.6).

The labelling of macromolecules with gold particles depends on the several interactions such as the electrostatic attraction between the positively charged gold particles and negatively charged sites on the protein molecule, adsorption phenomenon and the potential for covalent binding of gold to free sulphydryl groups (dative binding). Monodispersed colloidal gold suspensions are used for protein labelling which can be produced by a variety of chemical methods in which reductive processes on chlorouric acid ($HauCl_4$) are used to create the spheroidal gold particles.

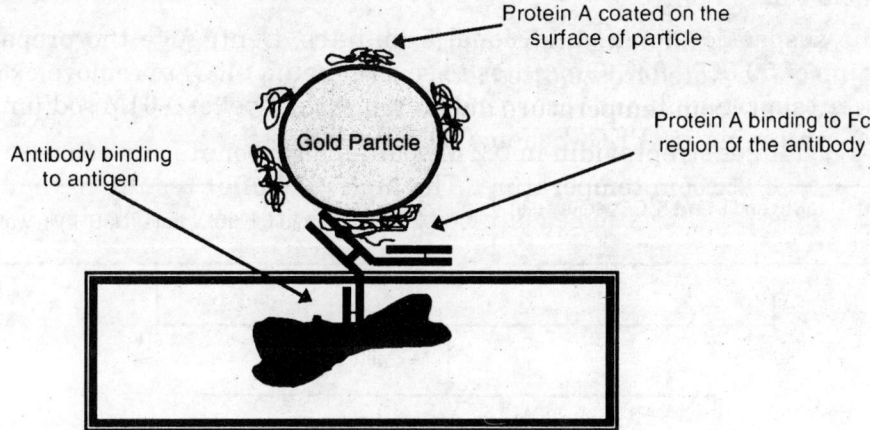

Fig. 20.6. *Schematic diagram showing protein A-gold complex for visualisation of tissue components in electron microscopy*

Materials and chemicals

Chlorouric acid
Polyethylene glycol
Potassium carbonate
Sodium borohydride
Sodium bicarbonate
Sodium phosphate

Procedure

Preparation of Gold Particle Sol

- Prepare 1 ml of 4% $HauCl_4$ solution in deionised water. 375 µl of chlorouric acid solution and 500 µl of 0.2 M K_2CO_3 to 100 ml deionised water, cool on ice to 4°C and mix well. Mix sodium borohydride ($NaBH_4$) in 5 ml of water at a concentration of 0.5 mg/ml. It should be freshly prepared.

- Add five 1ml aliquot of the sodium borohydride solution to the chlorouric acid/carbonate suspension with rapid stirring. As the reaction completes, the reddish-orange colour becomes visible. After the completion of sodium borohydride addition stir the suspension for 5 minutes.

Preparation of Complex

- The minimum amount of protein A required to stabilise the colloidal gold sol being used is determined. The suspension should be adjust, if needed, with 0.1 M K_2CO_3, to pH 6–7.

- Mix stabilising amount of protein A and an additional 10% with the appropriate volume of colloidal gold. After 1 minute, add 250 µl of 1% PEG (Mw 20,000) per 10 ml of gold sol.
- Stir the suspension for an additional 5 minutes. Centrifuge the preparation at a minimum of 50,000g for 30 minutes to several hours (4°C) to remove excess protein A. Discard supernatant and resuspend protein A-gold pellet 0.01M sodium phosphate, pH 7.4, containing 1% PEG (Scheme 20.4).

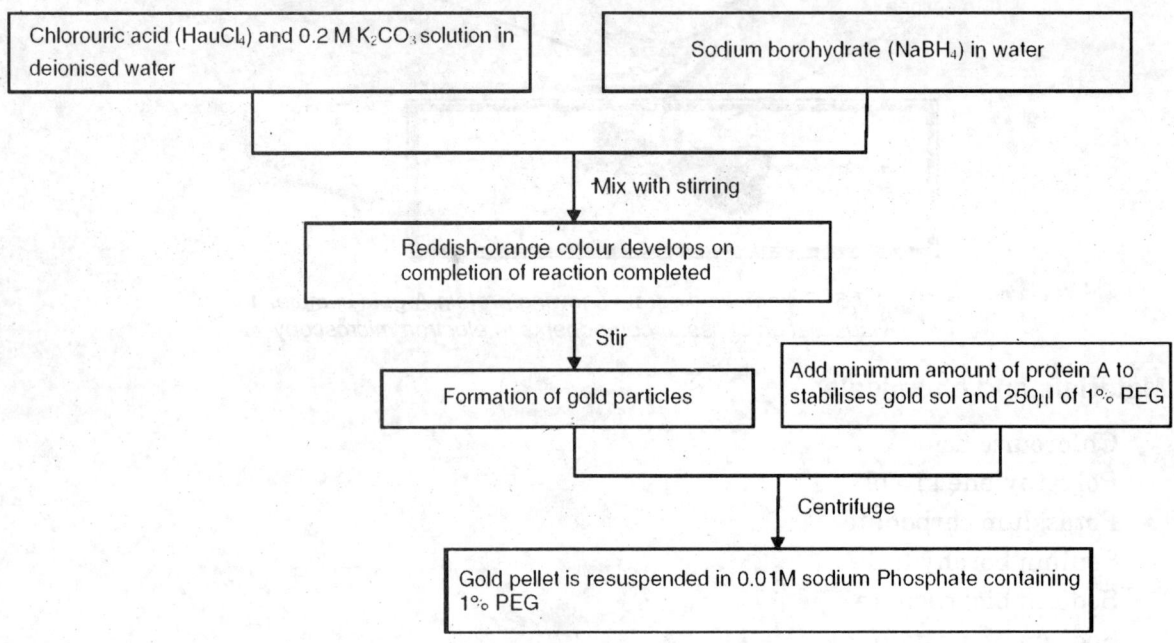

Scheme 20.4: Preparation of colloidal gold- labelled proteins

Radiolabelled Antibodies

Radioactive labels can be attached onto an antibody molecule, which is a powerful means of detection in immunoassay procedures, tracking of analytes, for *in vivo* diagnostic procedures, and for detection or therapy of numerous types of malignancies. Radioactive iodine can be labelled to an antibody using number of techniques. [125]I supplied as sodium salt, is used in most of the procedures by virtue of its comparably 60 days long half life, easy availability and relatively low-energy photon emission. It must be oxidised to electrophilic species capable of modifying molecules. Chloramine-T, Iodo-beads and Iodogen are commonly used oxidising agents causing an iodination reaction to occur at available tyrosine residues within the polypeptide chain. Some other crosslinking or modification reagents containing an activated aromatic ring may also be iodinated to label at other conjugation site within protein molecule, if tyrosine can not be labelled. For example, Bolton-Hunter reagent may be used to add radioactive iodine to antibody molecule by modifying the primary amines within the antibody. It can also be used in the absence of tyrosine residue on the molecule (Fig. 20.7).

PROTOCOL 20.6

Cascade Blue Conjugation of Antibodies

Cascade Blue, a UV-excitable dye, can be used for immunofluorescence labelling. When used with the 351/361 nm excitation lines of an Argon laser, it is not very bright; usually only extremely high density antigens can be well-resolved by Cascade Blue. However, when used with the 405 nm excitation line of a Krypton laser, it becomes a useful dye with a brightness approaching that of fluorescein. Emission is collected at 440 nm.

Conjugation Method

The conjugation can be performed in two steps:

    Covalent conjugation

    Preparation of Antibody

The antibody at a concentration of at least 2 mg/ml is also needed in addition to the materials given below. The extent of the dye conjugation to the antibody may depend on the concentration of antibody in solution. Therefore a consistent concentration of antibody should be used for consistent conjugation. One should know how to use a desalting column and how to take absorbance spectra.

    The reactive Cascade Blue molecule is unstable. Solution of the Cascade Blue is solubilised; it should be used almost immediately. When first conjugating an antibody, a range of Cascade Blue to antibody concentrations should be compared. The protocol suggests 150 µg per mg of antibody; for a first-time titration of Cascade Blue, try a range of 40 to 600 µg Cascade Blue per mg of antibody. Compare each conjugate by staining (a titration of antibody on cells for each reagent to determine the optimal staining concentration should be performed). Then the conjugate with the brightest "positive" cells should be chosen.

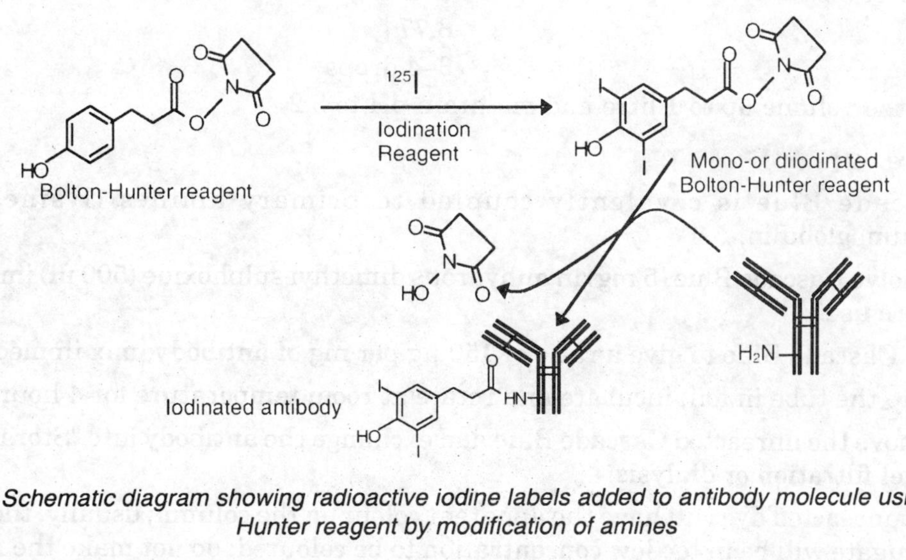

Fig. 20.7. *Schematic diagram showing radioactive iodine labels added to antibody molecule using Bolton-Hunter reagent by modification of amines*

Materials, Chemicals and Buffers

Materials

For column separations, one of the two types of pre-poured columns can be used:

For 1.25 ml to 2.5 ml sample volumes: PD-10 (Sephadex G-25M).

For 0.5 to 1.5 ml sample volumes: KwikSep dextran desalting columns.

Chemicals

Cascade Blue acetyl azide trisodium salt

pH 9–5 mg/ml Pentachlorophenol in 95% ethanol (use as 10,000X, or 3–4 drops per litre)

DMSO - Anyhydrous dimethyl sulphoxide

Note: Keep the DMSO absolutely dry at all times and the bottle in a dessicator. Pour out an amount of DMSO sufficient for the need and then pipette that; do not pipette directly into the bottle.

Sodium bicarbonate

Sodium chloride

TRIZMA 8.0 - Combination of Tris base and Tris HCl

Buffers

Two buffers are used:

B Reaction Buffer

NaHCO$_3$ 84 g

Make the volume to 1 litre with distilled water and maintain pH to 8.4.

Storage-Buffer

TRIZMA 8.0   1.42 g

NaCl   8.77 g

PH 9   3–4 drops

Make the volume up to 1 litre and maintain pH to 8.2

Procedure

- Cascade Blue is covalently coupled to primary amines (lysines) of the immunoglobulin.

- Dissolve Cascade Blue (5 mg) in anhydrous dimethyl sulphoxide (500 µl) immediately before use.

- Add Cascade Blue to give a ratio of 150 µg per mg of antibody; mix immediately.

- Wrap the tube in foil, incubate and rotate at room temperature for 4 hours.

- Remove the unreacted Cascade Blue and exchange the antibody into "Storage Buffer" by gel filtration or dialysis.

- The unreacted dye will have the apparent colour on the column; usually, the antibody conjugate will be in too low concentration to be coloured: do not make the mistake of collecting the antibody by colour visualisation. (a hand-held UV lamp in a darkened room should be used to visualise the conjugate, which will appear faintly blue in comparison to the buffer).

Preparation of Antibody

- Dialyse or exchange antibody over a column in the "B Reaction Buffer". Measure the antibody concentration after buffer equilibration. (1 mg/ml IgG has absorbance 1.4 at 280 nm).

- If the antibody concentration is less than 1 mg/ml, the conjugation will probably be suboptimal. If necessary, dilute the antibody to a concentration of 4 mg/ml (Scheme 20.5).

Note: It is critical that sodium azide be completely removed from any antibody.

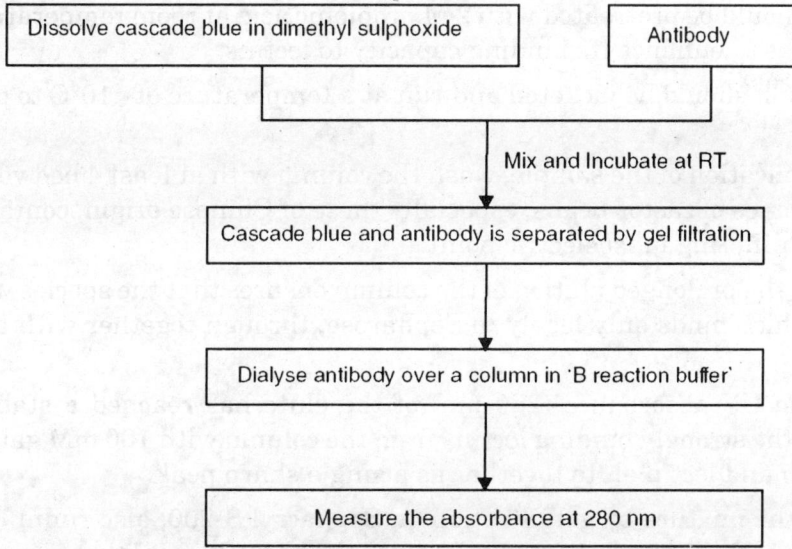

Scheme 20.5 *Formation blue conjugate of antibodies*

PROTOCOL 20.7
Preparation of Antibody- Toxin Conjugates

Purification of Toxins

Ricin

- The galactose-binding toxic lectin may be readily purified by a two-stage chromatographic process based on the method of Nicolson and Blaustein. Isolate galactose-binding proteins on an agarose matrix and then subject to a gel filtration step.

- Untoasted castor bean cake (pomace) may be obtained from castor bean processors.

- It should be further defatted by extraction three times with 5 volumes (v/w) 40-60°C petroleum ether.

- Extract the air-dried material (500 g) overnight by stirring it in 4 litres PBS (pH 7.4).

- Clarify the supernatant partially by filtration through nylon gauze followed by centrifugation at 1500 g for 1 hour.

- The supernatant is subjected to ammonium sulphate precipitation at 4°C, the fraction precipitating between 40 and 60% saturation being collected by centrifugation (1500 g, 1 hour), redissolve in about 500 ml PBS and dialyse against three changes of 6 litres PBS.

- This solution may be further clarified by centrifugation if necessary. It is then applied to a column (bed volume~800 ml) of Sepharose 4B running in PBS.

- The gel should be pretreated with 2 M propionic acid at room temperature for at least 2−3 weeks to enhance its binding capacity to lectins.

- The column should be jacketed and run at a temperature of <10°C to optimise lectin binding.

- After application of the sample, wash the column with at least 4 bed volumes of PBS. Some sources of castor beans, especially those of Chinese origin, contain two species of toxins differing in isoelectric point.

- Washing the prolonged elution of the column ensures that the species with higher pH (~8.2), which binds only feebly to Sepharose, through together with all nonbinding proteins.

- When the UV absorbance (280 nm) of the elute has reached a stable, low value, dispalce the strongly binding lectins from the column with 100 mM galactose in PBS. The toxin and lectin elute together as a single sharp peak.

- Resolve the mixture by gel filtration on Sephacryl S-200, also running in PBS. The sample size should be restricted to 3–4% of the bed volume of the column, under these conditions the lectin of molecular weight 120,000 and the toxin of molecular weight 60,000 are fully resolved and separated.

- The material recovered from the affinity column (second step) must be concentrated by ultrafiltration to ~20 mg/ml before applying to the gel filtration medium.

- Some sources of beans contain quantities of a material, which has a molecular weight about 90,000 and is both toxic and a haemagglutinin.

- Toxin fractions should be selected so as to avoid contamination with this material. Five hundred grams of defatted pomace should yield about 1250 mg toxin, $E_{1cm}^{1\%}$ 11.8, at 280 nm.

- Sterile solutions of holotoxin may be stored at 4°C for at least 12 months without any detectable loss of activity or deep frozen (−30°C) for several years.

Abrin

- Abrin may be purified from seeds of *Abrus precatorius* by essentially similar methodology.
- The seeds (500 g), which should be bright scarlet, ground and extract overnight with 4 litres of PBS at 4°C.
- The yield may be increased by reextracting the pellet of softened stroma from the first centrifugation with a further quantity (2 liters) of PBS for 4–6 hours at room temperature after homogenisation.
- Subject the combined extracts to ammonium sulphate precipitation, and collect the material precipitated between 40 and 70% saturation.
- Other procedures are identical to those for ricin, but it may be noted that material of intermediate molecular weight (i.e. 90,000) is not seen in the galactose-binding proteins of Abrus extracts. 500 g of ground beans will yield about 800 mg of toxin, $E^{1\%}_{1cm}$ 15.9 at 280 nm.

Diphtheria Toxin

- Partially purified diphtheria toxin may be purified by the method given by Collier and Kandel.
- Apply the dialysed solution of 500 mg crude diphtheria toxin in 0.01 M sodium phosphate buffer, pH 7.0, to a column (2.6 × 34 cm) of DADE-cellulose equilibrated in the same buffer.
- When the column is washed at 100 ml per hour with a sequence of sodium phosphate buffer (pH 7.0) of increasing molarity (300 ml of 0.01 M buffer, 300 ml of 0.05 M buffer, 700 ml of 0.1 M buffer and 300 ml of 0.25 M buffer respectively). The toxin elutes as a major peak with a trailing shoulder during the 0.1 M buffer step. The toxin may be identified by means of its precipitation reaction with horse antitoxin in Ouchterlony immunodiffusion assays.
- Concentrate the toxin solution by ultrafiltration to 25 ml and apply to a column (5 × 76cm) of Sephadex G-100 (super fine grade) equilibrated in 0.05 M sodium borate buffer, pH 8.5.
- Elution with the same buffer removes the toxin as a component (~90%) of approximate molecular weight 65,000.
- A minor component (~20%) of approximate molecular weight 130,000, probably dimeric toxin, may also be seen.
- The toxin should be concentrated to 20 mg/ml ($E^{1\%}_{1cm}$, 12.3 at 280 nm) and stored in aliquots at 30°C.

Isolation of Toxin A Chains

Abrin and Ricin

The A chains may be conveniently prepared by cleaving the disulphide bond while the toxins are immobilised on an agarose matrix via the binding site of the B chain.

Procedure

- Apply Toxin (100–150 mg) to a column of acid treated Sepharose 4B, bed volume 24 ml. This represents about half to maximal loading of the gel.
- Equilibrate sample and column with 0.1M phosphate buffer, pH 8.0, containing 0.1 mM EDTA.
- Immediately, after the sample has been run onto the column, allow it to run 15 ml buffer containing 5% 2-mercaptoethanol and allow the column to stand for 2 minutes at room temperature.
- Liberated A chain with the phosphate buffer, B chain and residual holotoxin being retained on the column. Dialyse the eluted peak against three changes of 0.1 M phosphate buffer, pH 8.0, containing 0.1 mM each of EDTA and dithiothreitol to prevent oxidation of the sulphydryl group.
- Remove the traces of B chain or holotoxin by absorption twice with asialofetuin immobilised on Sepharose: approximately 2 mg asialofetuin per millilitre of gel, 1 ml of settled gel per 20 ml of A chain solution. Yield of recovered A chain should be between 75 and 95% of theoretical yield.
- Free A chains should not be frozen (freesing tends to cause loss of enzymatic function) but rather stored at 4°C. They are particularly prone to surface denaturation and manipulations such as concentration by ultrafiltration should be avoided where possible.
- The addition of 20% glycerol is recommended to stabilise sample before transport. In general, it is desirable to prepare A chains as and when required.

Diphtheria Toxin

- To 1 ml of a 25 mg/ml solution of purified diphtheria toxin in 0.05 M borate buffer, pH 8.6, add 1 ml of a 2 µg/ml solution of trypsin in the same buffer containing 2 mM EDTA.
- Incubate the mixture for 2 hours at 25°C to cleave any single chain toxin proteolytic to its nicked (i.e. A and B chain) form; 500 µl of a 10 µg/ml solution of soyabean trypsin inhibitor is added to terminate the reaction.
- Reduce the nicked diphtheria toxin by addition of 500 µl of 0.6 M dithiothreitol and incubate for 90 minutes at 37°C.
- Liberated B chain sediments as a dense, elute the precipitate.
- Centrifuge and apply the clear supernatant to a column (2.6 × 50cm) of Sephadex-G-100 (Superfine grade) equilibrated with 0.05 M borate buffer, pH 8.5, containing 1 mM EDTA and 0.1M 20 ml mercaptoethanol.
- Eluting with the same buffer solution removes the A chain as the major peak (MW~22,000).
- Concentrate the A chain to 5 ml by ultrafiltration and further purify by gel filtration on a column (2.6 × 80 cm) of Sephadex G-75 equilibrated with the same buffer.

- Heat the A chain to 80°C for 10 minutes to destroy any residual traces of toxin or B chain (Scheme 20.6).

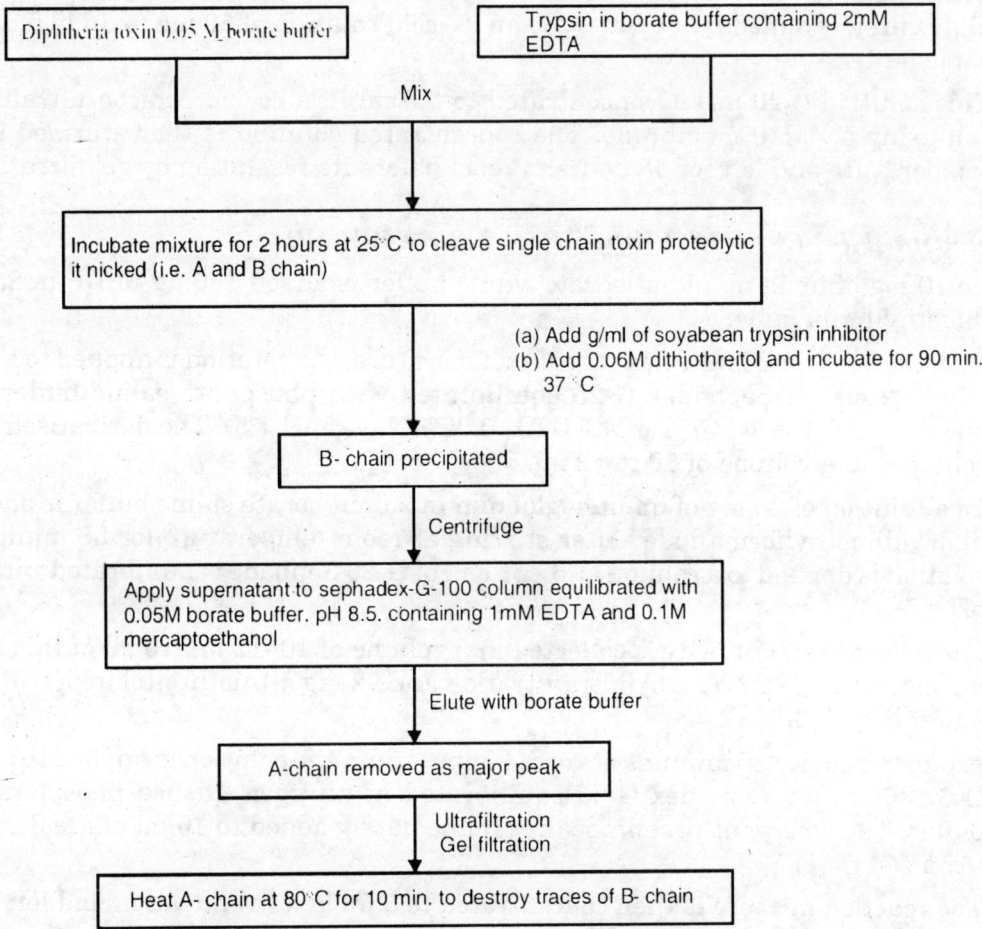

Scheme 20.6: *Isolation of A-chain of diphtheria toxoid*

Coupling of Antibodies and Intact Toxins

Heterobifunctional agents have two reactive groups that are different and which react with amino acids in proteins under different conditions. These reagents permit for greater control over the coupling reaction and reduce the risk of forming intra- and intermolecular crosslinks. Coupling reaction protocols for three such heterobifunctional reagents are as follows;

N-hydroxysuccinimidyl Ester of Chlorambucil

- To 30 mg immunoglobulin at a concentration of 10mg/ml in borate saline buffer (0.05 M borate, 0.3 M NaCl, 0.5% n-butanol, pH 9.0) is added 1 mg of the N- hydroxysuccinimidyl ester of chlorambucil dissolved in 0.5 ml dry dimethyl sulphoxide.

- After stirring on ice for 1 hour, the solution is applied to a jacketed column (1.6×36 cm) of Sephadex G-25 equilibrated with borate saline buffer and maintained at 4°C.

- The column is washed with borate saline buffer and the derivatised globulin, which elutes first, is added immediately to an ice cold solution of 50 mg toxin in 5 ml of the same buffer.

- This solution (~20 ml) is concentrated to 5.0 ml in a cooled Amicon ultrafiltration cell using a PM10 membrane. The concentrated solution is then warmed to room temperature and left for 48 hours to react before its resolution by gel filtration.

N-succinimidyl-3-(2-pyridyldithio)Propionate (SPDP)

- To 10 mg of toxin in 1.0 ml borate saline buffer is added 150 µg SPDP in 25 µl dry dimethylformamide.

- After stirring for 30 minutes at room temperature, the solution is applied to a column (1.6×22 cm) of Sephadex G-25 equilibrated with phosphate saline buffer (0.1 M phosphate, 0.1 M NaCl, 1 mM EDTA, 0.02% NaN_3, pH 7.5). The derivatised toxin is collected in a volume of 10 to 12 ml.

- To a solution of 25 mg of immunoglobulin in 2.5 ml borate saline buffer is added 185 µl dry dimethylformamide. After stirring at room temperature for 30 minutes, the solution is applied to a column (1.6×36 cm) of G-25 Sephadex equilibrated with NaN_3, pH 4.5.

- The derivatised antibody is collected in a volume of 10–12 ml. 10 ml of this solution is concentrated to 2.5 ml by ultrafiltration and 22 mg dithiothreitol in 500 µl acetate buffer is added.

- After stirring for 30 minutes at room temperature, the solution is applied to a column (1.6×36 cm) of Sephadex G-25 equilibrated in nitrogen flushed phosphate saline buffer. The emergent protein peak is immediately added to 10 ml of the derivatised toxin.

- The reaction mixture is then concentrated to 5 ml by ultrafiltration and left at room temperature for 18 hours before resolution by gel filtration.

N-hydroxysuccinimidyl Ester of Iodoacetic Acid

- To a solution of 20 mg ricin in 1.5 ml borate saline buffer is added 300 µg of the N-hydroxysuccinimidyl ester of iodoacetic acid in 200 µl of dry dimethylformamide.

- After stirring for 30 minutes at room temperature, the solution is applied to a column (1.6×22 cm) of Sephadex G-25 equilibrated with phosphate saline buffer and the derivatised ricin is collected in a volume of 10–12 ml.

- Immunoglobulin (45 mg) is derivatised with SPDP and then concentrated to 3.0 ml.

- This intermediate is reduced by the addition of 22 mg of dithiothreitol in 500 µl acetate buffer.

- After stirring for 30 minutes at room temperature, the solution is applied to a column (1.6 × 20 cm) of Sephadex G-25 equilibrated with nitrogen flushed phosphate saline buffer.
- The protein that elutes at the void volume is added immediately to 11 ml of the derivatised ricin solution.
- The reaction mixture is then concentrated to 5.0 ml by ultrafiltration and left at room temperature for 18 hours.
- N-ethylmaleimide (1 mg) dissolved in dimethylformamide is added to inactivate any remaining free sulphydryl groups and the reaction mixture stirred gently for an hour before resolution by gel filtration (Scheme 20.7).

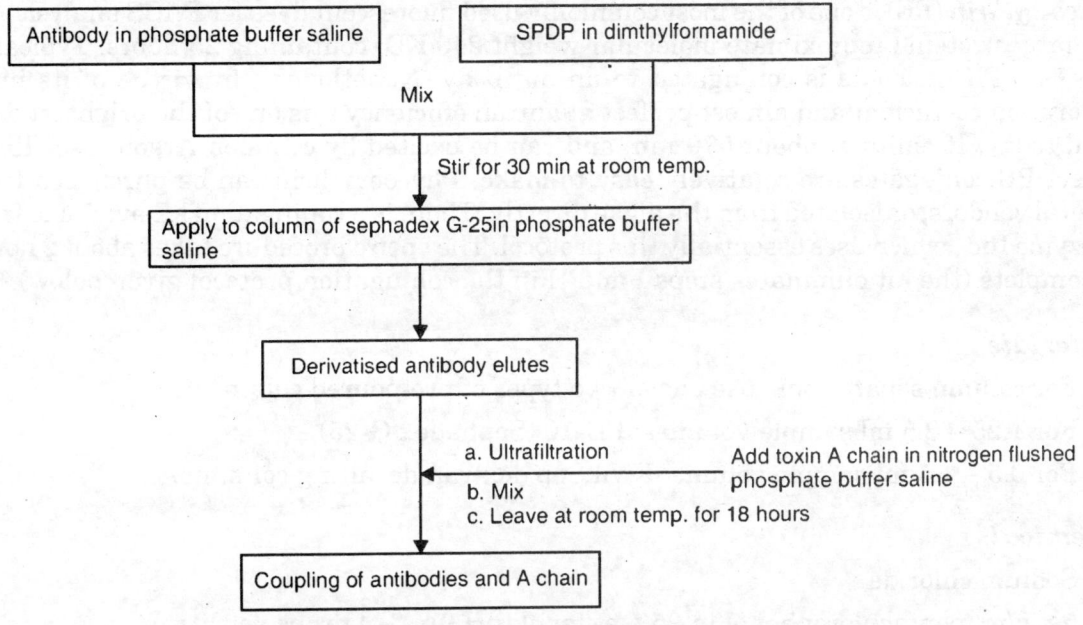

Scheme 20.7: Coupling of antibodies and toxin A-chain

Coupling of Antibodies and Toxin A Chains

- To 26 mg antibody at a concentration of 10 mg/ml in phosphate saline buffer is added 220 µg SPDP in 100 µl dry dimethylformamide.
- Stir for 30 minutes at room temperature and apply to a column (1.6 × 30 cm) of Sephadex G-25 equilibrated in the same buffer; the derivatised antibody elutes in the void volume in about 10–12 ml.
- Concentrate the product to about 3.5 ml by ultrafiltration.
- To it add 15 mg of toxin A chain in 7 ml of nitrogen flushed phosphate saline buffer and mix the solution for 10 minutes and then leave at room temperature for 18 hours before resolution by gel filtration.

Note: An antibody (i.e. immunoglobulin or Ig) is a protein molecule with two identical heavy (H) chains and two identical light (L) chains. Both the H and L chains consist of a variable (V) region that constitutes the antigen combining site and a constant (C) region that determined the isotype (e.g., IgG, IgM, IgA, IgD and IgE for H chains; κ, λ for L chains) of an antibody. T cell receptors (TcR) have a heterodimeric protein structure which exists either as a α/β or a γ/δ form, each (TcR) polypeptide subunit (i.e. α, β, γ, δ) also carries an antigen recognising V region and a C region of unknown function.

PROTOCOL 20.8

Phycoerythrin (PE) Conjugation of Antibodies

Phycoerythrin (PE) is one of the most commonly used fluorescent dyes for FACS analysis. PE is a large protein (approximate molecular weight 240 KD) containing 25 fluors. Typically, only one PE molecule is conjugated to an antibody. Nonetheless, by virtue of its huge absorption coefficient and almost perfect quantum efficiency it is one of the brightest dyes used today. It emits at about 570 nm, and can be excited by common Argon laser lines. Direct PE conjugates are relatively easy to make. Phycoerythrin can be purchased from several vendors, or isolated from the algae directly. There is a conjugation kit available from Prozyme Inc., which uses essentially this protocol. The entire procedure takes about 2 hours to complete (the kit eliminates steps I and II in the conjugation protocol given below).

Materials

For column separations, use one of two types of pre-poured columns:

For 1.25 – 2.5 ml sample volumes: PD-10 (Sephadex G-25),

For 0.5 – 1.5 ml sample volume: KwikSep dextran desalting columns.

Chemicals

Sodium chloride

5 mg/ml pentachlorophenol in 95% ethanol (pH 9), (3–4 drops per litre)

Succinimidyl 4-(N-maleimidomethyl) cyclohexane-1-carboxylate (SMCC)

Anyhydrous dimethyl sulphoxide (DMSO)

Dithiothreitol (DTT)

Ethylenediaminetetraacetic acid (EDTA), (Disodium salt: dihydrate)

[2-(N-morpholino)ethanesulphonic acid] (MES)

TRIZMA 8.0 - Combination of Tris base and Tris HCl

Buffers

Dialysis Buffer (50 mM Sodium phosphate, 1 mM EDTA, pH 7.0)

Sodium phosphate dibasic ($7H_2O$)   13.41 g

EDTA   0.37 g

Make the volume up to 1 litre with distilled water.

Exchange Buffer (50 mM MES, 2 mM EDTA, pH. 6.0)

MES	10.90 g
EDTA	0.74 g

Make the volume up to 1 litre with distilled water and adjust the pH to 6.0

Storage Buffer (10 mM Tris, 150 mM NaCl, pH 9, pH 8.2)

TRIZMA 8.0	1.42 g
NaCl	8.77 g
pH 9	3-4 drops

Make the volume up to 1 litre with distilled water and adjust the pH to 8.2

Conjugation Methods

Preparation of PE
Derivatisation of PE
Reduction of IgG
Covalent conjugation

Procedure

The entire conjugation can be performed in a single day. However, dialysis of stored PE prior to conjugation can take 24–48 hours. In addition, a solution of antibody at a concentration of at least 2 mg/ml is also required for conjugation.

Preparation of PE

- Dialyse or exchange the PE into "Dialysis Buffer". PE concentration before derivatisation is typically 5–10 mg/ml.

  Note: PE is most stable as a SAS (sodium ammonium sulphate) precipitate prior to coupling. If the PE is stored as a SAS precipitate, it must be extensively dialysed prior to use.

- Dialyse against 2 changes of 1 litre per ml PE of PBS before dialysing against 1 litre per ml of "Dialysis Buffer".

- Use 3.5 mg of PE per mg of IgG to be modified; this includes an extra 10% for loss during buffer exchanges.

- To check the PE purity and concentration, measure the absorbance at 280, 565 and 620 nm. (1 mg/ml of PE has an optical density at 565 nm of 8.2). A 565/620 ratio > 50 indicates adequate removal of contaminating phycocyanin; a 565/280 ratio > 5 indicates adequate removal of all other proteins.

Derivatisation of PE

- The amino groups on the phycoerythrin (PE) react with the succinamide to yield a maleimide-labelled PE.

- Prepare a 10 mg/ml stock solution of SMCC in dry DMSO immediately prior to use.

- Add 11 µl of SMCC per mg of PE while vortexing.
- Wrap the reaction tube in aluminum foil and rotate at room temperature for 60 minutes.
- Pass the derivatised PE over a gel filtration column pre-equilibrated with "Exchange Buffer".
- The SMCC-derivative is stable and may be stored at 4°C for several weeks; a high concentration of PE (> 4 mg/ml) is desirable for such longer-term storage.

Note: For conjugations, which fail or are poor, it may help to increase or decrease the amount of SMCC with respect to PE, or to use an alternative heterobifunctional cross linking reagent.

Reduction of IgG

The hinge disulphide bonds are reduced to yield free sulphydryls.

- Prepare a fresh solution of 1 M DTT (15.4 mg/100 µl) in distilled water. IgG solutions should be at 4 mg/ml or higher for best results.
- The reduction can be carried out in almost any buffer; MES, phosphate, and TRIS buffers (pH range 6 to 8) have been used successfully.
- The antibody should be concentrated if the concentration is less than 2 mg/ml. Include an extra 10% for losses on the buffer exchange column.
- Make each IgG solution 20 mM in DTT by adding 20 µl of DTT stock per ml of IgG solution while mixing.
- Allow it to stand at room temperature for 30 minutes without additional mixing (to minimise reoxidation of cysteines to cystines).
- Pass the reduced IgG over a filtration column pre-equilibrated with "Exchange Buffer". Collect 0.25 ml fractions off the column; determine the protein concentrations and pool the fractions with the majority of the IgG. This can be done either spectrophotometrically or colorimetrically.
- Carry out the conjugation as soon as possible after this step.

Note: For conjugations, which are poor or fail, it may help to reduce the DTT concentration.

Covalent Conjugation

- The PE is covalently coupled to the IgG through reaction of the maleimide groups with the free sulphydryl on the IgG. Do not delay this step since the IgG sulphydryls will reoxidise.
- Add 3.2 mg of SMCC-PE per mg of IgG. Wrap the reaction tube in aluminum foil and rotate for 60 minutes at room temp.

Note: These molar ratios (~2 PE per IgG) have worked very well. For conjugations, which fail or are poor, different other molar ratios may help.

- After 60 minutes, unreacted free sulphydryls on the IgG must be blocked.

- Prepare a fresh solution of 10 mg NEM in 1.0 ml dry DMSO.

- Add 34 µg (3.4 µl) per mg of IgG. Wrap and rotate for 20 minutes at room temperature.

- The product can be either dialysed or exchanged over a column into an appropriate buffer (e.g. storage buffer). It is best to keep the product at high concentration (> 1 mg/ml) for optimal stability. Never freeze the conjugates. It may be useful to spin PE conjugates prior to use in staining, especially if background seems to be a problem (e.g., at 10,000g in a microcentrifuge, at 4°C).

Antibody-Toxin Conjugates

Cell-type-specific cytotoxic agents have been constructed in several laboratories by linking highly potent toxins or their subunits to antibody molecules. The toxins most widely used have been diphtheria toxin (the endotoxin from *Cornebacterium diphtheriae*) and the plant toxins ricin (from *Ricinus communis*) and abrins (from *Abrus precatorius*). Abrin, ricin and diphtheria toxin are composed of two polypeptide subunits, A and B joined by a disulphide bond. All three toxins have similar mode of cytotoxic action. They bind by means of recognition sites on the B chain to the component of plasma membrane of virtually all cell types in sensitive species of animals: abrin and ricin recognise galactose terminating glycoproteins and glycolipids whereas the receptor for diphtheria toxins have not yet been identified.

The A chains then penetrates (or is transported across) the plasma membrane or the membrane of an endocytic vesicle and kills the cells by inactivating its machinery for protein synthesis.

There are two ways of constructing antibody-toxin conjugates with the cell types specificity. First is to link the antibody by a disulphide bond to the isolated A chain moiety or alternatively to one of the single chain plant peptides such as gelonin from *glonium multiflorum*, whose damaging action on the eukaryotic ribosomes is apparently identical to that of the A chain of abrin and ricin. The second is to link the intact toxin to the antibody and block the cell recognition site on the B chain to prevent the conjugate from binding to and killing cells non-specifically.

Step 1. Purification of Toxins

Ricin

The galactose-binding toxic lectin may be readily purified by a two stage chromatographic process based on the method of Nicolson and Blaustein. Galactose-binding protein are first isolated on an agarose matrix and are then subject to gel filtration step.

Purification of Ricin

- Untoasted castor bean cake (pomace) may be obtained from castor bean processor.

- It should be further defatted by extraction three times with 5 volume of petroleum ether at 40–60°C.

- Extract the dry material (500g) overnight by stirring it in 4 litre phosphate buffer saline (PBS 0.15N NaCl, 0.01M Phosphate pH 7.4).

- Supernatant is partially clarified by filtration through nylon gauge followed by centrifugation at 1500g for 1 h to produce a clear solution suitable for chromatographic procedures.

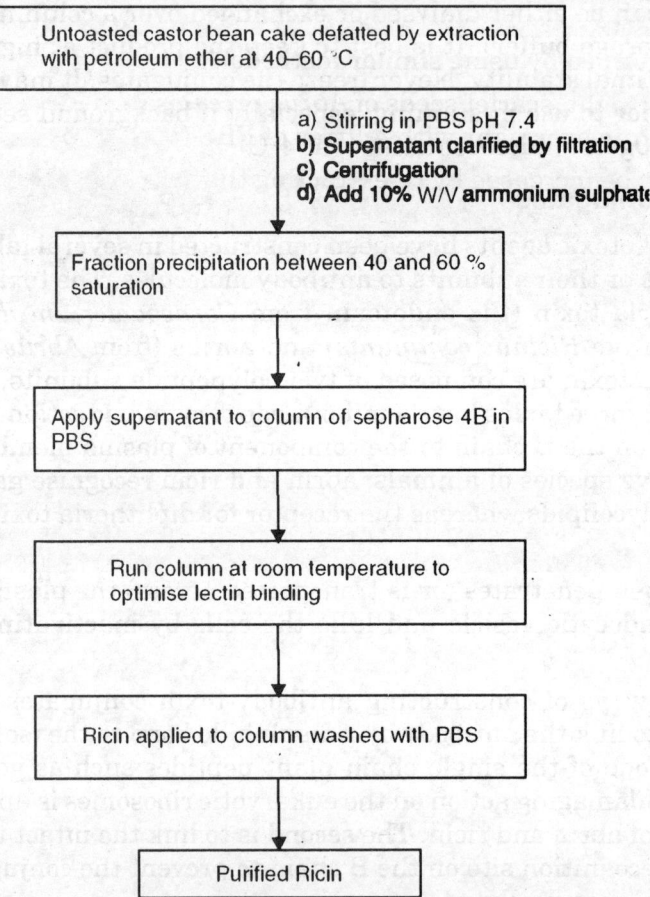

Scheme 20.8: Purification of Ricin

- Add the 10% w/v ammonium sulphate to the supernatant for precipitation at 4° C. The fraction precipitating between 40 and 60% saturation being collected by centrifugation (1500 g at 1 h) and re-dissolve in about 500ml PBS and dialyse against three changes of 6 litres PBS.

- Clarify this solution by further centrifugation, if necessary. Apply the supernatant to a column (volume ~800ml) of sepharose 4B running in PBS.

- Treat the gel with 1.0 M propionic acid at room temperature for at least 2–3 weeks to enhance its binding capacity for lectins.

- Run the column at room temperature of <10°C to optimise lectin binding. Sample is applied to the column and washed with at least 4 bed volumes of PBS (pH 7.4).

- Resolve this mixture by gel filtration on sepahacryl S-200, also running in PBS.
- The sample size should be restricted to 3–4 % of the bed volume of the column (Scheme 20.8).

Purification of Abrin

Abrin may be purified by using similar methodology from seeds of *Abrus precatorious*.

- Take 500g of bright, scarlet seeds of *Abrus precatorious* and grind in a coffee grinder before extracting overnight with 4 litres of PBS (pH 7.4) at 4°C.
- The yield may be increased by re-extracting the pellets of stroma with 2 liters of PBS at room temperature after homogenising in a waring blender (2 min).
- Add ammonium sulphate to the combined extract to obtain precipitates, and collect the material precipitating between 40 and 70% saturation.

Purification of Diphtheria Toxins

- Prepare the solution of 500 mg crude diphtheria toxin in 0.01 M sodium phosphate buffer (pH 7.0).
- Apply to a column (2.6 × 34 cm) of DADE-cellulose equilibrated in the same buffer.
- Wash the column with sodium phosphate buffer (pH 7.0) of increasing molarity at the flow rate 100 ml/hr and the sequence of molarity as follows- 300 ml of 0.05 M buffer, 600 ml of 0.1 M buffer, and 300 ml of 0.25 M buffer.
- The toxin elutes as a major peak with a trailing shoulder during the 0.1 M buffer step.
- The toxin may also be identified by means of its precipitation reaction with horse antitoxin by ouchterlony immunodiffusion assay.
- The toxin solution is concentrated by ultra filtration to 25 ml and applied to a column (5 × 76 cm) of Sephadex G-100 (Superfine grade).
- Equilibrate in 0.05 M Sodium borate buffer (pH 8.5). Elute the column with the same buffer and remove the toxin as a major component (~90%) of approximate molecular weight 65,000.
- A minor component of approximate MW 130,000 probably dimeric toxin may also be obtained and collected similarly as stated above.
- The toxin should be concentrated to 10 mg/ml and stored in aliquot at –30°C.

Step 2. Isolation of Toxin A Chain from the Toxin

Principle: Method of preparation of toxin A chains involve reductive cleavage of the disulfide bond and then followed by separation of the subunits. Special measures are necessary to ensure removal of all traces of holotoxin from the desired product.

Isolation of Toxin A Chain of Abrin or Ricin

- Prepare a column of Sepharose 4B (5 × 45 cm, pretreated with acid, bed volume 25 ml). Equilibrate the sample and column with 0.1M phosphate buffer pH 8.0, containing 0.1mM EDTA.

- Apply the toxin solution to a Sepharose 4B column. This represents about half the maximal loading of the gel. Immediately after the run into the column, it is followed by 15 ml of the running buffer containing 5% 2-mercaptoethanol.
- Then stop the flow and allow the column to stand for 2 h at room temperature.
- Elute the liberated A chain with the phosphate buffer (pH 7.0) and B chain and residual holotoxin being retained on the column.
- Dialyse the eluted peak against three changes of 0.1M phosphate buffers pH 8.0 containing 0.1mM each of EDTA and dithiothreitol to guard against oxidation of the sulphydryl group.
- Remove the traces of B chains or holotoxins by adsorption twice with asialofetuin immobilised on sepharose: approximately 2 mg of asialofetuin per milliliter of gel, 1 ml of settle gel per 20 ml of A chain solution.
- Store the free A chain (freesing tends to cause loss of enzymatic function) at 4°C. The addition of 20% glycerol is recommended to stabilised sample before transport (Scheme 20.9).

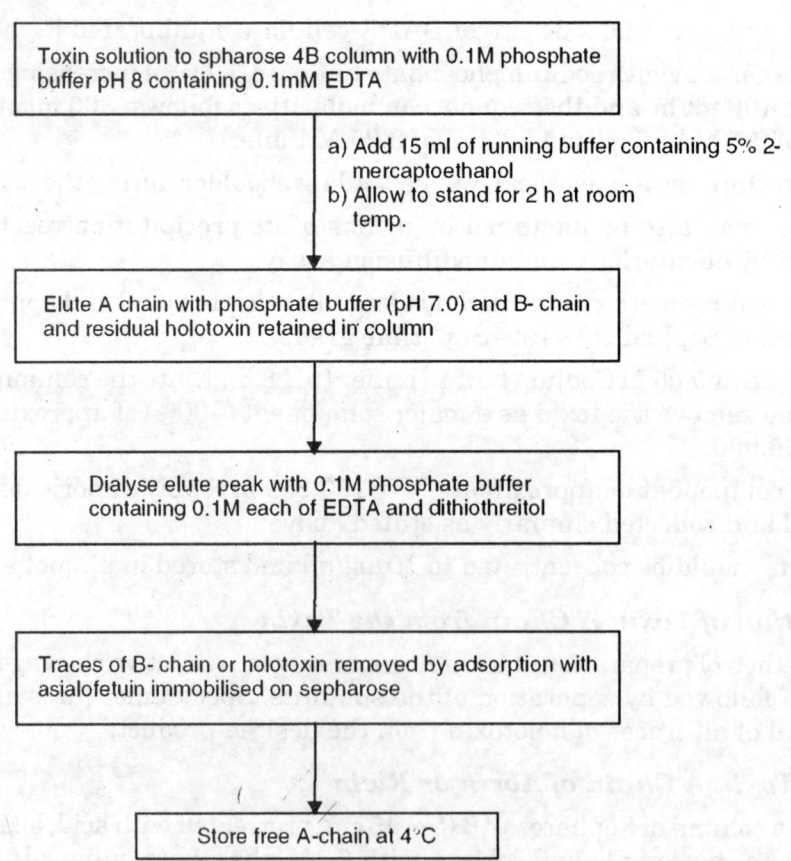

Scheme 20.9: *Isolation of A-chain from toxin*

Isolation of Toxin A Chain from Ricin

This method for isolating both polypeptide chains of ricins derives from the procedure described by Olsnes and Pihl.

- Take ricin toxin at a concentration of 5 mg/ml in 0.1M Tris-HCl (pH 8.5) to make 0.5 M with respect to galactose and 2% to 2- mercaptoethanol.
- Adjust the pH to 8.5 with 0.1N NaOH and incubate the samples overnight at room temperature and then followed by 2–3 h at 37°C.
- Then apply the sample to a column of DEAE-Sepharose equilibrated with 0.1 M Tris buffer, pH 8.5. Take 1.0 ml of Sepharose for each 5 mg of ricin.
- Wash the column with 0.1 M Tris-HCl buffer (pH 8.5) until all the unbound material-essential pure A chain has been eluted.
- Finally wash the column with 0.1 M Tris-HCl; pH 8.5 containing 0.1M galactose, which remove only bound ricin.

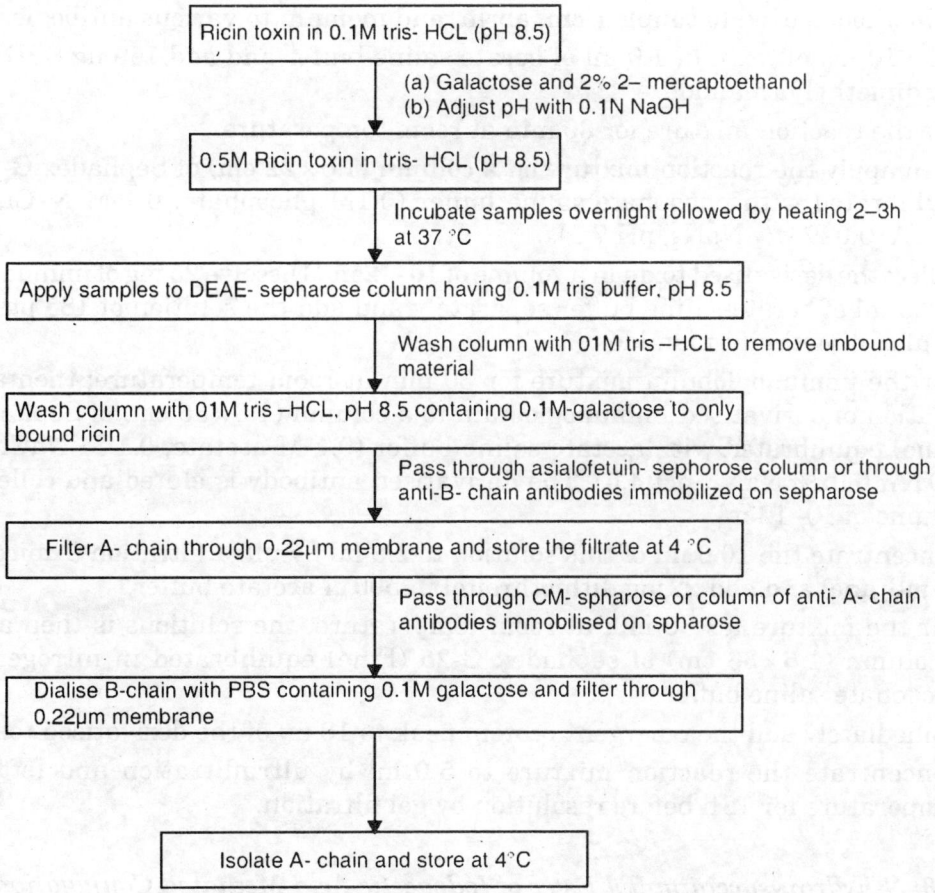

Scheme 20.10: *Isolation of toxin A chain from ricin*

- To remove any contaminating ricin from the A chain, pass down the material through 2.0 ml asialofetuin-sepharose column (2–3 mg asialofeutin per millilitre of gel) or through 2.0 ml column of anti-B-chain antibodies immobilised on sepharose.

- Then filter the A chain through a 0.22µm membrane and store the filtrate at 4°C.

- To enhance the purity of B chain fraction pass down through a CM-Sepharose column equilibrated with 5 mM phosphate, pH 6.5 containing 0.1M galactose-approximately 10 ml of gel per 25 mg of protein.

- Alternatively (or additionally) a column of anti-A-chain antibodies immobilised on sepharose can be used.

- Dialyse the B chain with PBS containing 0.1 M galactose and filter through a 0.22µm pore size membrane filter and store at 4°C (Scheme 20.10).

Method 2: N-succinimidyl-3- (2-pyridyldithio) Propionate (SPDP) Mediated Conjugation

This method is used to couple ricin, abrin, and melanin to various antibodies.
- Take 10 mg of toxin in 1.0 ml of borate saline buffer and add 150 µg SPDP in 25µl dry dimethylformamide.
- Stir the reaction mixture for 30 min at room temperature.
- Then apply the reaction mixture on a column (1.6 × 22 cm) of Sephadex G-25 (Fine) equilibrated with phosphate saline buffer (0.1M phosphate, 0.1 M NaCl, 1.0 mM EDTA, 0.02%w/v NaN$_3$, pH 7.5).
- Collect the derivatised toxin in a volume of 10–12 ml. Dissolve 25 mg of immunoglobulin in 2.5 ml of borate-saline buffer separately and add the solution of 185 µg SPDP in 30 µl of dimethylformamide.
- Stir the immunoglobulin mixture for 30 min at room temperature; then apply the solution of derivatised immunoglobulin to a column (1.6 × 36 cm) of Sephadex G-25 (Fine) equilibrated with acetate saline buffer (0.1 M acetate, 0.1 M NaCl, 0.1 mM EDTA, 0.02% NaN$_3$, pH 4.5). The derivatised antibody is eluted and collected in a volume of 10–12 ml.
- Concentrate the 10.0 ml of this solution to 2.5 ml by ultra filtration (Amicon PM 10 membrane) and add 22 mg dithiothreitol in 500 µl acetate buffer.
- Stir the mixture for 30 min at room temperature, the solutions is then applied to a column (1.6 × 36 cm) of sephadex G-25 (Fine) equilibrated in nitrogen flushed phosphate saline buffer.
- Immediately add the emergent protein peak to 10 ml of the derivatised toxin
- Concentrate the reaction mixture to 5.0 ml by ultrafiltration and left at room temperature for 18 h before resolution by gel filtration.

Method 3: N-hydroxysuccinimidyl Ester of Iodoacetic Acid Mediated Conjugation

- Prepare the solution of 20 mg ricin in 1.5ml borate-saline buffer.

- Add the 300µg of the N-hydroxysuccinimidyl ester of iodoacetic acid in 200µl dry dimethylformamide

- Stir the reaction mixture for 30 min at room temperature; then apply the solution to a column (1.6 × 22cm) of sephadex G-25 (Fine) equilibrated with phosphate saline buffer. Elute the derivatised ricin and collect in a volume of 10–12ml.

- Derivatised the immunoglobulin with SPDP [N- Succinimidyl-3-(2-pyridyldithio) propionate] and then concentrate to 3.0 ml.

- Reduce this solution intermediately by the addition of 22 mg of dithiothreitol in 500µl of acetate buffer. Stir the reaction mixture for 30 min at room temperature.

- Then this solution is applied on a column of sephadex G-25 (Fine) equilibrated with nitrogen flushed phosphate-saline buffer.

- The protein that elutes at the void volume is added immediately to 11ml of the derivatised ricin solution.

- The reaction mixture is then concentrated to 5.0 ml by ultra filtration (Amicon PM 10 membrane) and left at room temperature for 18h.

- Dissolve N-ethylmaleimide (1mg) in dimethylformamide (2 ml) and add to the reaction mixture of immunoglobulin and toxin to inactivate any remaining free sulphydryl groups. Stir the reaction mixture gently for a 2 h before resolution by gel filtration.

Coupling of Antibodies and Toxin A Chains

Toxin A chain contains a free thiol group which can react with a 2-pyridyl disulphide-substituted antibody molecule to form a disulphide linkage.

Procedure

This method is used for conjugation of antibodies to the A chain of abrin, ricin, and diphtheria toxin. We routinely attach two pyridyl disulfide groups to the antibody and allow the product to react with a 2 to 3-fold molar excess of the A chain. Toxin conjugates with the yields upto 50% of the 1:1 conjugates obtained by this method.

Dissolve 26 mg antibody at a concentration of 10 mg/ml in phosphate-saline buffer and add 100µl solution of 220µg SPDP in dry dimethylformamide. Stir the reaction mixture for 30 min at room temperature. Apply the reaction mixture on a column (1.6 × 36cm) of Sephadex G-25F equilibrated with the same buffer. Elute the derivatised antibody in the void volume and collect in volume 10–12 ml.

Concentrate the reaction product to about 3.5 ml by ultrafiltration (Amicon PM 10 membrane). Then add 15 mg of toxin A chain in 7 ml of nitrogen flushed phosphate-saline buffer (pH 7.4). Gently mix the solution with occasional stirring for 10 min and then leave the mixture at room temperature for 18 h before resolution by gel filtration.

Purification and Storage of Conjugates

The unreacted toxin and polymeric material is readily removed by gel filtration on the polydextran gels. The unreacted holotoxins elute later than would be predicted from their molecular weight, probably because they have a weak affinity for the carbohydrate residues of the gel. The toxin A chain are sufficiently low molecular weight that they, too, are clearly separated from the conjugates. Column of the sephadex G-200 (superfine) or the faster running Sephacryl S-300 (3.2 × 80cm) provide adequate separation for holotoxin conjugates. Sephacryl S-200 column gives a satisfactory separation. The fraction containing the 1:1 conjugates are identified from the elution volume and by the radioactivity associated with the toxin moiety. Further purification of holotoxin conjugates can be achieved by returning the product of 210,000–215,000 (1:1 antibody toxin) on the gel filtration column.

Purified conjugates from any of the procedures described above can be stored at 4°C for several months after filtration sterilisation without detectable loss of activity. Alternatively, samples may be rapidly frozen in a solid CO_2-ethanol mixture, or in liquid nitrogen and stored at −70°C or below. Conjugates recovered from the frozen state manifest unchanged activity and this method is the most suitable for long-term storage.

Protein Conjugates of Fungal Toxins

Nearly all fatal cases of poisoning by mushrooms in man are due to three *Amanita* species (*A. phalloides, A. verna, A. virosa*), which contain two families of toxic cyclopeptides, amatoxins and phyllotoxins. Conjugation of amatoxins and phallotoxins to protein was performed for two purposes:

To obtain a selective killing of cells, which display high uptake of the protein, attach to the toxins.

To induce the production of toxin specific antibodies in animals or cultured hybrid cells. Such antibodies provided the tool for detection of toxins in biological fluids by radioimmunoassay. Another aim of these experiments was to obtain a serum useful in the treatment of human amanita poisoning.

PROTOCOL 20.9

Coupling of Amatoxins with the Proteins by Carbodiimides

Materials

β-Amanitin

Albumin protein

1-ethyl-3- (dimethylamino propyl) carbodiimide (ECDI)

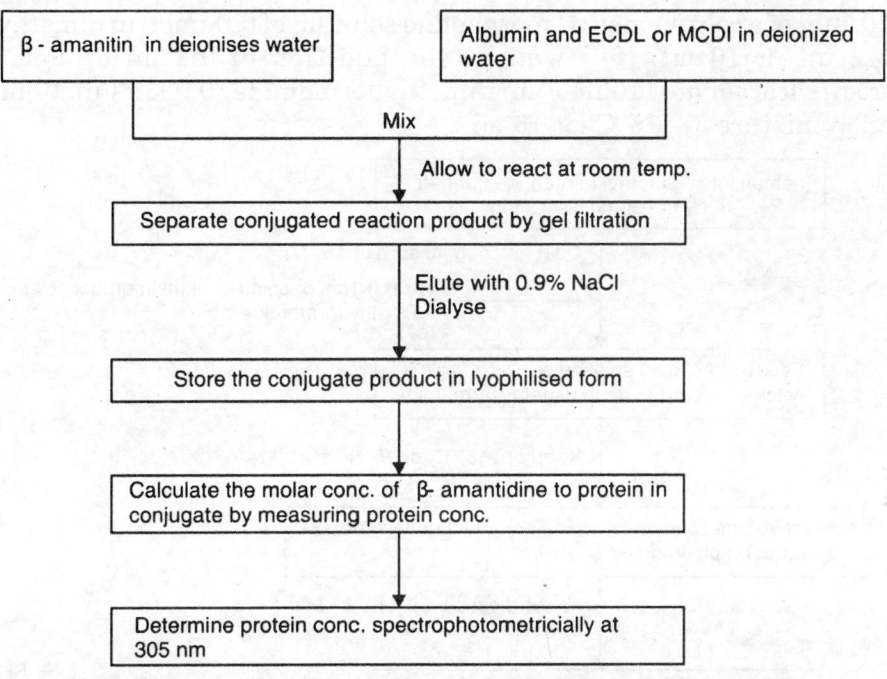

Scheme 20.11: *Coupling of amatoxins with protein by carbodiimides*

Procedure

- Dissolve 10 mg of β-amanitin (βA, 11μmol) in 1 ml of deionised water and mix with 20 mg of albumin (0.29μmol) and 5 mg of 1-ethyl-3- (dimethylamino propyl) carbodiimide (ECDI, 26μmol) or with 8 mg of 1-cyclohexyl-3-[2-morpholinyl-(4)-ethyl] carbodiimide (MCDI, 18.9μmol) in 1 ml of deionised water and allow to react at room temperature for 24h.

- Separate the conjugated reaction product from free β-amanitin and urea derived from carbodiimide by gel filtration through column (1.2 × 100cm) of Sephadex G-75 pre-equilibrated and eluted with 0.9% NaCl.

- Dialyse the reaction product against water and store the conjugate products by keeping them in frozen state or in lyophilised form.

- Calculate the molar ratio of β-amanitin to the protein in the conjugate by measuring protein concentration according to the Lowry *et al* and determine the β-amanitin concentration spectrophotometrically at 305nm (Scheme 20.11).

PROTOCOL 20.10

Coupling of Amatoxins via Mixed Anhydrides

- Dissolve 8.0 mg of β-amanitin (~9μmol) in 0.2 ml of dimethylformamide purified from water and dimethylamine by fraction distillation. Cool the reaction mixture to −15°C.

- Add 0.1 ml of a cold N- methyl morpholine solution of (10µmol) in dimethylformamide (0.112 ml in 10 ml), followed by the addition of 0.1 ml of cold solution of chloroethylcarbonate (10µmol) in dimethylformamide (0.095ml in 10 ml). Keep the reaction mixture at –15°C for 15 min.

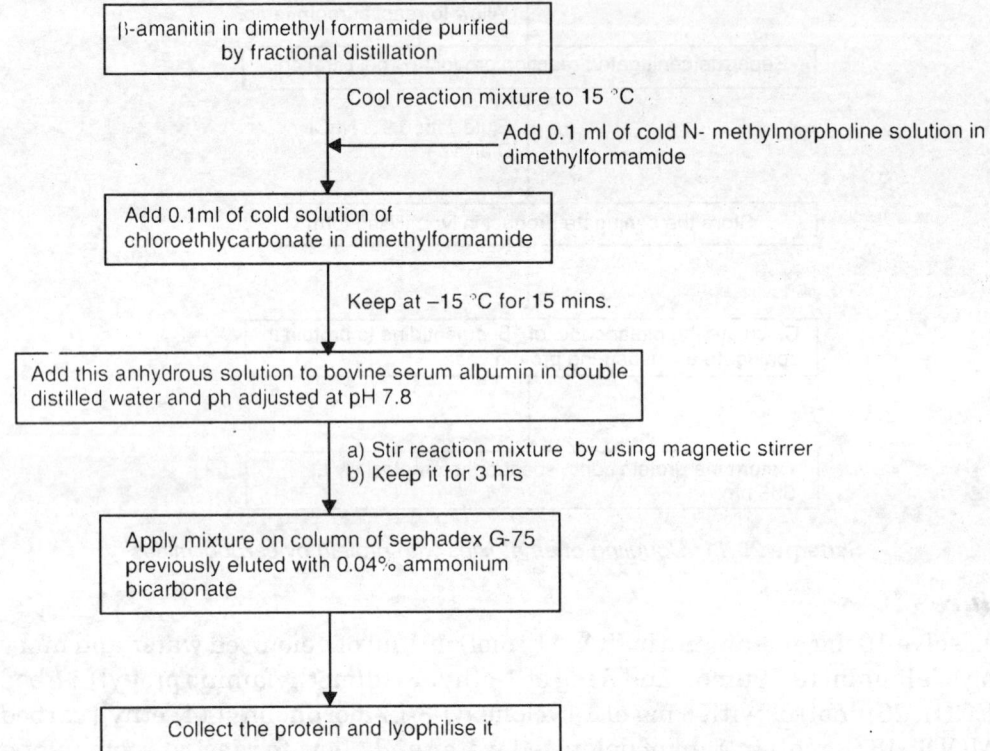

Scheme 20.12: Coupling of amatoxins via anhydrides

- Add this anhydride solution to a solution of 32 mg (0.46 µmol) of bovine serum albumin in 1.2 ml of double distilled water and adjust the pH 7.8 with 0.1N NaOH, and stir the reaction mixture gently using magnetic stirrer.
- Leave the mixture for approximately 3 hr to come to room temperature and then apply on a column of Sephadex G-75 (2.4 × 80 cm) previously equilibrated and eluted with 0.04% ammonium bicarbonate (NH_4HCO_3).
- Elute the protein in the first peak, collect it and then lyophilise. During the lyophilisation most of the buffer salt is removed as a result of its volatility.
- Remove the residual ammonium salt if necessary, by dialysis against NaCl solution (Scheme 20.12).

PROTOCOL 20.11

Phallotoxins Fungal Toxin to Proteins

Using either carbodiimide or mixed anhydrides coupling method, four different phyllotoxins-bovine serum albumin conjugates have been prepared with the same procedures as described for the amatoxins (Table 20.1). Phallacidin (PC) is the most abundant phallotoxin with a native carboxylic groups in a side chain, which allow the formation of amide bond with the amine group of the protein however, the carboxylic group is very close to the peptide backbone, and thus its coupling can affect the biological activity of the toxin. Therefore a functional group has been introduced into the dihydroxy-L-leucine side chain of phallocidin (PD-C).

Table 20.1: *Phallotoxin coupling to bovine serum albumin by various methods*

Compounds	Molar Ratio	Coupling Method	Remarks
Bovine serum albumin-PC	2.7	ECDI	No affinity to actin
Bovine serum albumin-PD-C	9.6	Mixed anhydride (MA)	Affinity to actin ~5%
Bovine serum albumin-PD-C	2.4	ECDI, MCDI	Affinity to actin ~5%
Bovine serum albumin-PD	2.3	ECDI	-

PROTOCOL 20.12

Antibody-drug Conjugates for Transferrin Receptor

Preparation of Ricin Toxins

- Purify the ricin toxin from locally obtained castor bean seed as follows– decorticated castor beans are grounded in 1 litre PBS (0.15M NaCl, 0.01M sodium phosphate buffer, pH 7.3) in a waring blender.

  Caution: This step should be performed with extreme care in a fume hood, as the aerosol produced is very toxic. After grinding, the aerosol should be allowed to settle for at least 10 min before filtering out the ground through cheesecloth.

- Centrifuge the extract in 500-ml bottles at 10000g for 30 min in a centrifuge.

- The homogenate will separate into an aqueous layer and a lipid layer.

- Decant off the aqueous layer through 9xx gauge nylon cloth and repeat the centrifugation step.

- Add 60% w/v ammonium sulphate or saturated solution to obtain precipitate. Collect the precipitate by centrifugation at 10000g for 30 min.

- Dissolve the precipitate in 100 ml of PBS and dialyse exhaustively against PBS.

- Load the dialysed extract onto a column (30 × 5cm) of sepharose 6B and elute all unbound protein with PBS.

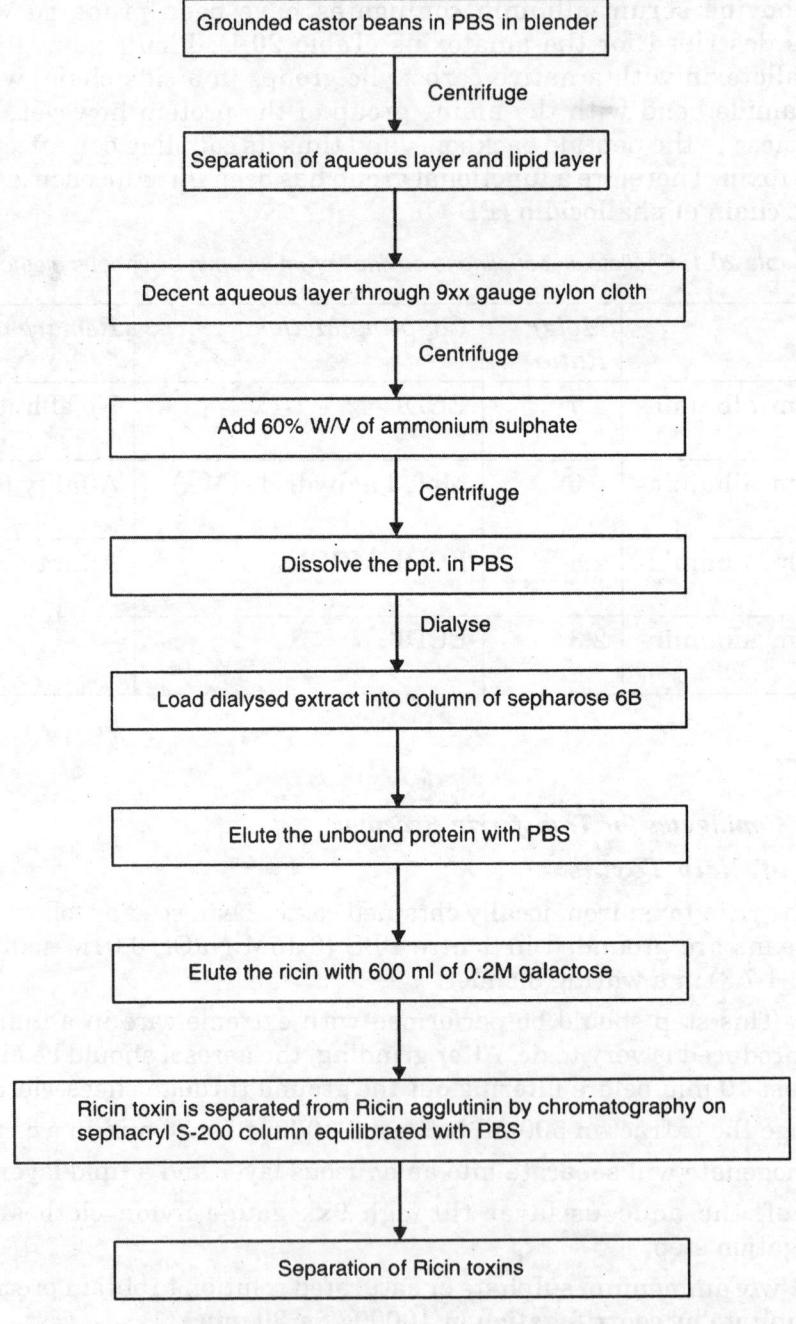

Scheme 20.13: *Preparation of ricin toxin*

- Then elute ricin with 600 ml of 0.2 M galactose or lactose in PBS; collect the 10ml fractions and concentrate it.

- Castor beans contain approximately equal amount of ricin toxin and ricin agglutinin.

- Separate the toxin from the agglutinin by chromatography on a Sephacryl S-200 column (65 × 3.5 cm) equilibrated with PBS.

- Finally, collect the fractions, elute the ricin toxins as the second of two well resolved protein peaks (Scheme 20.13).

Isolation of Chain A of Ricin Toxin

- Ricin toxin subunit (A chain) is isolated from the binding subunit (B chain) as described by Olsnes and Pihl.

- Dissolve 50 mg of ricin toxin in 3 ml of 0.5 M lactose containing 0.1M Tris-HCl, (pH 8.5). Add 5% (v/v) 2-merceptoethanol to reduce the toxin and incubate for 16 h at room temperature with continuous stirring using magnetic stirrer.

- Apply this reduced ricin on a DEAE-cellulose column (25 × 1.0 cm) equilibrated with 0.1M Tris-HCl (pH 8.5). Partially purified ricin A chain elutes slightly before 2-mercaptoethanol addition. The fraction containing ricin A chain can be identified by electrophoresis on a 10% SDS-polyacrylamide gel.

- Elute the ricin B chain from the column with 0.1M NaCl in the same buffer. Dialyse the fraction containing ricin A chain against 5 mM sodium phosphate buffer (pH 6.5) containing 0.01M lactose, 0.1% 2-mercaptoethanol. Then apply this solution on a CM-cellulose column (9.0 × 1.0 cm) equilibrated in same buffer (Scheme 21.14).

Chemical Modification of the Anti-Transferrin Receptor Antibody

- Prepare a 20 mM stock solution of SPDP in absolute alcohol (99.9% pure alcohol).

- Add 10 μl of this stock SPDP solution to the antibody solution containing 5 mg antibody in 1 ml of PBS with magnetic stirring at room temperature.

- Incubate the reaction mixture for 30 min at room temperature.

- Separate the excess SPDP from the antibody by gel filtration using sephadex G-25 superfine column (15 × 1.5 cm) equilibrated previously with PBS.

Coupling of Ricin A Chain to Anti-Transferrin Receptor Antibody

- Incubate ricin A chain (4–5 mg in 1 ml of CM-cellulose elution buffer) with fresh 0.1% 2-merceptoethanol for 30 min at room temperature to ensure complete reduction.

- Separate ricin A chain from the reducing agent by filtration on a sephadex G-25 column (15 × 1.8 cm) in PBS.

- Add this Ricin A chain solution (~3 mg in 4 ml of PBS) slowly with the 5 mg of SPDP-derived antibody (3 mol of pyridyldisulfide per mole of antibody) in 4 ml of PBS at 4°C (ricin A chain to antibody molar ratio 3) under magnetic stirring condition.

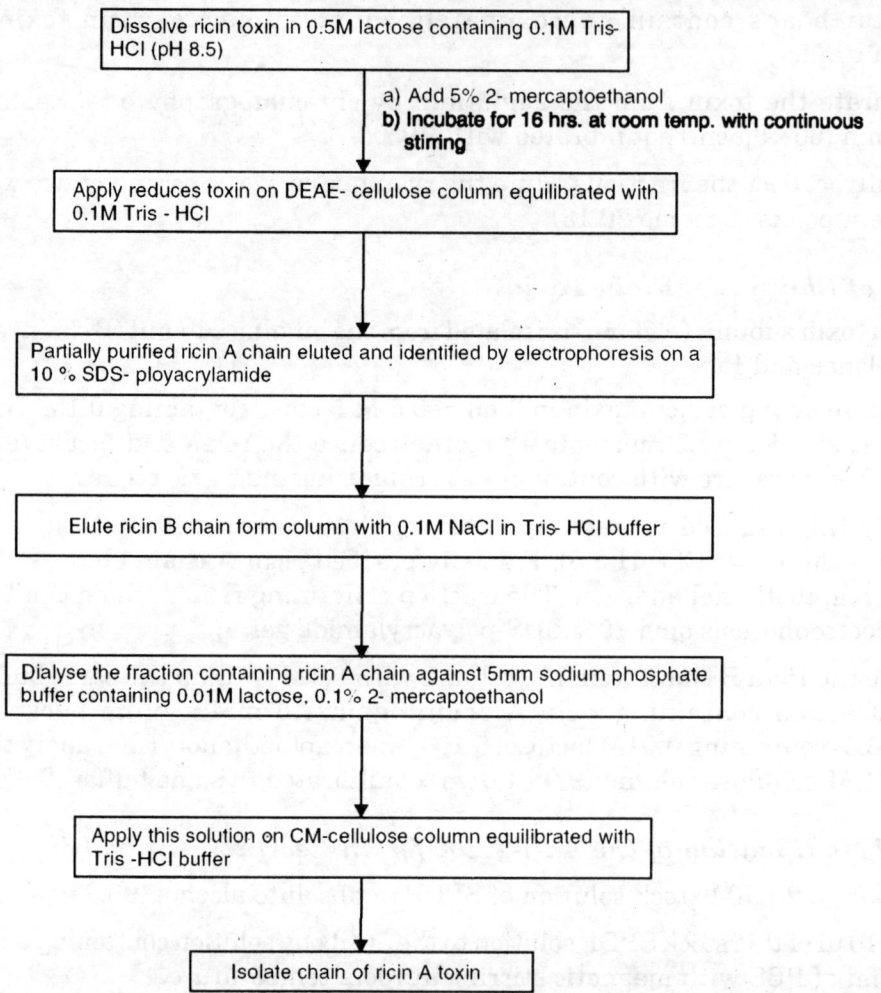

Scheme 20.14: *Isolation of chain A of ricin toxin*

- Keep the reaction mixture for 5 min in ice and then incubate the mixture overnight at 37°C.
- Concentrate the mixture to 1–2 ml using amicon ultrafiltration apparatus or by vaccum dialysis and separate the conjugates from unreacted ricin A chain by gel filtration on a Sephacryl S-200 column (120 × 1.5cm) equilibrated previously with PBS (pH 7.4).
- Analyse the antibody- ricin A conjugates under nonreducing condition on a 5% SDS-polyacrylamide gel (Scheme 20.15).

Hormone-Drug Conjugates

The impetus for preparation of hormone-drug conjugates are the finding that the biologically active peptides such as melanotropins (MSH) epidermal growth factor (EGF) and insulin are internalised by their target cell.

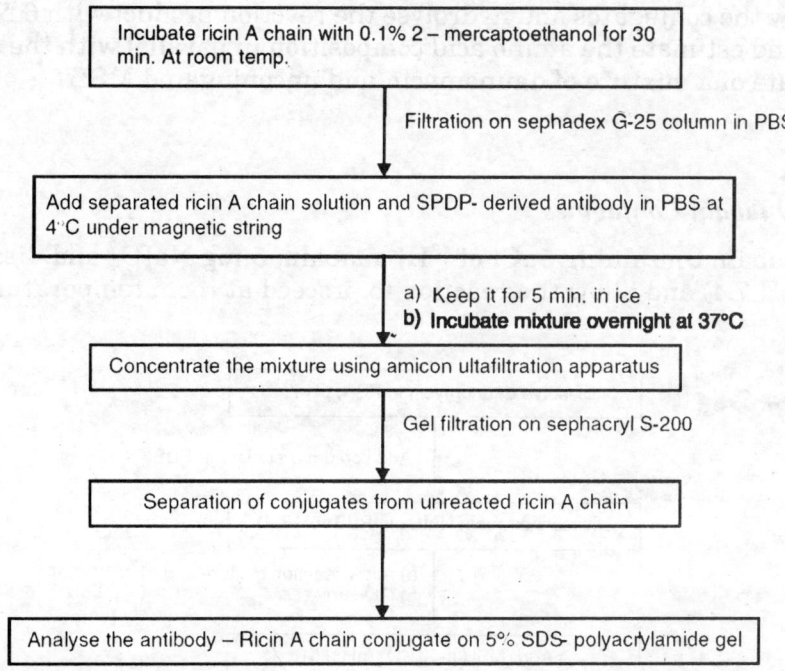

Scheme 20.15: Coupling of Ricin A chain to anti-transferrin receptor antibody

---

PROTOCOL 20.13

Melanotropin-Daunorubicin Conjugates

Melanotropin-Daunorubicin conjugates are prepared by Hurwitz *et al* for the covalent binding of daunomycin to antibodies. Free amino groups of procine β MSH (N- terminal Asp and the ε amino groups of Lys-6 and Lys-17) were substituted with an oxidised derivative of daunomycin.

- Dissolve the daunomycin (10mg, 19µmol) in 0.75 ml phosphate-buffered saline (PBS, pH 7.4).
- Add 27 µmol sodium periodate (5.8mg) in PBS.
- Adjust the pH 9.5 with 1N NaOH. Incubate the reaction mixture in the dark for 1h at room temperature.
- Add the glycerol to obtain a final concentration of 50 mM to consume excess periodate.
- Add the HPLC purified procine β melanotropin (15mg, 8 µmol) containing 1µCi of ^{125}I-labelled βMSH in 0.5ml $\cdot$ 0.15 M K_2CO_3 (pH 9.5).
- Incubate the reaction at 22°C for 1h. Reduce the schiff base by addition of $NaBH_4$ (0.3 mg/ml) at 37°C for 2h.
- Apply the reaction mixture on a sephadex G-25 (90 × 1cm) column and elute with the PBS.
- The appearance of red colour in the void volume coincident with the major peak of ^{125}I-βMSH indicates the presence of peptide-toxin conjugate.

- Freeze dry the conjugates and hydrolyse the reaction product with 6 N HCl at 110°C for 18 h and estimate the amino acid composition in parallel with the analysis of the hydrolysate of a mixture of daunomycin and unconjugated MSH.

PROTOCOL 20.14

Melanotropin-Ouabain Conjugates

- 10 mg ouabain containing 5μCi of [³H] ouabain, 5 mg NaIO₄ and dissolve in 0.5 ml of PBS (pH 7.4) and allow the reaction to proceed at room temperature for 1h.

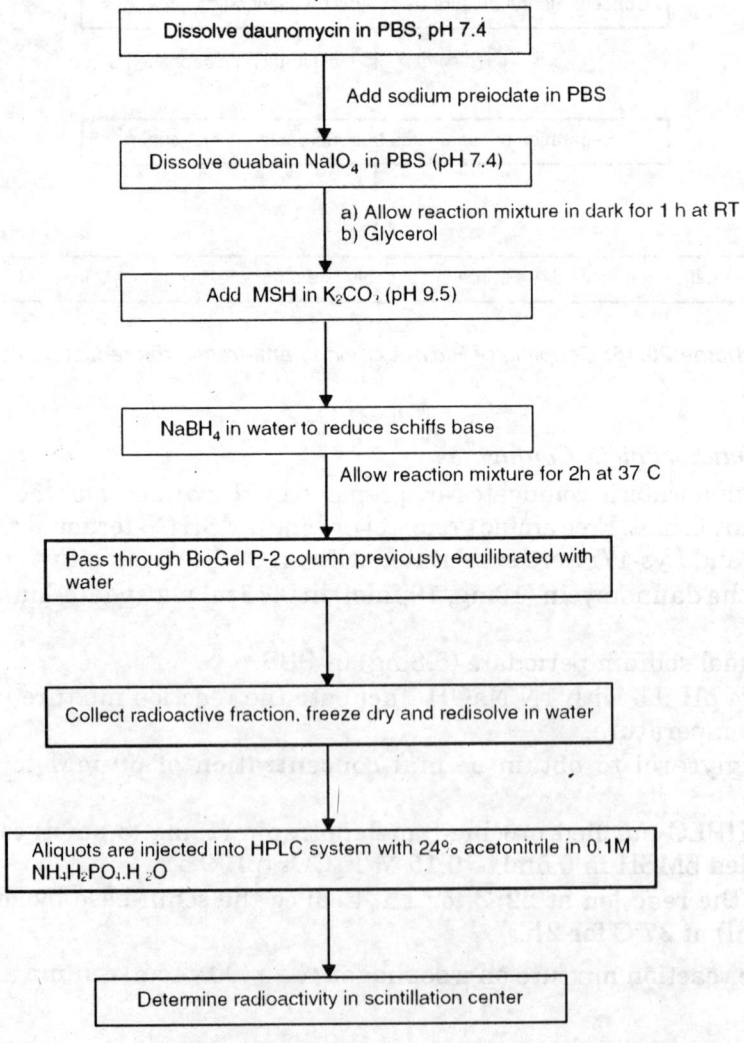

Scheme 20.16: *Formation of melanotropin- ouabain conjugates*

- Neutralise the unreacted periodate by addition of glycerol to a final concentration of 50mM.

- Add 15mg βMSH in 0.5 ml of K_2CO_3 (pH 9.5). Keep the reaction mixture for 1 h at room temperature.

- Reduce the Schiff's base by addition of 0.5 mg $NaBH_4$ in 0.1 ml water and allow the reaction mixture to react at 37°C for 2h.

- Then pass the mixture through a BioGel P-2 column (20 × 0.8 cm), previously equilibrated with water.

- Collect the radioactive fraction appearing in the void volume, freeze-dry and re-dissolve in water.

- Aliquots are injected into water HPLC system operated in the isocratic mode with 24% acetonitrile in 0.1M $NH_4H_2PO_4.H_2O$ (pH 8.0). Determine the radioactivity in a scintillation counter (Scheme 20.16).

PROTOCOL 20.15

Thyrotropin-daunomycin Conjugates

The thyrotropin-daunomycin conjugates are generally prepared by Kaneko *et al* using the method described for the preparation of MSH-daunomycin.

PROTOCOL 20.16

Polylysine-6-aminonicotinic Acid Conjugates

Preparation of 6-aminonicotinamide –⁶N-succinic Acids

- To prepare polylysine-6-aminonicotinic acid conjugate, first the 6-aminonicotinic acid derivative 6-aminonicotinamide –⁶N-succinic acid is prepared as follows-

- Take 20 g 6-aminonicotinamide (0.146 mol) with 23.0 g succinic anhydride (0.23 mol) in 200 ml dimethylsulfoxide (DMSO) and allow to react for several hours at 100°C and then followed by overnight incubation at 70°C.

- Observe the progress of the reaction by thin layer chromatography using cellulose plates with the solvent system of Ether: Methanol: Water: Concentrated NH_4OH (13:6:1:1).

- After completion of the reaction, pour the reaction mixture into 300 ml of ice-cold water.

- Filter the precipitate and dry in the air. Then grind the precipitate with diethyl ether and re-filter.

- Determine the yield of the prepared compound 6-aminonicotinamide -⁶N-succinic acid and confirm the structure of reaction product by FTIR, ¹H–NMR, Mass spectroscopic method (Scheme 20.17).

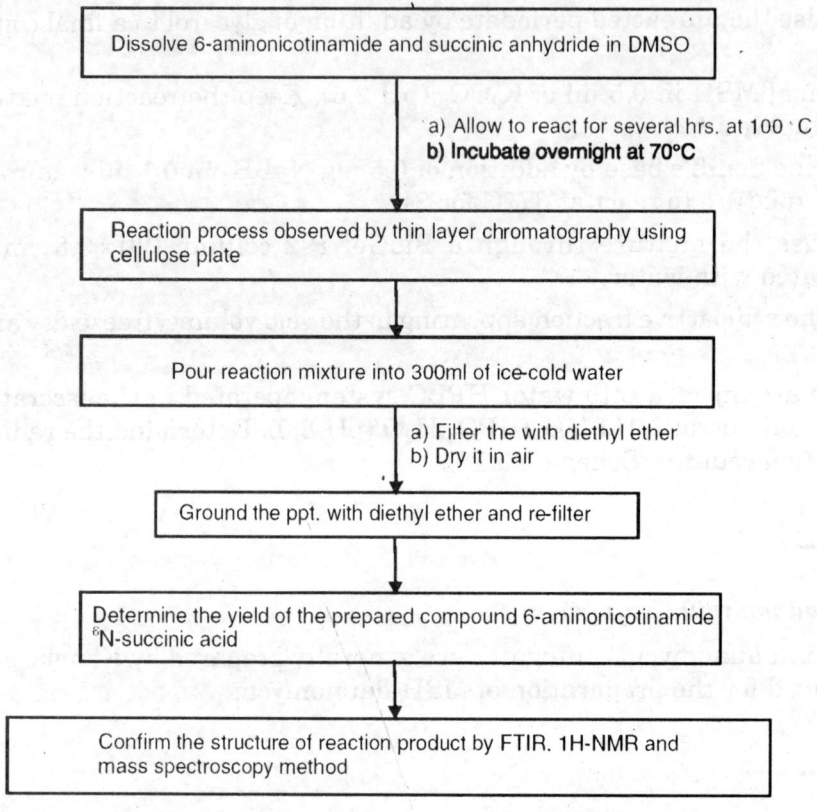

Scheme 20.17: *Preparation of 6-aminonicotinamide acid conjugate*

Preparation of 6-aminonicotinic Acid-polylysine Conjugate by Carbodiimide Method

- Take 400 mg (2.1mmol) of 1-ethyl-3-(3-dimethyl aminopropyl)carbodiimide, 200mg 6-aminonicotinamide $-^6$N-succinic acid (0.85mmol) in 10 ml water and heat the solution nearly to boiling, then add small amount of K_2HPO_4.

- Cool the reaction mixture and adjust the pH to 7.0 with 1.0 N NaOH.

- Then add 200 mg of poly (L-lysine) HBr and incubate the reaction mixture for 1h, adjust the pH once again to 7.0 with 1.0 N NaOH.

- Keep the reaction mixture for further reaction for about 1h with occasional heating at 70–80°C.

- Dialyse the reaction mixture and purify further using a 1.5 × 45 cm BioGelP-2 column with dilute HCl (pH 2) as an eluent (Alternatively, 6-Aminonicotinamide -N^6-succinic acid was also coupled to polylysine with 1-ethyl-3- (3-dimethylaminopropyl) carbodiimide as a catalyst in DMSO and pyridine) (Scheme 20.18).

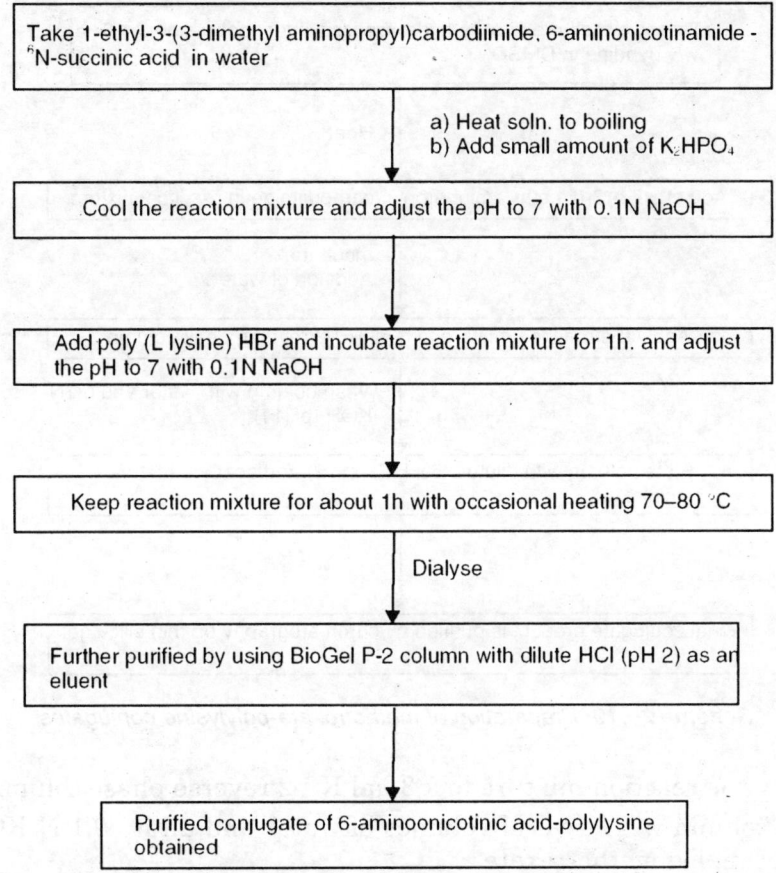

Take 1-ethyl-3-(3-dimethyl aminopropyl)carbodiimide, 6-aminonicotinamide - ^{n}N-succinic acid in water

a) Heat soln. to boiling
b) Add small amount of K_2HPO_4

Cool the reaction mixture and adjust the pH to 7 with 0.1N NaOH

Add poly (L lysine) HBr and incubate reaction mixture for 1h. and adjust the pH to 7 with 0.1N NaOH

Keep reaction mixture for about 1h with occasional heating 70–80 °C

Dialyse

Further purified by using BioGel P-2 column with dilute HCl (pH 2) as an eluent

Purified conjugate of 6-aminoonicotinic acid-polylysine obtained

Scheme 20.18: *Preparation of 6-aminonicotinic acid-polylysine conjugate by carbodiimide method*

PROTOCOL 20.17

Methotrexate-polylysine Conjugates

The methotrexate-polylysine conjugates can also be prepared by condensing glutamate residue of methotrexate with the ε-amino groups of polylysine.

Procedure

- Take 7.0 mg of methotrexate (0.015 mmol), 5mg N-hydroxysuccinimide (0.043 mmol), and 15mg polylysine and dissolve in 2 ml of 10% w/v pyridine in DMSO.
- Heat the reaction mixture at 50°C to dissolve any solid material, add 15 mg of 1-ethyl-3-(3-dimethylaminopropyl) carbodiimide (0.078 mmol) in the reaction mixture.
- Incubate the reaction mixture 5–30 min, followed by the addition of 5 volume of water.

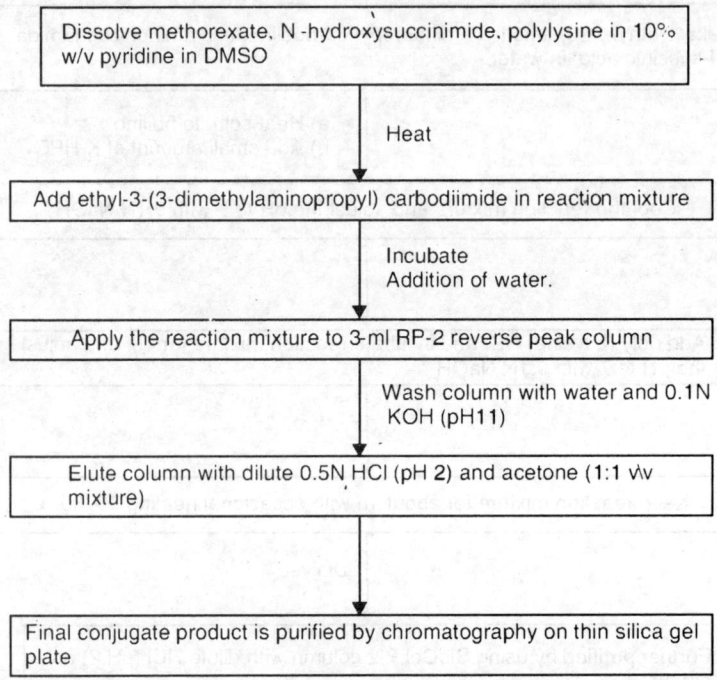

Scheme 20.19: Preparation of methotrexate-polylysine conjugates

- Then apply the reaction mixture to a 3–ml RP-2 reverse phase column.
- Wash the column with several volumes of water and dilute 0.1 N KOH (pH 11) to remove uncoupled methotrexate.
- Elute the column with dilute 0.5 N HCl (pH 2) and the acetone (1:1 v/v) mixture.
- Determine the purity of the conjugated final product by the chromatography on thin-layer silica gel plates using an ascending solvent system of methanol: water: NH$_4$OH (con.) (40:10:1) (Scheme 20.19).

PROTOCOL 20.18

Doxorubicin/Daunomycin-Polylysine Conjugate

Principle

- The conjugates of anthracylines with polylysine can also be prepared by using succinate to link between the amino group of the anthracylines and the ε-amino groups of polylysine.

Procedure

- Dissolve the 14 mg N-hydroxysuccinimide (0.125 mmol), 5 mg succinic anhydride (0.05 mmol) and 96 mg of 1-ethyl-3-(3-dimethylaminopropyl) carbodiimide (0.5 mmol) in the 3 ml DMSO and allow to react for 20 min at room temperature.

- Then add daunomycin hydrochloride (1.2 mg, 0.002 mmol) previously dissolved in 0.5 ml DMSO into the reaction mixture and vortex occasionally for 1 h.

- Then cool the reaction mixture to 0°C, then mix 2 ml of chloroform and 2 ml cold 0.1M K_2HPO_4, (pH 7.0). Keep the reaction mixture for 1h then evaporate the chloroform phase.

- Pool the chloroform extracts and extract back once with 2.0 ml cold 0.1M K_2HPO_4, (pH 7.0), and wash three times with 2 ml cold water.

- Evaporate the chloroform phase to leave the daunomycin succinate N-hydroxysuccinimide ester as a residue. Then dissolve the residue in 2 ml water, and add 25 mg poly (L-lysine). HBr (M_r 35,000) in 1 ml water immediately.

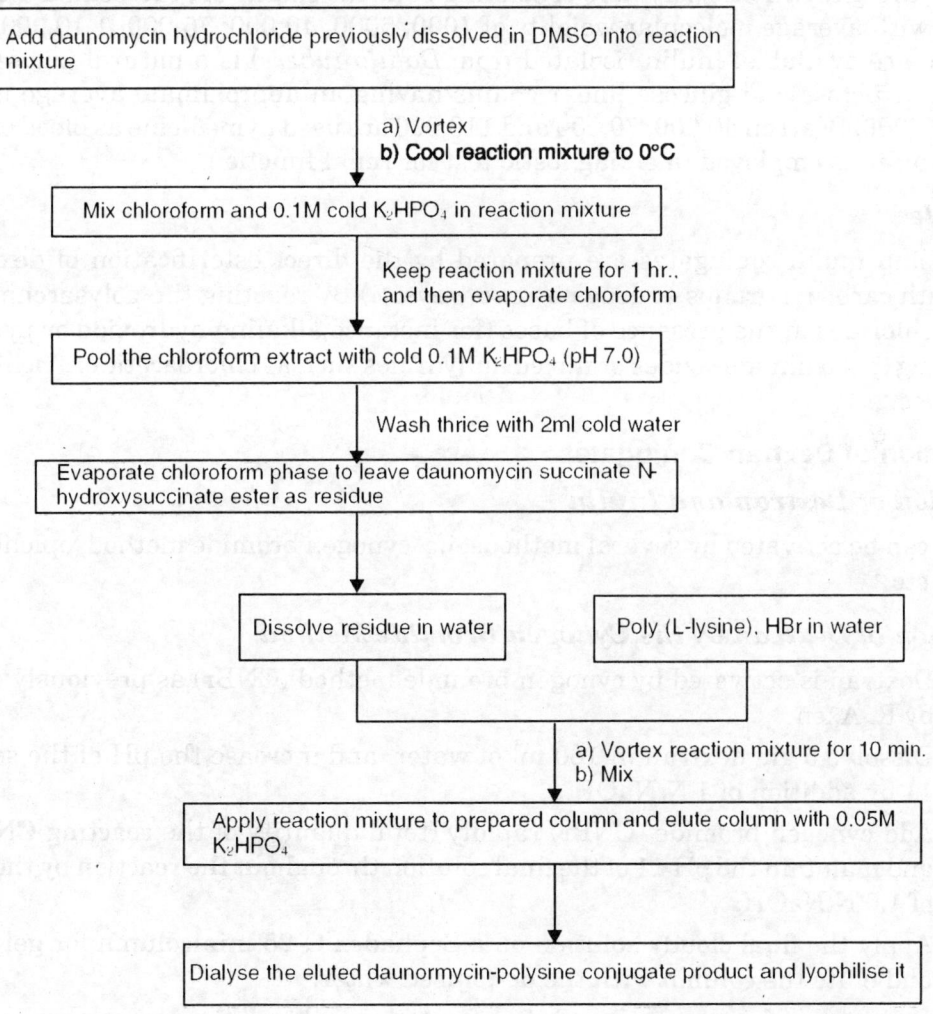

Scheme 20.20: *Preparation of doxorubicin\ daunomycin-polylysine conjugate*

- Vortex the reaction mixture continuously for 10 min and subsequently mixed occasionally for 2 h. Prepare a DE-52 column and wash with 10% K_2HPO_4, pH 7.0 followed by washing with water. Then apply the reaction mixture to this prepared DE-52 column and elute this column with an isocratic gradient of 0.05 M K_2HPO_4.
- The daunomycin-polylysine conjugates elute first and free unconjugated daunomycin derivatives elute later. Then dialyse the final conjugate product against PBS and lyophilise the conjugates for further use (Scheme 20.20).

PROTOCOL 20.19

Dextran and Inulin Conjugates as Drug Carriers

Dextrans are biosynthetic polymers consisting of linear chains of glucose in a 1:6 linkage. Dextran with average molecular weights of 1000, 5000, 40,000, 75,000, 1,10,000, 700,000 and more are available. Inulin (isolated from *Dahila tubers*) is a natural polysaccharide formed by fructose and glucose linear chains having an approximate average molecular weight of 5000. Dextran 40,000, 70,000 and 110,000 are used in medicine as blood expanders and the inulin is employed in a diagnostic test for renal function.

Principle

Dextran and inulin conjugates are prepared by the direct esterification of dextran and inulin with carbonyl groups of drugs by two ways: (i) By reacting the polysaccharide with the acid chlorides in the presence of bases (for instance alkaline hydroxide or pyridine) or (ii) by using carbodiimide, azides or mixed anhydrides such as chloroacetic or trichloroacetic anhydrides.

Preparation of Dextran Conjugates

Activation of Dextran and Inulin

Dextran can be activated by several methods, i.e. cynogen bromide method, epichlorhydrin method, etc.

Activation of Dextran by the Cynogen Bromide Method

- Dextran is activated by cynogen bromide method (CNBr) as previously described by R. Axen.
- Dissolve 5 gm dextran in 160 ml of water and increase the pH of the solution to 11 by addition of 1 N NaOH.
- Add cynogen bromide (CNBr) rapidly (total quantity of the reacting CNBr, 2.5g) and maintain the pH 11 of the final solution throughout the reaction by the addition of 1.0 N NaOH.
- Apply the final cloudy solution on a Sephadex G-25 minicolumn for gel filtration and elute the column with the de-ionised water.
- Collect the dextrorotatory-eluted fractions and use them directly for coupling reaction.

Activation of Dextran or Inulin by Epichlorhydrin

- In a 250ml round bottom flask well equipped with a reflux condenser and a stirrer, dissolve the 10 g of dextran in 25 ml of water.

- Add 50 ml epichlorhydrin, and 10 ml of 25%w/v solution of $Zn(BF_4)_2$ in water. Warm this mixture on a steam bath for 5 h and then pour into the 700 ml of acetone.

- Filter the precipitate, wash with acetone and dry. Then dissolve the dried crude product in a minimum amount of water and add acetone to re-precipitate.

- Repeat this procedure twice in order to obtain pure chlorohydroxypropyl dextran (a dextran derivative).

- Alternatively UV light of 254 nm can also act as an alternative catalyst to prepare chlorohydroxypropyl dextran under same basic synthesis condition (10g of polysaccharide, 25ml of water, and 50 ml epichlorhydrin); however the longer retension time of 48 hr is required.

- These reaction produces chlorohydroxy propyldextran or chlorhydroxy propylinulin with the chlorine content of 5–6%, a content corresponding to an activated hydroxyl group with every two or three glucosidic residue.

Coupling of Activated Dextran with the Drugs

Primary amino groups of drugs can easily react with iminocarbonate dextran (as obtained from CNBr or organic cynates activation).

Sodium Borate Mediated Coupling

- The activated polysaccharides are dry powders, which may be stored as long as several years.

- Activated dextran or activated inulin (chlorohydroxy propyl dextran or chlorohydroxy propyl inulin respectively) can be conjugated with the amino groups containing drugs using 2% sodium borate ($Na_4B_2O_7 . 10H_2O$), pH 9.2 at 5°C for 48 hr.

- The same mild conditions (pH 9.2 at 5°C for 48 h) can also be used for conjugation of amino group containing drugs with the activated dextran.

Reduction of Schiff's Bases

- Dissolve the chlorohydroxy propyldextran and the drugs (weight ratio of drug to activated dextran 1:1) in borate buffer solution and adjust the pH at 9.2 with the 1N NaOH and allow to react for 48h at 5°C.

- The conjugation of polyaldehyde dextran with the primary amino groups of drug can also be carried out at room temperature in the dark for 12 h in a phosphate buffer solution, pH 7.2.

- The resulting schiff base is reduced with $NaBH_4$ at about 40°C for 2 h.

Coupling by Hydrazine Method

- The preparation method of conjugate of formyl rifamycin SV with dextran is given as— prepare a hydrazine derivative of polysaccharide by reacting this chlorohydroxy propyl dextran with hydrazine in 1:1 molar ratio.

- After reaction with the drug, a hydrazone is formed which when reduced forms a hydrazine.

- Chlorohydroxy propyl dextran (chlorine content, 6 %) is dissolved in a 2% sodium borate buffer solution, is treated with an excess of hydrazine (NH_2-NH_2) in water.

- Keep the reaction mixture overnight at room temperature.

- Dialyse the sample against water and lyophilise the final product, a white powder is obtained (nitrogen content 2.3%).

- Dissolve the hydrazine hydroxypropyl dextran (1.0 g) in 10 ml of 10% of the sodium acetate and add 1 gm of formyl drug dissolved in 10 ml of the same solvent.

- Incubate the solution for 2h at room temperature and then react with 50mg of sodium borohydride to reduce the hydrazone bond to a more stable hydrazine (Scheme 20.21).

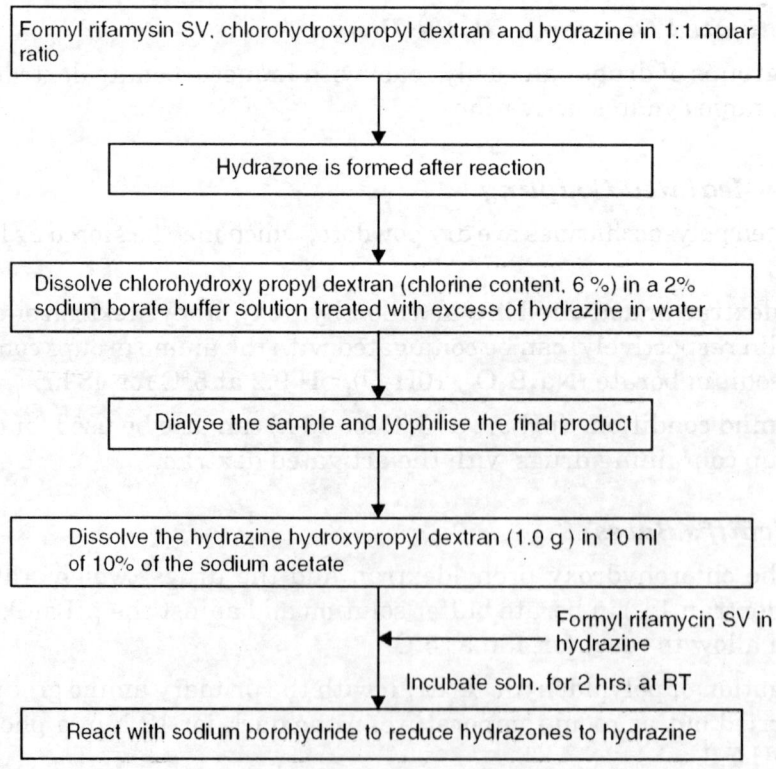

Scheme 20.21: *Coupling of activated dextran with the drugs*

PROTOCOL 20.20

Lectin as Carrier

Preparation and Purification of Concanavalin A —Trypsin Conjugates

Lectins are a group of proteins with the characteristic ability to bind saccharides moieties at two or more binding sites on the molecules. This structure endows lectins with the ability to agglutinate red blood cells and cultured cells by agglutinate red blood cells and cultured cells by crosslinking cell surface saccharides structures. The majority of the lectins, which have been characterised, are derived from plant seeds and they have been extensively studied under the name of phytohaemagglutinins. Some lectins are used in blood typing a variety of them have been used as experimental tools to investigate biological roles of cell surface glycoproteins. Some lectins (e.g. wheat germ agglutinin, concanavalin A) specifically agglutinate tumour cells but not normal control cells under defined experimental conditions, thereby providing the valuable tools for investigating biochemical changes associated with oncogenic transformation.

Advantages of Lectins as a Carrier of Drugs and Enzymes Include–

- Lectins are readily purified by simple affinity chromatography techniques that are useful both in the initial isolation of the lectins and in purifying conjugates, which contains lectins.
- Lectins can tolerate higher coupling frequencies without loss of binding activity as compared to antibodies.

Disadvantages of lectins as a carrier include-

- Retention for longer period at the site of injection in a variety of tissues
- Lower specificity
- Many lectins are toxic and potent inducers of inflammation

PROTOCOL 20.21

Preparation of Concanavalin A —Trypsin Conjugates

Materials

Concanavalin A

Tris acetate saline buffer, TAS

Crystalline bovine trypsin

25% v/v aqueous glutaraldehyde solution

Procedure

Preparation of Concanavalin Affinity Column

- Affinity purification on Con A containing species was carried out on columns of swelled Sephadex G-200 in TAS.
- Wash the column with 2 bed volumes of TAS buffers.
- Then elute the column with 1.5-bed volume of 0.2 M α-methylmannoside in TAS.

Trypsin Affinity Column

- Trypsin containing species can also be purified on an affinity column prepared essentially by p-(ε-aminocaproylamido) benzamidine couple to cynogen bromide activate Sepharose 4B. This ligand is prepared in two-step:

Step 1. Preparation of p-(ε-aminocaproylamido) Benzamidine. 2HCl

- Dissolve 5 g p-aminobenzamidine.2HCl, 6.65 N-benzyloxycarbonyl-6-amidocaproic acid, and 11.65 g 1-cyclohexyl-3-(2-morpholinoethyl) carbodiimide metho-p-toluenesulfonate in a mixture of 10 ml pyridine and 150 ml acetonitrile and stir the mixture overnight at room temperature.

- Evaporate the solvent and dissolve the residue in ethyl acetate: butanol mixture (1:1).

- Extract the solution by 1N hydrochloric acid, water, and 5% aqueous $NaHCO_3$.

- Separate the organic and aqueous phase. Dry the organic layer over anhydrous sodium sulfate, concentrate under reduced pressure, and triturate with ether to produce 6 g of product.

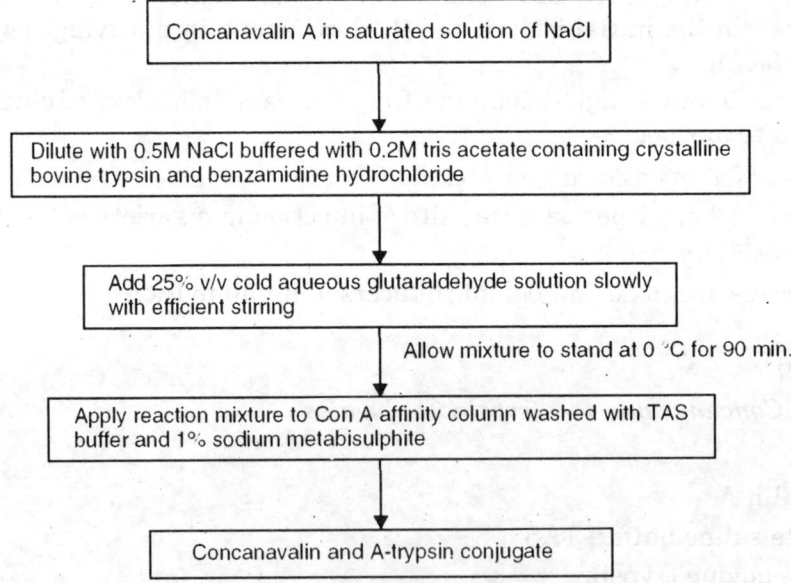

Scheme 20.22: *Preparation of concanavaline A-trypsin conjugate*

- Heat the product at 90–95°C for 30 min in 40 ml of trifluoroacetic acid to remove the benzyloxycarbonyl-protecting group.

- Evaporate the trifluoroacetic acid under reduced pressure, and dissolve the residue in excess of methanol saturated with anhydrous HCl.

- Evaporate the mixture under reduced pressure; and wash with ether and crystallise the product by dissolving in a mini column of methanol and bringing the mixture to the incipient cloud point by addition of ether. p- (ε-aminocaproylamido) benzamidine. 2HCl obtained with the melting point 286°C.

Step 2. Preparation of Cynogen Bromide Activated Sepharose 4B

- Suspend the 100 ml sepharose 4B in 70 ml of 0.1M NaHCO$_3$ buffer, pH 10.
- Mix with the 35 ml of an aqueous solution containing 1g of p- (ε-aminocaproylamido) benzamidine and adjust the pH to 10 with aqueous NaOH.
- Maintain the temperature of reaction mixture at 4°C with occasional remixing for 24 h and wash with the water on a sintered glass funnel, and store until used in 1 M NaCl containing 0.02% sodium azide.

Preparation of Concanavalin A-trypsin Conjugates

- Take 100 mg concanavalin A in 2 ml saturated solution of NaCl and dilute this solution up to 10 ml with 0.5 M NaCl buffered with 0.2 M Tris acetate (Tris acetate saline buffer, TAS, pH 5.0) containing 100 mg crystalline bovine trypsin and 10mM benzamidine hydrochloride to prevent trypsin from attacking the Con A during the coupling reaction.
- Add 0.4 ml of 25% v/v cold aqueous glutaraldehyde solution slowly with efficient stirring and allow the mixture to stand at 0°C for 90 min.
- Terminate the coupling reaction by applying directly the reaction mixture to the Con A affinity column (100 ml of sephadex G-200) washed with 10 ml of TAS buffer, 20 ml 1% sodium metabisulphite and an additional 200ml of TAS (Scheme 20.22).

Purification of Concanavalin A-trypsin Conjugates

The coupling reaction mixture contains random mixture of Con A-trypsin conjugates plus Con A, aggregated Con A, trypsin, aggregated trypsin, and unreacted glutaraldehyde oligomers.

Assay Procedures

Method 1: Trypsin Assay

- Trypsin activity can be determined spectrophotometrically in a Gilford recording spectrophotometer using tosyl-L-arginine methyl ester as substrate and crystalline bovine trypsin as standard.
- Trypsin activity monitored by the change in absorbance at 247nm using 1mM tosyl-L-arginine methyl ester, 40 mM Tris-HCl buffer, pH 8.
- Add 3–7 µg of trypsin in same buffer in 1 ml cuvettes.
- Determine the amount of substrate hydrolysed by monitoring the absorbance at 247 nm for 3 min.
- Determine the amount of trypsin activity by interpolation from a standard curve.

Method 2: Trypsin Assay

- Trypsin activity can also be determined in the purified conjugates using azocasein as substrate and monitoring production of peptides, soluble in 5% w/v aqueous trichloroacetic acid.

- Incubate the 0.5 ml of 1 mg/ml of azocaseinin 40 mM Tris-HCl, pH 8.1 at 25°C with 0.5–1.5 μg of crystalline trypsin or equivalent for 10 min.
- Stop the reaction by adding 0.5ml of 10% w/v aqueous trichloroacetic acid.
- Sediment the precipitate in clinical centrifuge and the absorbance of the supernatant fluid measured at 340nm.
- Determine the amount of trypsin activity by interpolation from a standard curve.

Hemagglutination Activity Determination

- Hemagglutination activity of concanavalin A in Con A-trypsin conjugates can be determined in triplicates using a Takasty microtiter apparatus.
- Take 25-μl test samples and add 25.0-μl aliquots of phosphate buffered saline (0.14 M NaCl, 0.01 M Potassium Phosphate pH 7.4) per well as a diluents to make 2 fold dilutions. Then add 25-μl of suspension of 2×10^8 sheep red cells per milliliter pretreated with 0.05% trypsin in PBS for 30 min at 25°C and then wash with the same buffer.
- Then estimate the Con A content in ConA-trypsin preparations by comparison of serial dilution end point concentration (i.e. maximum concentration that does not cause agglutination) with standard concentrations of unconjugated Con A.

Glycoproteins as Drug Carriers

Glycoproteins are well-known carrier for drug targeting to specific cell types, by virtue of the range of plasma membrane receptors for glycoprotein. Some of these receptors are listed in the Table 20.2. In general they mediate entry into cells by endocytosis and so are valuable in directing molecules to endosomes, lysosomes, and other structures with which such vesicles fuse. In addition, small permeable molecules may be deposited inside particular cells by such mean and then, after hydrolysis of their carrier, be freed to diffuse throughout the cell, thus reaching cytosolic and other locations non-selectively. Glycoproteins have also found application as spacer molecules, thereby allowing larger amounts of a drug to be linked to antibodies (which are used to target the drugs) than is possible to antibody alone. Glycoproteins may also be used to direct liposomes erythrocyte ghosts or viral envelopes to specific cell types with whose cell surface they fuse, thereby depositing their soluble contents into the interior of the cell.

Table. 20.2: Some cellular receptors for glycoproteins and their respective location

Receptor	*Respective locations*
Serum glycoproteins with carbohydrate termini	
Galactose terminated glycoproteins	Hepatocytes
Other serum glycoproteins	
Transferrin	Reticulocytes
2-Macroglobulins	Macrophages, fibroblasts

Table. 20.2: *Some cellular receptors for glycoproteins and their respective location*

Contd..

Receptor	Respective locations
Lysosomal enzymes	
Mannose terminated enzymes	Macrophages
Mannose 6-phosphate terminated enzymes	Fibroblasts
Hormones and growth factors	
TSH	Thyroids
Gonadotropins	Gonadal cells
Cellular growth factors such as epidermal growth factors	Fibroblast
Opsonins	
Complement components	Leukocytes
Antibodies	Leukocytes

PROTOCOL 20.22

Galactose Terminated Feutin as Carriers for Pepstatin

Pepstatin is a group specific inhibitor of aspartic proteinases and has some clinical applications already. Although directing pepstatin to the liver is not difficult, the first pepstatin glycoprotein carrier, which has been made, asialofeutin (galactose terminated)-pepstatin, has been designed to achieve selectivity towards hepatocytes. The conjugation involves purification of the serum glycoprotein fetuin (from commercial samples) and its enzymatic (or chemical) desialylation- to expose terminal galactose residues.

Procedure

- The coupling of pepstatin to asialofeutin can be performed through the ε-amino groups of the proteins to the N-hydroxy succinimide ester of pepstatin.
- Dissolve 18.0 μmol of pepstatin in 1ml of dimethylformamide.
- Then add 36.0 μmol of 1-ethyl-3- (3-dimethylaminopropyl) carbodiimide and 36.0 μmol of N-hydroxysuccinimide.
- Allow the reaction to proceeds for 2 h at room temperature.
- After 2 h, add the resultant mixture drop wise to 30.0 ml of 0.1M sodium bicarbonate solution containing 3.0 μmol of asialofeutin.
- Keep the reaction mixture for 2 h at room temperature.
- Separate the reaction product by using a column of LH-20 (3.5 × 50 cm) eluted with 0.9% NaCl. The conjugate elutes in the void volume while free pepstatin is retarded by gel (Scheme 20.23).

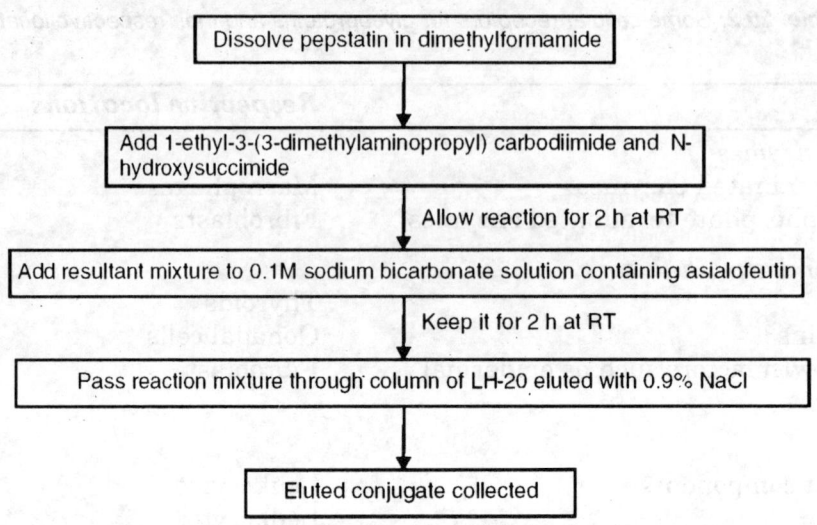

Scheme 20.23: *Formation of Galactose terminated fetuin as carriers for pepstatin*

SUGGESTED READINGS

- Annemiek, J.M.L., van Rensen, Wauben, M.H.M., Stulemeyer, M.C.G., van Eden, W. and Cromelin, D.J.A. (1999) Pharm. Res. 16, 198.
- Avrilionis, K. and Boggs, J.M. (1996) Cell. Immunol. 168, 13.
- Bayer, E.A. and Wilchek, M. (1990) In: Methods in Enzymology, vol. 184, Wilchek, M. and Bayer, E.A., (eds.), San Diago Academic Press, 174.
- Bartling G. J., Brown H. D. and Chattopadhyoy S.K.(1973) Nature, 243, 432.
- Chu, B.C.F., Kramer, F.R. and Orgel, L.E. (1986) Nucleic Acid Res. 14, 5591.
- Gao, X. and Huang, L. (1996) Biochemistry 35, 1027.
- Garagiola, D.M., Huard, T.K. and Lo Buglio, A.F. (1979) Blood 54, 84.
- Galardy R.E. *et al* (1978) J. Med. Chem., 21,1279.
- Ghose S.S., Kao, P.M. and Kwoh, D.Y., (1989) Anal. Biochem., 178, 43.
- Ghose S.S., Kao P.M., Mecue A.W., Chappelle H.L. (1990) Bioconjugate Chem, 1,71.
- Hermanson, G.T. (1996) Bioconjugate Techniques, New York: Academic Press, 10.
- Hoare, D.G., Ksohland D.E., (1966) J. Am. Chem. Soc., 88, 2057.
- Hearn M. J. W., Bethell, G. S., Ayers J. S. and Hancock W. S. (1979) J. Chromatography. 185,463–470.
- Haisma, H.J., Boven, M., Vanmuijen, M., Dejong, J., Vander Vijgh, W.J.F. and Pinedo, H.M. (1992) Br. J. Cancer 66, 474.
- Hartman, F.C. and Wold, F. (1966) J. Am. Chem. Soc. 88, 3890.
- Hege, K.M., Daleke, D.L., Waldmann, T.A. and Matthay, K.K. (1989) Blood 74, 2043.
- Kraehenbuhl, J. P., Galardy, R.E. and Jamieson, J.D. (1979) Fab. J. Exp. Med., 139, 208.
- Kotite, N.I., Staros, J.V. and Cunningham, L.W. (1984), Biochemistry, 23,3099-3104.

- Kedar, E., Rutkowski, Y., Braun, E., Emanuel, N. and Barenholz, Y. (1994) J. Immunother. Emphasis Tumor Immunol. 16, 47.

- Khaw, B.A., Torchilin, V.P., Vural, I. And Narula, J. (1995) Nature Med. 1, 1195.

- Kim, Y.W., Fung, M.S.C., Sun, N.C., Sun, C.R.Y., Chang, N.T. and Chang, T.W. (1990) J. Immunol. 144, 1257.

- Kinsky, S.C. (1972) Biochim. Biophys. Acta. 265, 1.

- Kitagawa, T. and Aikawa, T. (1976) J. Biochem. 79, 233.

- Ludwig F.R. and Jay F.A. (1985) Eur. J. Biochem. 151, 53.

- Peng L., Calton G. J. and Burnett J.W. (1987) Appl. Biochem. Biotechnol., 14, 91.

- Sheehan J.C., Cruickshank P.A. and Boshart G.C.(1961) J. org. Chem., 26,2525.

- Sheehan, J .C., Preston J. and Cruickshank P.A. (1965) J.Am. Chem. Soc., 87,2492.

- Tan, Y., Sun, X., Xu, M., An, Z., Tan, X., Han, Q., Miljkovic, D.A., Yang, M. and Hoffman, R.M. (1998) Protein Extra. Puruf. 12, 45.

- Tanaka, T., Kaneo, Y., Miyashita, M. (1996) Biol. Pharm. Bull. 19, 774.

- Till, M.A., Ghetie, V., Gregori, T., Patzer, E.J., Porter, J.P., Uhr, J.W., Capon, D.J. and Vitetta, E.S. (1988) Science 242, 1166.

- Wagner, E., Zatloukal, K., Cotton, M., Kirlappos, H., Mechtler, K. and Curiel, D.T. (1992) Proc. Natl. Acad. Sci. USA 89, 6099.

- Wagner, E., Curiel, D. and Cotton, M. (1994) Adv. Drug Deliv. Rev. 14, 113.

- Weissner, J.H. and Hwang, K.J. (1982) Biochim. Biophys. Acta. 689, 490.

- Wright, S. and Huang, L. (1989) Adv. Drug Deliv. Rev. 3, 343.

- Wu, D., Yang, J. and Pardridge, W.M. (1997) J. Clin. Invest. 100, 1804.

- Wu, M., Fan, J., Gunning, W. and Ratnam, M. (1997) J. Membr. Biol. 159, 137.

- Vitetta, E.S. (1990) J. Clin. Immunol. 10, 515.

21

Cyclodextrin Complexes
Dextran Complexes, Cyclodextrin Complexes

INTRODUCTION

Cyclodextrins are cyclic oligosaccharides typically containing 6(α-CD), 7(β-CD), or 8(γ-CD) glucopyranose units. This cyclic orientation provides a truncated cone structure that is hydrophilic on the exterior and lipophilic on the interior. Cyclodextrin complexes are formed when a guest molecule is partially or fully contained in the interior of the cavity (Table 21.1). The parent α-, β-, and γ-cyclodextrins (particularly β) have limited aqueous solubility and show toxicity when given by injection. Therefore, the parent cyclodextrin structure has been chemically modified to generate a parenterally safe CD-derivative. The modifications are typically made at one or more of the 2, 3, or 6 position hydroxyls (Fig. 21.1).

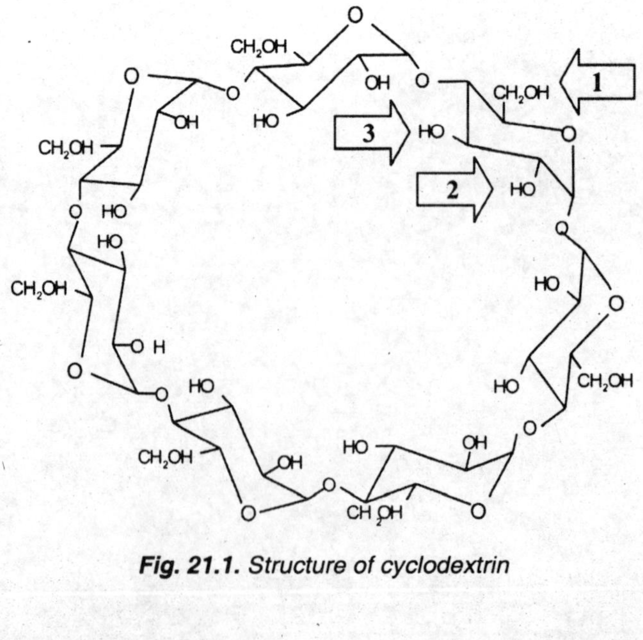

Fig. 21.1. *Structure of cyclodextrin*

MECHANISM OF DRUG CYCLODEXTRIN COMPLEXATION

The kinetics of drug cyclodextrin interaction and subsequent complexation could be explained on the basis of hydrophilic and hydrophobic interaction possibilities of cyclodextrin with water and drug molecules respectively.

- The displacement of polar water molecules from the apolar cyclodextrin cavity
- The increased number of hydrogen bonds formed as the displaced water returns to the larger pool
- A reduction of the repulsive interactions between the hydrophobic guest and the aqueous environment
- An increase in the hydrophobic interactions as the guest inserts itself into the apolar cyclodextrin cavity.

The ability of a cyclodextrin to form an inclusion complex with a guest molecule depends on two key factors. The first is steric and depends on the relative size of the cyclodextrin to the size of the guest molecule or certain key functional groups within the guest. If the size of guest molecule is not appropriate, the steric fit into the cyclodextrin cavity could not be brought about. The second critical factor is the thermodynamic interactions between the different components of the system (cyclodextrin, guest, solvent) where a favourable net energetic driving force is essential to pull the guest into the cyclodextrin.

While this initial equilibrium to form the complex is very rapid (often within minutes), the final equilibrium can take much longer to reach. Once inside the cyclodextrin cavity, the guest molecule makes conformational adjustments to take maximum advantage of the weak van der Waals forces that exist.

Table 21.1: *Cyclodextrin characteristics*

Cyclodextrin Type	α	β	γ
Number of glucose units	6	7	8
Cavity diameter (Å)	4.7–5.3	6.0 – 6.5	7.5 – 8.3
Cavity height (Å)	7.9	7.9	7.9
Cavity volume (Å^3)	174	262	427
Appearance	White crystalline powder	White crystalline powder	White crystalline powder
Molecular weight	973	1135	1297
Bulk density, g/cm^3	0.4 – 0.7	0.4 – 0.7	0.4 – 0.7
Water solubility (25 °C), g/100 mL	14.5	1.8	23.2
Content (dry basis)	>98%	>98%	>98%
Specific rotation in aqueous Solution [α] D,20	+147° to +152°	+160° to +164°	+174° to +180°

Table 21.1: *Cyclodextrin characteristics* Contd...

Cyclodextrin Type	α	β	γ
Water	<10%	<14%	<11%
Heavy metals	<5 ppm	<5 ppm	<5 ppm
Residue on lgnition	<0.1%	<0.1%	<0.1%
Volatile organics	<20 ppm	<5 ppm	<50 ppm
Micro-organisms	<1000/g	<1000/g	<1000/g

Comparative specification of commercial cyclodextrins of CAVAMAX® Pharma

PHARMACEUTICAL APPLICATIONS OF DRUG CYCLODEXTRIN COMPLEXES

Cyclodextrins increase the water solubility of poorly soluble drugs to improve their bioavailability. Light, thermal and oxidative stability of bioactives can be improved through the formation of cyclodextrin complexes. Cyclodextrins have also been used to reduce dermal, gastrointestinal or ocular irritation, mask unpleasant tastes or odours, prevent adverse drug-ingredient interactions and convert oils/liquids into powders to improve handling.

The most stable three-dimensional structure of cyclodextrins is a typical toroid with the larger and smaller openings presenting hydroxyl groups to the external environment and mostly hydrophobic functionality lining the interior of the cavity (Fig. 21.2). It is this unique configuration that gives cyclodextrins their interesting properties and creates the thermodynamic driving force needed to form host-guest complexes with apolar molecules and functional groups.

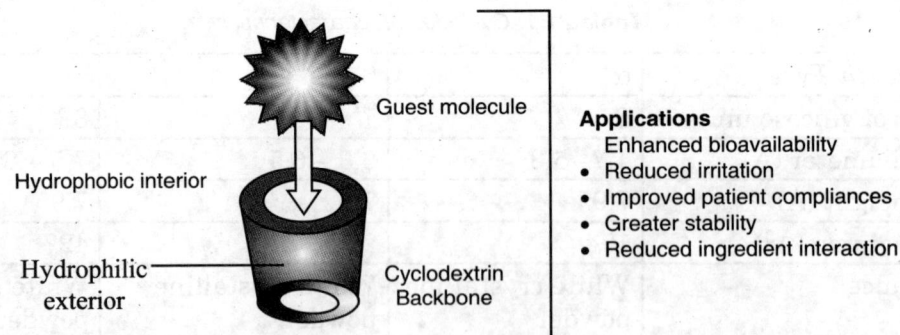

Fig. 21.2. *Multiple benefits exist for cyclodextrin complexes in pharmaceutical formulations*

BIOAVAILABILITY ENHANCEMENT

Drugs with poor bioavailability generally possess low water solubility and/or tend to be highly crystalline. As shown, cyclodextrins are water-soluble and form inclusion complexes with apolar molecules or functional groups in water insoluble compounds. The resulting complex hides most of the hydrophobic functionality in the interior cavity of the cyclodextrin while the hydrophilic hydroxyl groups on its external surface remain exposed to the environment. The net effect being a water-soluble cyclodextrin-drug complex. In addition to improving solubility, cyclodextrins also prevent crystallisation of active ingredients by complexing individual drug molecules so that they can no longer self-assemble into a crystal lattice.

Active Stabilisation

For an active molecule to degrade upon exposure to radiation, heat, oxygen or water, chemical reactions must take place. When a molecule is constrained within the cyclodextrin cavity, it is difficult for reactants (water or oxygen) to diffuse into the cavity and react with the protected guest. In the case of thermal or radiation induced degradation, the bioactive must undergo molecular rearrangements. Again, due to the steric constraints on the guest molecule within the cavity, it is difficult for the active to fragment upon exposure to heat or light or if it does fragment, the fragments do not have the mobility needed to separate and react before a simple recombination takes place.

Odour or Taste Masking

Through encapsulation within the cyclodextrin cavity, molecules or specific functional groups that cause unpleasant tastes or odours are hidden from the sensory receptors. The resulting formulations have no or little taste or odour and are much more agreeable to the patient.

Compatibility Improvement

Often one would like to combine multiple ingredients or drug actives within a single formulation due to the potential for synergistic benefits. However, different drugs are often incompatible with each other or another inactive ingredient within a formulation. Encapsulating one of the incompatible ingredients within a cyclodextrin molecule stabilises the formulation by physically separating the components in order to prevent chemical interaction.

Preparation of Cyclodextrin Drug Complexes

Complexes can be formed by a variety of techniques that depend on the properties of the drug, the equilibrium kinetics, the other formulation ingredients and processes and the final dosage form desired. Preparation of complexes is accomplished by using either of three general methods depending upon the physicochemical properties of material to be complexed as well as purpose of the complexation. However, each of these processes depends on a small amount of water to help drive the thermodynamics. Among the methods used are simple dry mixing, mixing in solutions and suspensions followed by a suitable separation, the preparation of pastes and several thermo-mechanical techniques.

Dissociation of the inclusion complex is a relatively rapid process usually governed by a large increase in the number of water molecules in the surrounding environment. The resulting concentration gradient shifts the equilibrium towards left. In highly dilute and dynamic systems like the body, the guest may account difficulty finding another cyclodextrin to reform the complex and is left free in solution.

PROTOCOL:21.1

Complexation in Solution

Material

Cyclodextrin (α, β, or γ-)

Drug

Procedure

- Prepare aqueous solution of α, β, or γ-cyclodextrin (Concentration 10g/100 ml, 1.5g/100ml and 23g/100ml respectively) at room temperature.
- Add an equimolar amount of drug or guest molecules that is to be encapsulated and stir the mixture at ambient temperature for 12–24 hours. In some cases time may be extended up to 3 days.
- Complex formation is indicated by precipitation of a white solid. In addition the complexation can be deduced from the disappearance of the guest molecules.
- Separate the solid complex by filtration, wash with distilled water and dry under vacuum (if the guest compound is not too volatile) at elevated temperature (e. g. 50°C).
- Dry the complexes with volatile guests in a desiccator over silica gel.
- Grind finally, the material to obtain the complex as a powder.
- Then estimate the amount of drug encapsulated in cyclodextrin complexes by the general analytical methods, i.e. HPLC, UV, and NMR, etc. (Scheme 21.1).

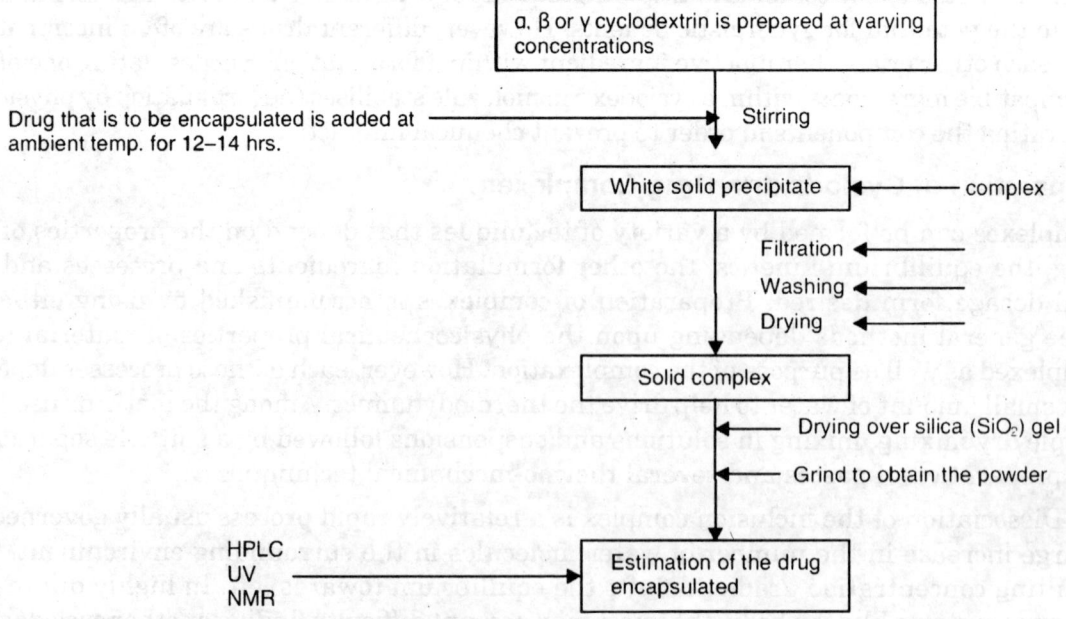

Scheme 21.1: *Preparation of cyclodextrin complexes*

PROTOCOL: 21.2

Complexation in Suspension —Complexation by Kneading Method

The suspension method is especially used for the complexation with the β-cyclodextrin due to its relatively low solubility in water.

Materials

Cyclodextrin (α, β, or γ-)

Drug (guest molecule)

Procedure

- Prepare an aqueous cyclodextrin paste by intensive mixing of typically 0.5 mole of α, β, or γ-cyclodextrin and 200-500 ml of water in a kneading machine. Smaller amount of paste can also be prepared upto 100g using the pastle and mortar.
- To prepare 1:1 stoichiometric complexes, add 0.5 mole of pure guest compound or drug with the continuous stirring of the paste for 3–4 h.
- Solid guest compound can also be used in a soluble form in a co-solvent (e.g. ethanol max 10 % of the water used) before they are added to the cyclodextrin paste.
- The increasing viscosity of the mixture indicates complex formation.
- It may be necessary to add some more water during the complexation procedure in order to keep the paste kneadable.
- After the paste has been dried under vacuum at elevated temperature (i.e. 50°C), grind the material to obtain a powdery complex (Scheme 21.2).

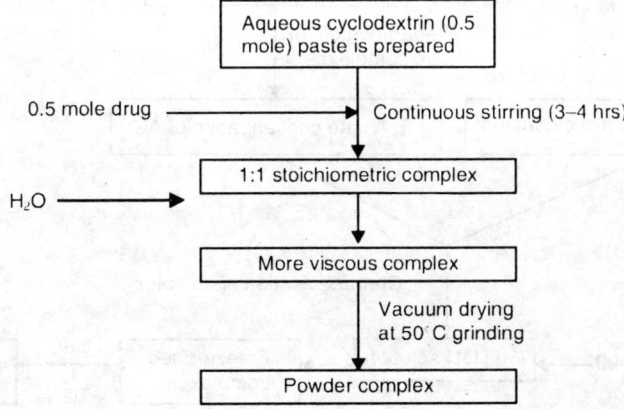

Scheme 21.2: *Preparation of cyclodextrin complexes by kneading method*

PROTOCOL:21.3

Cyclodextrin Complexation with Acyclovir in Aqueous and Solid Phase
Materials

β-cyclodextrin

Acyclovir (ACV)

Procedure

Preparation of the Complexes in Solution

- Mix β-cyclodextrin solution of different concentration $(13.2–281/10^{-3})$ mM to supersaturated solution of acyclovir and shaken at room temperature $(22\pm1^{\circ}C)$ for 36 hours.

- Filter the solution when equilibrium is reached.

- Estimate the concentration of ACV in the filtrate spectrophotometrically at 290nm with reference to suitably constructed standard curve (Scheme 21.3).

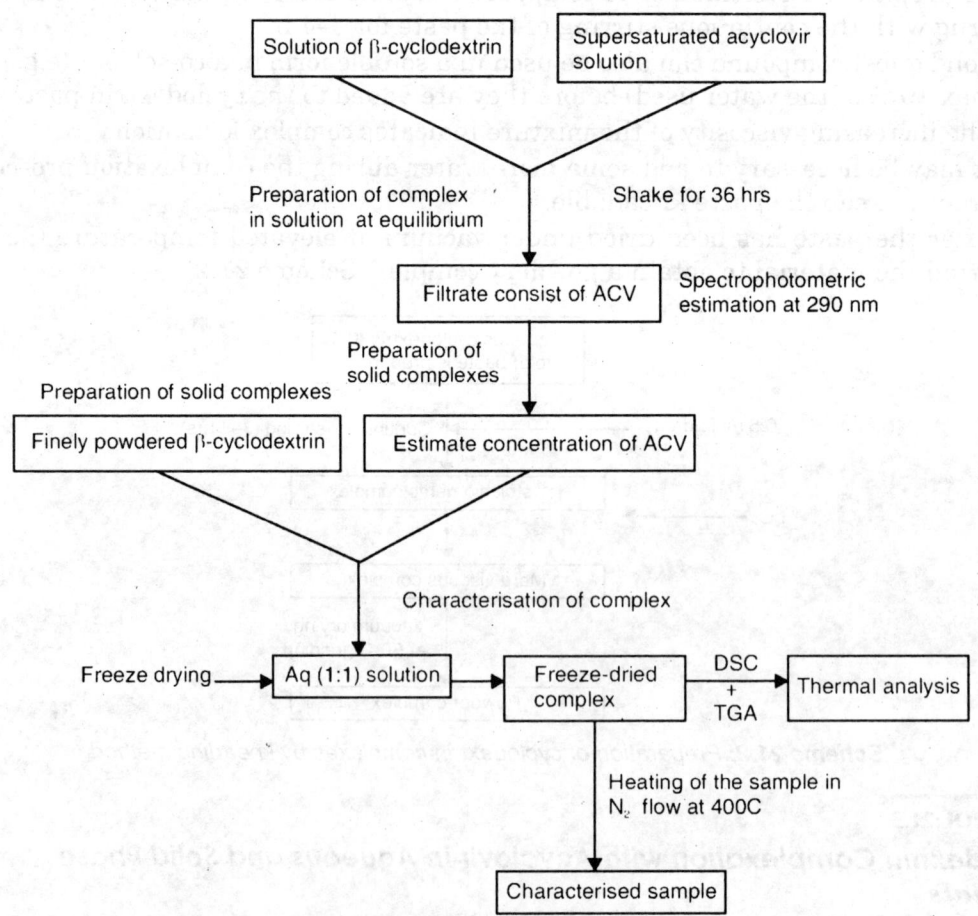

Scheme 21.3: *Preparation of Cyclodextrin complex with acyclovir*

Preparation of the Solid Complexes

- Weigh and mix the finely powdered β-cyclodextrin with acyclovir (1:1 molar ratio).
- Prepare a freeze-dried complex by drying an aqueous solution containing acyclovir and β-cyclodextrin in 1:1 molar ratio in freeze dryer.

Characterisation of Cyclodextrin Complexes

Thermal Analysis

Thermal analysis is performed on solid and freeze dried complexes by Differential Scanning Calorimetry (DSC) and thermal gravimetric analysis (TGA). Heat the samples (2–6 mg) in sealed aluminum pan under nitrogen flow (50 cm^3 min^{-1}) at heating rate of 10°C min^{-1} from 0–400°C.

X-ray Diffraction Studies

Powder diffraction patterns are recorded using X-ray crystallographer.

Dissolution Studies

Paddle dissolution method USP XXIII

PROTOCOL:21.4

Preparation of Solid Complex of Sparfloxacin with β-CD

Materials

HP-β-CD

Sparfloxacin

Procedure

- Accurately weigh 0.345 g HP-β-CD and place into a 50 ml conical flask and add 30 ml distilled water, stir using magnetic stirrer.
- Take 0.098 g sparfloxacin into a 50 ml beaker and add 20 ml of distilled water and put over a electromagnetic stirrer to stir until it is dissolved.
- Then slowly pour the HP-β-CD solution into stirred sparfloxacin solution, continually stir for 12 h at room temperature.
- Keep the reaction mixture into refrigerator for 24 h to obtain white crystalline precipitate.
- Filter the precipitate using G4 sand filtering funnel, and wash with distilled water.
- After drying in oven at 80°C, white powdered products may be separated as inclusion complex of sparfloxacin with HP-β-CD obtained (Scheme 21.4).

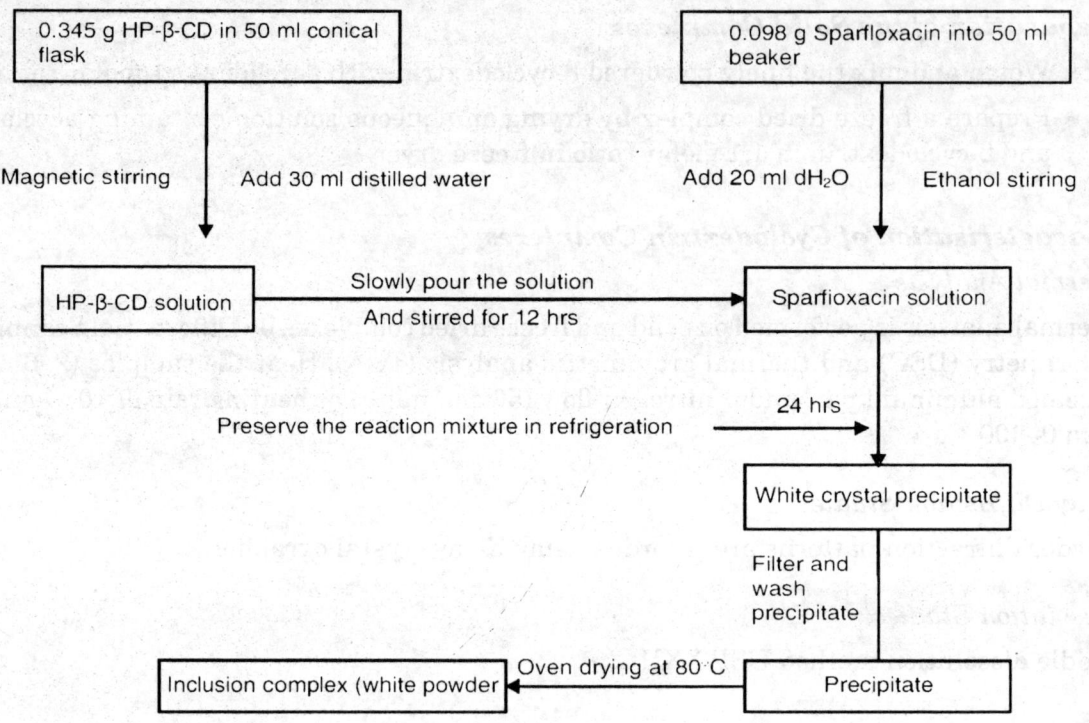

Scheme 21. 4: *Preparation of solid complex of sparfloxacin with β-CD*

SUGGESTED READINGS

- Ammeraal R (1988). US Patent 4 738 923.
- Armbruster F (1970) .US Patent 3 541 077
- Biwer A, Antranikian G, Heinzle E (2002),. Appl Microbiol Biotechnol,59:609–17.
- Bar R (1996) In: Atwoods J et al (eds) Comprehensive supramolecular chemistry, vol 3.. Pergamon, Oxford, pp 423–440.
- Blackwood A, Bucke C (2000) Enzyme Microb Technol 27:704–708.
- Brunet C, Lamare S, Legoy M (1998). Biocatal Biotransfor 16:317–327.
- Buschmann H, Knittel D, Jonas C et al (2001) t. Lebensmittelchemie 55:54–56.
- Choi J, Lee J, Choi K (1996) US Patent 5 492 829.
- Grull D, Stifter U (2001). US Patent 6, 235 505
- Hokse H, Kaper F, Wijpkema J (1984). US Patent 4, 477 568
- Horikoshi K, Nakamura N (1979). US Patent 4 135 977
- Kim T, Kim B, Lee H (1997) Enzyme Microbial Technol 20:506–509
- Lima H, De Moraes F, Zanin G (1998) Appl Biochem Biotechnol 70/72:789–804
- Stanier C. A., Connell M J O, Anderson H. L. and Clegg W. (2001). Chem. Commun. (5): 493–494.
- Villiers A., Sur, L.A. (1981), Compt. Rend. Fr. Acad. Sci.,435–8

Combination Systems

ARTIFICIAL CELLS CONTAINING MULTIENZYME SYSTEM

An artificial cell is a spherical ultra-thin membrane of cellular dimensions enveloping biologically active materials. The enveloping membranes of each artificial cells form the external environment. A typical artificial cell has an ultra-thin membrane of 20 nm thickness, an equivalent pore radius of about 1.8nm, and a large surface/volume relationship (2.5 cm^2 in 10 ml of 20µm diameter microcapsules). This allows for an extremely rapid equilibrium of external permeant molecules at a rate, which is 400 times faster than that of a standard haemolysis machine. Therefore proteins, enzymes, and other macromolecules or particulate matters can be retained within the artificial cells to act as artificial cells that equilibrate rapidly with external permeant molecules. It is possible to enclose almost any combination of enzymes, multienzyme, systems, cofactors-regarding enzyme systems; cell extracts whole cells proteins, adsorbents, surfactants, magnetic materials and multi-compartmental systems.

Methods of Preparation

The basic methods used for preparation of artificial cells are, in fact of physical examples for demonstrating the principle of artificial cells. Many new physical systems are being developed to demonstrate the same principle.

Reagents

- *Haemoglobin solution:* Dissolve 15gm of haemoglobin in 100ml of distilled water, and then filter through Whatman no. 42 filter paper. Adjust the final concentration of haemoglobin in the filtrate to 10g/100ml.

- *Enzyme solution*: Dissolve enzyme (single, multiple, insolublised cell extract or other materials) the haemoglobin solution. Make suitable adjustment to maintain a final concentration of 10gm of haemoglobin per 100ml. Also maintain a minimum pH of 8.5 by use of tris buffer.

- *Organic solution:* Saturate 100ml of ether (analytical grade) with distilled water in a separating funnel, and then discard the water layer.

- *Cellulose nitrate solution:* Prepare by completely drying 100ml of collodion (USP 4gm of cellulose nitrate in a 100ml of mixture of one part alcohol and three part of ether) into a thin sheet, then dissolve to its original volume by using a solution consisting of 82.5ml of ether and 17.5ml of alcohol. This exact composition is required for membrane preparation.

- *N butyl benzoate*

- *Tween20 solution:* Prepare 50% Tween 20 solution by dissolving 50ml of Tween 20, an oil/water emulsifying agent in an equal volume of distilled water. Prepare 1% Tween 20 solution by dissolving 1ml of Tween 20 in 99ml of distilled water. Adjust the pH in both the solution using buffer to 7.

PROTOCOL 22.1

- Add 25 ml of organic solvent to a 2.5 ml of Tris-buffered haemoglobin solution with the constant stirring at a speed of 1200 rpm.

- Add 25 ml of cellulose nitrate solution and stir further for 60 sec. at 40°C and allow to stand for 45 minutes.

- Sediment the prepared microcapsules by adding 30 ml of butyl benzoate with stirring at 1200 rpm followed by standing for 45 minutes.

- Transfer microencapsulated enzyme form organic phase to aqueous phase for this add 5% tween 20 and centrifuge suspension 1200rpm for 30 sec remove the supernatant and add 25ml of water.

- Repeat washing with 1%tween until butyl benzoate is removed completely since it may affect the permeability of semipermeable microcapsule.

- Suspend final preparation in 0.9gm NaCl/100ml water or in suitable buffer solution.

PROTOCOL 22.2
ISCOM—Preparations

Principle

Immunostimulating complex (ISCOM) is particulate cage-like structure, typically 40 nm in diameter, comprising saponin, phospholipid and cholesterol. ISCOM vaccines are generated by incorporating antigen during formulation or alternatively by associating the antigen with the ISCOMATRIX adjuvant (IMX), a process that can be achieved using a number of association strategies.

Materials

Ovalbumin
Palmitoyloxysuccinimide
Sodium deoxycholate

50mM Tris buffer
Cholesterol
Saponin

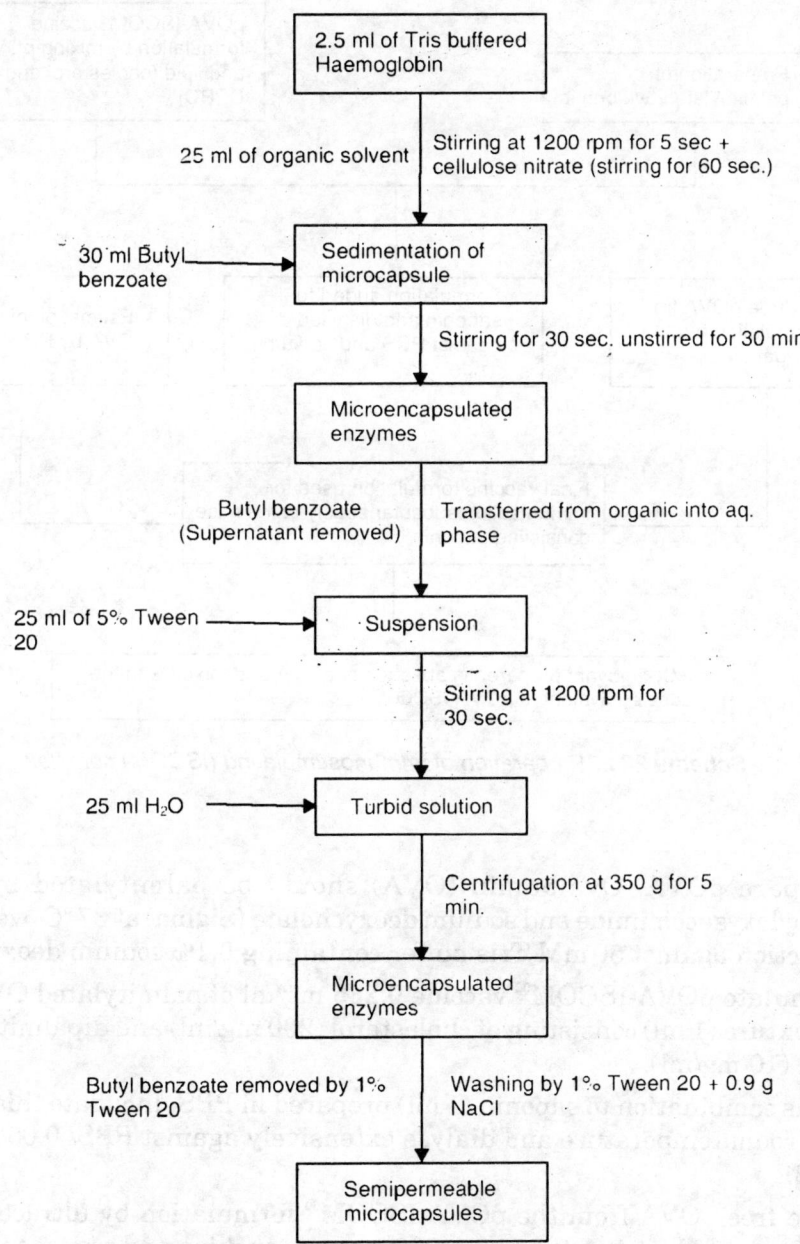

Scheme 22.1: *Preparation of semipermeable microcapsules*

Sodium azide
Di palmitylphosphatidyl choline (DPPC)
PBS (pH 7.2)

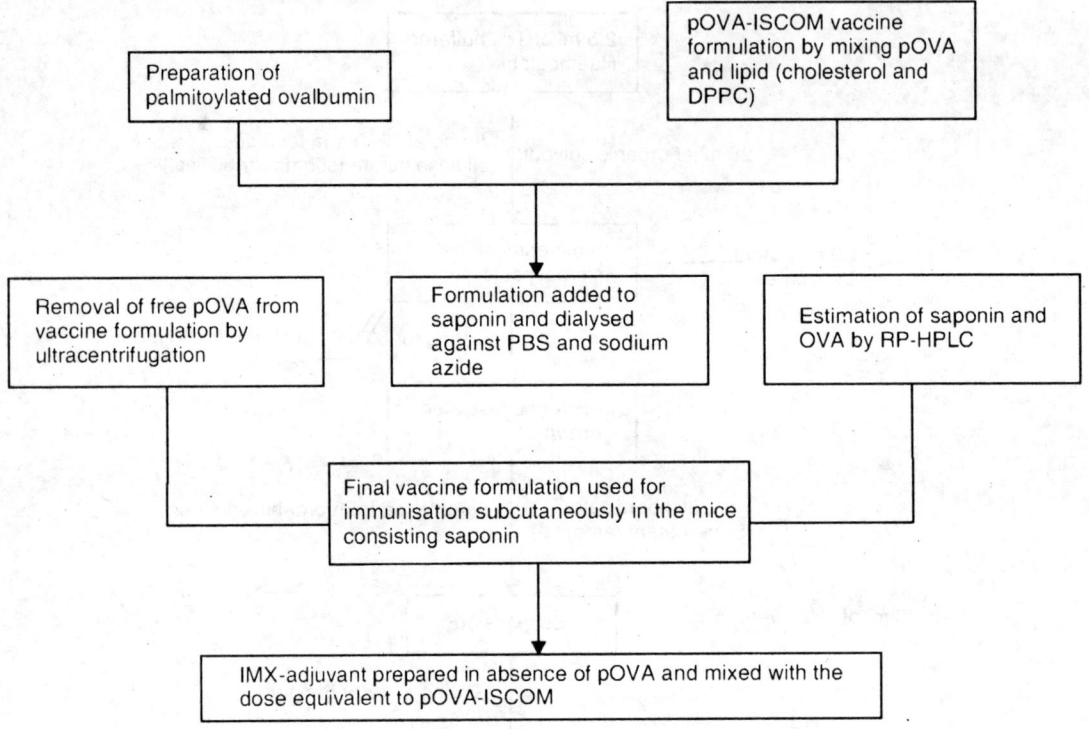

Scheme 22.2: *Preparation of immunostimulating (ISCOM) complex*

Procedure

- To prepare pOVA, Ovalbumin (OVA) should be palmitylated by mixing with palmitoyloxysuccinimide and sodium deoxycholate (Sigma) at 37°C overnight. Dialyse the reaction against 50 mM Tris buffer containing 0.1% sodium deoxycholate.

- To formulate pOVA-ISCOM® vaccine 0.235 mg/ml of palmitylated OVA (pOVA) to a lipid mixture (1 ml) consisting of cholesterol (200 mg/ml) and dipalmitylphosphatidyl choline (10 mg/ml).

- Add this combination to saponin (1 ml) prepared in PBS. Incubate this solution for 90 min at room temperature and dialyse extensively against PBS/ 0.05% sodium azide (pH 7.2).

- Remove free pOVA from the pOVA-ISCOM® formulation by ultracentrifugation at 200,000 g for 16 h at 4°C, through a 20% sucrose cushion and resuspend in PBS/0.05% sodium azide.

- Determine the saponin and OVA content of pOVA-ISCOM vaccines by reverse phase HPLC and quantitative protein analysis by HPLC, respectively.

- Inject the final pOVA-ISCOM vaccine formulation in mice contained saponin at 2.98 mg/ml and OVA at 0.2 mg/ml. Administer this vaccine to mice subcutaneously at doses equivalent to 5μg saponin per mouse, which corresponds to an OVA dose of 0.5μg.

- Prepare ISCOMATRIX adjuvant (IMX) in the absence of pOVA and mix with OVA at doses equivalent to the pOVA-ISCOM vaccine.

PROTOCOL 22.3
β-cyclodextrin-protein Complex Loaded Alginate Microspheres
Materials

Sodium alginate salt

Chitosan

Protein

β-Cyclodextrin

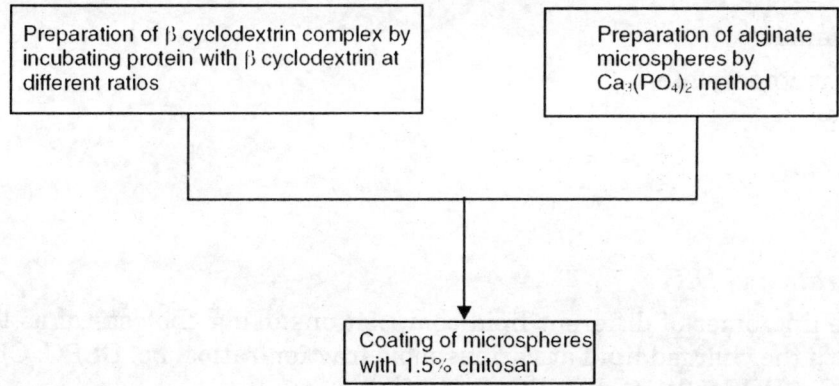

Scheme 22.3: β-cyclodextrin-protein complex loaded alginate microspheres

Procedure

- *Preparation of β-cyclodextrin-protein complexes:* Incubate the protein solution (100mg/ml in phosphate buffer saline pH 7.4) with 100, 200, 400 mg β-cyclodextrin to obtain 1:1, 1:2, and 1: 4 ratios respectively. Stir the mixture overnight at room temperature and lyophilise the prepared complexes.

- *Preparation of alginate microspheres:* Prepare 2%w/v solution of sodium alginate in distilled water, and dissolve the sodium tripolyphosphate (Na-TPP) and 1.9g $CaSO_4$. Emulsify this aqueous phase containing sodium alginate Na-TPP and $Ca_3(PO_4)_2$ into 300 ml double filtered groundnut oil under constant stirring at 2000 rpm at room temperature for 1h to obtain microspheres. Then filter the microspheres and wash with acetone and dry to store at 4°C.

- Finally coat the prepared microspheres with the 1.5% w/v chitosan solution as follows-suspend the prepared microspheres previously weigh (5mg) in the 1.5% chitosan solution and allow to stand at room temperature for 2 h.

PROTOCOL 22.4
Development of a Mini Capsular Extrusion System for Enteric Delivery of Metronidazole Bearing Liposomes

Materials

Phosphatidylcholine (PC)

Distearoylphosphatidylcholine (DSPC)

Cholesterol (Ch)

Dicetylphosphate (DCP)

Stearylamine (SA)

Cellulose acetate

Polyacrylamide

Polyethyl methacrylate

Chloroform

Methanol

Procedure

Step 1. Preparation of DRVs

- Prepare liposomes of different lipid compositions using cholesterol as the principal lipid with the charged lipid at various mole fraction ratios, i.e. DSPC: Ch: SA (7:2:1), DSPC: Ch: DCP 7:2:1 and DSPC: Ch (7:3).
- Dissolve lipids in chloroform in a round bottom flask. Evaporate chloroform using a rotary flash evaporator leaving an uniform film on the wall of the flask.
- Hydrate the dried lipid film using an aqueous solution of metronidazole for 45 minutes at 45°C under moderate occasional agitation.
- Then sonicate the liposomes at 15000 Hz frequency for 3 minutes, where every 30 second sonication period followed by a 5 second pause period.
- After sonication, centrifuge the liposomal suspension at 6000 rpm for 15 minutes..
- Discard the sediment and the liposomes in the supernatant are freeze dried with 2%w/v glycerin as cryoprotectant.
- Store the prepared liposomes under nitrogen at 4°C until used.

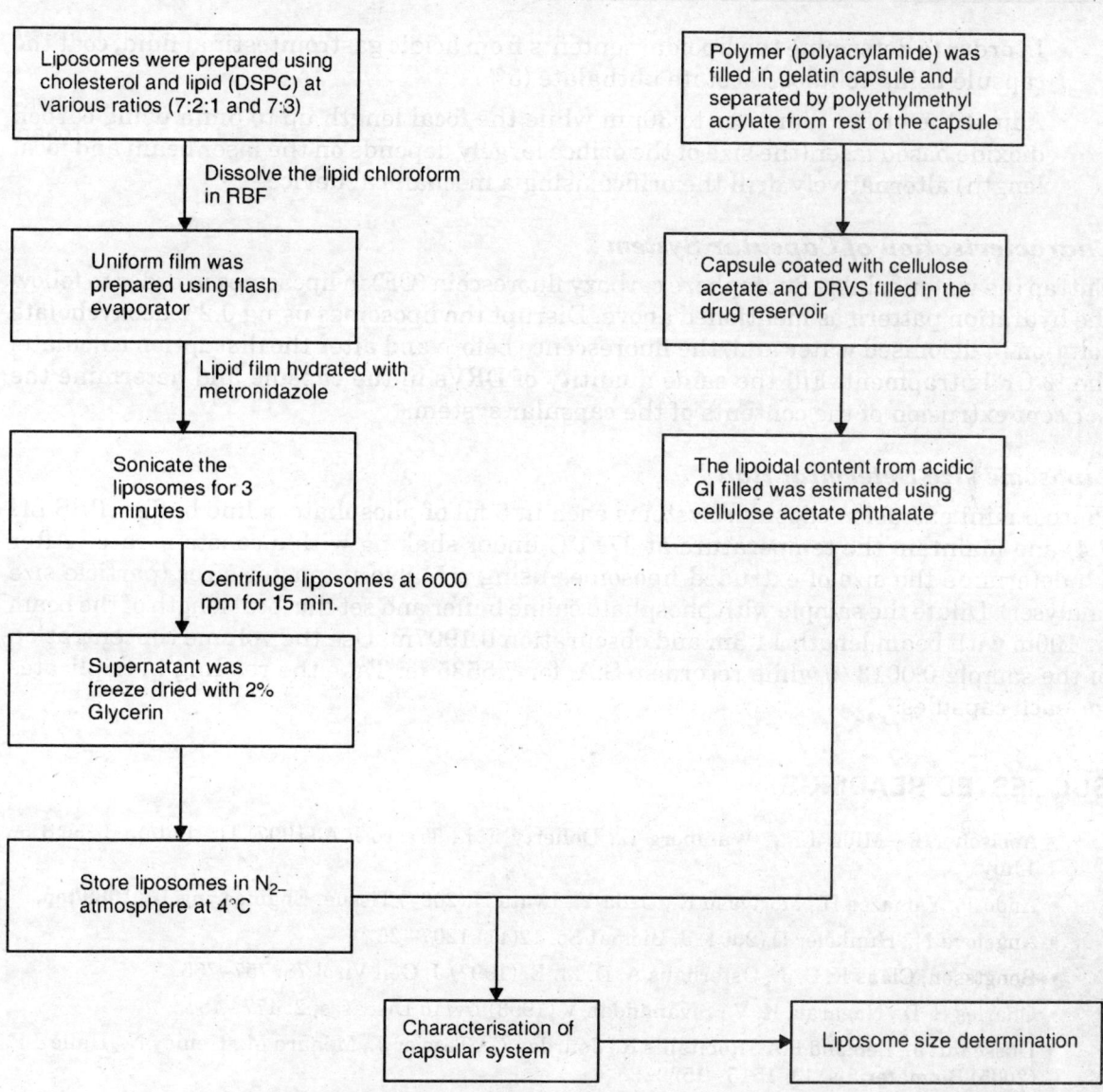

Scheme 22.4: *Preparation of minicapsular extrusion system*

Step 2. Designing of Capsular System

- Fill the one-third part of a gelatin capsule with a swellable polymer (polyacrylamide) and separate it with the help of a polyethyl-methacrylate vestibule from the rest of the capsule body.
- Fill the drug reservoir compartment with metronidazole DRVs. Seal the capsule and coat with cellulose acetate lamella.
- An orifice is laser drilled as a delivery port in the drug reservoir compartment.

- In order to determine the lipoidal contents from acidic gastrointestinal fluid, coat the capsule using cellulose acetate phthalate (5%).
- Adjust the orifice diameter to 30µm while the focal length up to 5mm using carbon dioxide based laser (the size of the orifice largely depends on the laser beam and focal length) alternatively drill the orifice using a mechanical device.

Characterisation of Capsular System

Entrap the water-soluble fluorophore carboxy fluorescein (CF) in liposomes in order to follow the hydration pattern as mentioned above. Disrupt the liposomes using 0.2% deoxycholate solution in deionised water and, the fluorescence before and after the disruption calculate. the % CF entrapment. Fill the same quantity of DRVs in the capsule and determine the per cent extrusion of the contents of the capsular system.

Liposome size Determination

Place 5 mini extrusion capsular systems each in 5 ml of phosphate saline buffer (PBS pH 7.4) and maintain the temperature at 37±1°C under shaking with a constant rate. After 1h determine the size of extruded liposomes using a Malvern master sizer (particle size analyser). Dilute the sample with phosphate saline buffer and set the focal length of the beam at 100m with beam length 14.3m and obscuration 0.1907m. Use the volume concentration of the sample 0.0013 % while record sp S.A. for 7.5535 m. Take the reading in triplicates for each capsules.

SUGGESTED READINGS

- Aebischer P., Mills J.F., Wahlberg L., Doherty E.J., Tresco P.A.(1997) US Patent Issued on 1July
- Ando T., Yamazoe H., Moriyasu K., Ueda Y., Iwata H.(2007) Tissue Engineering 10. 1089/ten.
- Angelova N., Hunkeler D.(2001) J. Biomat Sc. 12(11):1207–25.
- Bengtsson, Claas E. C. J., Osterhaus A. D. M. E. (1997) J. Gen Virol 78: 757–765.
- Charles S. D., Nagaraja K. V., Sivanandan V.(1993) Avian Diseases, 2: 477–484 .
- Dusseault J., Leblond F.A., Robitaille R., Jourdan G., Tessier J., Ménard M., Henley N., Hallé J.P. (2005) Biomaterials. 13: 1515–1522 .
- Erturk M, Hill TJ, Shimeld C, Jennings R. (1992) Arch Virol. 125 (1–4): 87–101.
- Green D.W., Leveque L., Walsh D., Howard D., Yang X., Partridge K., Mann S., Groot M. D., Schuurs T., Schilfgaarde Van R.(2004) Surgical Res. 121 (1): 141–150.
- Heng B. C., Yu Y. -J. H., S. C. Ng. S. (2004). J. Microencp. 4: 455 – 467.
- Hu K.F., Elvander M., Merza M., Akerblom L., Brandenburg A., Morein B.(1998) Clin Exp Immunol. 113(2): 235–243.
- Le TT, Drane D, Malliaros J, et al. (2001)Vaccine 19: 4669–75.
- Mowat AM, Smith RE, Donachie AM, Furrie E, Grdic D, Lycke N.(1999) Immunol Lett 65: 133–40.

- Moses L.R., Dileep K.J., Sharma P.C.(2000) Journal of Applied Polymer Science. 75 (9) 1089-1096.

- Pham H.L., Shaw P.N., Davies N.M.(2006) Int. J. Pharm, 310 (1−2) 196−202 .

- Rimmelzwaan G. F., Baars M., R. van Beek, G. van Amerongen, K. Los vgren- Oreffo O.R.C. (2005) Biomaterial 15: 917 − 923.

- Shen F., Legrand P.C., Somers S., Slade A., Yip C., Duft M.A., Winnik M.F., Chang P.L. (2003) Biotechnology and Bioengineering. 83(3) 282-292.

- Paveli E., Nata A., Ivan K.B., Enjak J.(2004) Acta Pharm. 54 319−330.

- Silva M.C., Ribeiro J.A., Figueiredo F.V., Gonçalves R.A., Veiga F.(2006) International Journal of Pharmaceutics. 1-2: 1-10.

- Sihorkar V., Vyas S.P. (2001) Pharmaceutical Research. 18 (9): 1247− 54 .

- Wang J.L., Jiang X.J., Wang Q., Hou L.J., Xu D.W., Wang J., Zhao X.F. (2007) BMC Dev Biol. 7: 76.

Index

Reader's Notes

Reader's Notes